Obstructive Sleep Apnea in Adults

Advances in Cardiology

Vol. 46

Series Editor

Jeffrey S. Borer New York, N.Y.

Alain Lurie

Obstructive Sleep Apnea in Adults

Relationship with Cardiovascular and Metabolic Disorders

95 figures in color, 37 tables, 2011

KARGER

Basel · Freiburg · Paris · London · New York · New Delhi · Bangkok · Beijing · Tokyo · Kuala Lumpur · Singapore · Sydney

To my wife Liora and
my children Alexandra and David
for their patience and tolerance

In memory of my mother and father

Dr. Alain Lurie
Laboratoire du Sommeil
Centre d'Exploration, de Réanimation et
d'Intervention Cardio-Vasculaire
Centre Médico-Chirurgical Ambroise Paré
25–27 Boulevard Victor Hugo
F–92000 Neuilly-sur-Seine (France)

Disclosure Statement
A.L. has participated in speaking engagements for Linde Healthcare and Pfizer. He has no financial conflicts of interest with the subject matter discussed in this book.

Library of Congress Cataloging-in-Publication Data

Lurie, Alain.
Obstructive sleep apnea in adults : relationship with cardiovascular and metabolic disorders / Alain Lurie.
p. ; cm. -- (Advances in cardiology, ISSN 0065-2326 ; v. 46)
Includes bibliographical references and index.
ISBN 978-3-8055-9645-9 (hard cover : alk. paper) -- ISBN 978-3-8055-9646-6 (e-ISBN)
1. Sleep apnea syndromes. 2. Cardiovascular system--Diseases. 3. Metabolism--Disorders. I. Title. II. Series: Advances in cardiology ; v. 46. 0065-2326
[DNLM: 1. Sleep Apnea, Obstructive--complications. 2. Cardiovascular Diseases--etiology. 3. Metabolic Diseases--etiology. W1 AD53C v.46 2011 / WF 143]
RC737.5.L87 2011
616.2'09--dc23

2011021810

Bibliographic Indices. This publication is listed in bibliographic services, including Current Contents® and PubMed/MEDLINE.

www.karger.com
Printed in Switzerland on acid-free paper by Reinhardt Druck, Basel
ISSN 0065–2326
ISBN 978–3–8055–9645–9
e-ISBN 978–3–8055–9646–6

Contents

Preface

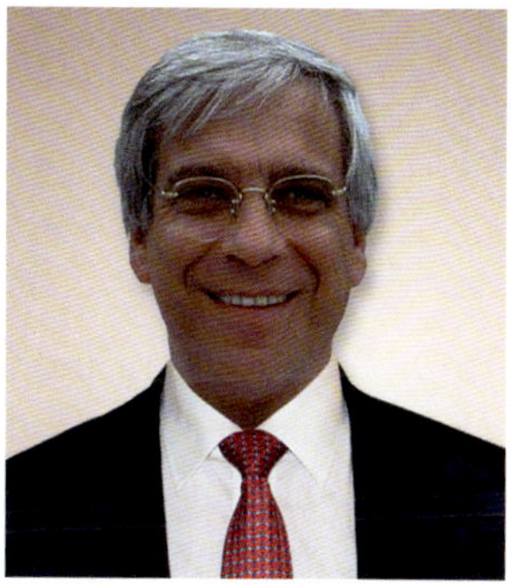

The relationship between obstructive sleep apnea (OSA) and cardiovascular and metabolic diseases is a topical subject of concern to a wide range of specialists and general practitioners. In the last 2 decades, significant advances have been made in the understanding of factors contributing to, and the complications of, OSA. With the increase in the population levels of obesity (the greatest risk factor for OSA), the effects of OSA are likely to increase in the coming years; therefore, there is a corresponding need for wider education concerning this disease. The goal of this peer-reviewed book is, therefore, to provide a comprehensive and clear review of the current knowledge of the relationship between OSA and cardiovascular and metabolic diseases.

Separate chapters describe the definition, symptoms and sequelae of OSA in adults, and the diagnostic strategies and treatment options for adults with OSA according to the American Academy of Sleep Medicine (chapter 1). The pathogenic mechanisms by which OSA may contribute to the development and progression of cardiovascular and metabolic disorders, including inflammation, oxidative stress and thrombosis, are also explored (chapter 2). In addition, special emphasis has been given to the relationship between OSA and obesity, alterations in glucose metabolism, and metabolic syndrome and liver injury (chapter 3). The evidence for a relationship between OSA, endothelial dysfunction, autonomic dysfunction and cardiovascular disorders is also presented, and the results of studies investigating the effect of treatment for OSA on the concomitant cardiovascular disease are discussed (chapters 4–6). The chapters tend to emphasize human rather than basic animal data; nevertheless, animal data are cited, particularly, for example, with reference to the difficulties associated with unraveling the mechanisms of metabolic dysfunction in obese populations, in which the prevalence of comorbidities and potential confounding factors is high.

Each chapter summarizes the essential information and is illustrated by tables and figures, many of which are drawn from the articles cited in the text. It is my hope that these easy-to-read tables and figures will aid the readers in their understanding of the complex systemic interactions involved in this disease.

Alain Lurie, Paris

Acknowledgements

To Dr. Pierre Squara and the reviewers for their insightful comments and fruitful suggestions that have critically contributed towards the writing of this book.

To the sleep technicians Bérengère Guillaume Beulé, for her helpful assistance in editing the manuscript, and Theo Sokphon Teng and Caroline Lafif, for their assistance during the writing of this book.

To editor L.C. (www.editage.com) for his efforts in providing excellent-quality English editing assistance.

Obstructive Sleep Apnea in Adults: Epidemiology, Clinical Presentation, and Treatment Options

1

Chapter 1

Obstructive Sleep Apnea in Adults: Epidemiology, Clinical Presentation, and Treatment Options

Abstract

Obstructive sleep apnea (OSA) is characterized by repetitive episodes of complete and partial obstructions of the upper airway during sleep. The diagnosis of OSA requires the objective demonstration of abnormal breathing during sleep by measuring the respiratory disturbance index (RDI, events per hour of sleep), i.e. the frequency of apnea (complete upper airway obstruction), hypopnea (partial upper airway obstruction) and arousals from sleep related to respiratory efforts. OSA is defined by combining symptoms and an RDI ≥5 or by an RDI ≥15 without symptoms. The apnea-hypopnea index (AHI), the frequency of apnea and hypopnea events per hour of sleep, is widely used to define OSA (many clinical and epidemiological studies use this metric). In the general adult population, the prevalence of OSA defined by ≥5 apnea and hypopnea events per hour of sleep associated with excessive sleepiness is approximately 3–7% in men and 2–5% in women. The prevalence of OSA is much higher, e.g. ≥50%, in patients with cardiac or metabolic disorders than in the general population. Risk factors for OSA include obesity (the strongest risk factor), upper airway abnormalities, male gender, menopause and age (the prevalence of OSA associated with a higher risk of morbidity and mortality increases with age and peaks at approximately 55 years of age). OSA is associated with symptoms during sleep (snoring, choking and nocturia) and wakefulness (excessive sleepiness, fatigue and lack of energy) and with sequelae such as psychological changes, alterations in the quality of life, and social, familial and professional performance including vehicle and industrial accidents. The identification of OSA may be a difficult task for the clinician, even in populations in which OSA is highly prevalent such as patients with cardiovascular disorders because they may not present the cardinal signs of the disease, e.g. excessive sleepiness and obesity. Guidelines have been developed to tailor OSA therapy to patients according to the results of their disease evaluation and their preferences.

1 Definitions

Obstructive sleep apnea (OSA) is characterized by repetitive episodes of complete or partial obstructions of the upper airway during sleep [1]. The spectrum of these obstructive respiratory events during sleep occurs as a continuum ranging from flow limitation to full apnea. These all lead to an increase in airway resistance and respiratory effort, and may produce oxygen desaturation, central nervous system arousal and sleep fragmentation. According to the International Classification of Sleep Disorders [1, 2], alternate names include OSA syndrome, sleep apnea, sleep apnea syndrome, obstructive apnea, mixed sleep apnea, sleep-disordered breathing (SDB), sleep hypopnea syndrome and upper airway obstruction. Sleep-related breathing disorder is a widely used but rather imprecise term that applies to all types of breathing abnormalities that may occur during sleep, including central sleep apnea syndromes, OSA syndrome, sleep-related hypoventilation/hypoxemia syndromes and sleep-related hypoventilation/hypoxemia due to a medical condition. The International Classification of Sleep Disorders recommends that upper airway resistance syndrome be included as part of OSA and not considered as a separate entity [1]. The diagnosis of upper airway resistance syndrome is a proposed diagnosis for patients with respiratory effort-related arousal (RERA) episodes who do not also have events that fulfill the definitions of apnea and hypopnea [1]. RERA episodes may be responsible for unrefreshing sleep, excessive sleepiness and fatigue as they have the same underlying pathophysiology as apnea and hypopnea. The definitive treatment for OSA, i.e. continuous positive airway pressure (CPAP) treatment, has been shown to significantly improve excessive sleepiness and other outcomes in upper airway resistance syndrome patients [3].

The frequency of apnea, hypopnea and RERA episodes per hour of sleep (respiratory disturbance index, RDI; events per hour of sleep) is used to quantify the severity of OSA (table 1, fig. 1). According to the International Classification of Sleep Disorders, a diagnosis of OSA can be made for an RDI ≥15, independently of the occurrence of symptoms, or whenever an RDI >5 is associated with any of the symptoms described in table 2. The severity of OSA is defined as mild for an RDI ≥5 and <15, moderate for an RDI ≥15 and ≤30, and severe for an RDI >30 [4]. The apnea-hypopnea index (AHI), the frequency of apnea and hypopnea events per hour of sleep, is a widely used index to define OSA, including many epidemiological studies [5–7].

Obesity hypoventilation syndrome (OHS) is different from OSA [8]. It is defined as daytime hypercapnia and hypoxemia (arterial carbon dioxide pressure >45 mm Hg and arterial oxygen pressure <70 mm Hg at sea level) in obese patients (body mass index, BMI, ≥30) with SDB in the absence of any other cause of hypoventilation, e.g. severe obstructive airways disease, severe interstitial lung disease, severe chest wall disorders such as kyphoscoliosis, severe hypothyroidism, neuromuscular disease and congenital central hypoventilation syndrome [8]. OSA is the SDB associated with OHS in approximately 90% of patients, while it is sleep hypoventilation in the remaining 10%. Sleep hypoventilation is defined by an increase in arterial carbon dioxide pressure of >10 mm Hg above that of wakefulness or significant oxygen desaturations, neither of which is the result of obstructive apneas or hypopneas [8]. Sleep hypoventilation patients are characterized by an AHI <5. Categorization of SDB in OHS patients is performed during an overnight polysomnography (PSG) examination.

Table 1. Definition of apnea, hypopnea and RERA according to the 2007 American Academy of Sleep Medicine recommendations [255]

Apnea	A respiratory event is scored as apnea when all of the following criteria are met: there is a drop in the peak oral and nasal thermal sensor excursion ≥90% of baseline, and at least 90% of the event's duration meets the amplitude reduction criteria for apnea
Obstructive apnea	Obstructive apnea meets the apnea criteria and is associated with continued or increased inspiratory effort throughout the entire period of absent airflow
Mixed apnea	Mixed apnea meets the apnea criteria and is associated with a lack of inspiratory effort in the initial portion of the event (no thoracic and abdominal movements), followed by the resumption of inspiratory effort in the second portion of the event (persistent thoracic and abdominal movements)
Central apnea	Central apnea meets the apnea criteria and is associated with absent inspiratory effort throughout the entire period of absent airflow
Hypopnea	A respiratory event is scored as hypopnea when nasal pressure excursion drops by (1) ≥30% of baseline and there is a ≥4% desaturation from the pre-event baseline, or (2) ≥50% of baseline and there is a ≥3% desaturation from the pre-event baseline or the event is associated with arousal. In both cases, at least 90% of the event's duration must meet the amplitude reduction of the criteria for hypopnea
RERA	A respiratory event is scored as RERA if a sequence of breaths characterized by increasing respiratory effort or flattening of the nasal pressure waveform leads to an arousal from sleep and does not meet the criteria for apnea or hypopnea

All these events have to last for at least 10 s.

2 Prevalence and Incidence of Obstructive Sleep Apnea

Studies of the prevalence of OSA in middle-aged adult populations assessed using in-laboratory PSG produced consistent estimates [9], despite study limitations including variability in measurements, definitions, sample construction and statistical techniques used for analyses (for a review on this aspect of epidemiology studies, see the article of Young et al. [10]). It is of note that studies using the RDI have higher estimates of prevalence than those using the AHI, including mostly desaturations. In the general adult population, the prevalence of OSA associated with excessive sleepiness is approximately 3–7% in men and 2–5% in women (table 3) [5, 11–15]. Despite its high prevalence rate, OSA often goes undetected. For example, in the general population of the Wisconsin Sleep Cohort Study, 82% of men and 93% of women with moderate or severe OSA had not been clinically diagnosed [16, 17]. Unrecognized OSA is a heavy health burden for society, and cost-effectiveness studies support the value of the diagnosis and treatment of OSA [18–23]. An economic model developed after

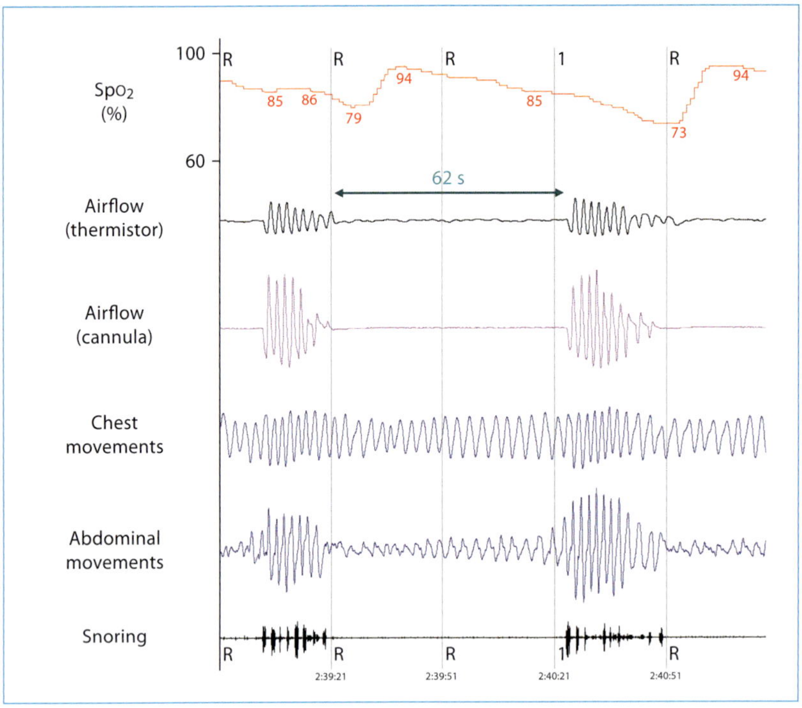

Fig. 1. Example of an obstructive apnea. This tracing shows obstructive apnea for 62 s while respiratory effort is ongoing, as indicated by the persistent chest and abdominal movements. Oxygen desaturation falls to 73% following the apnea. The drop to 79% is from a preceding apneic event. Spo_2 = Peripheral oxygen saturation.

a literature review of cost-effectiveness studies for CPAP therapy revealed that CPAP administration was associated with higher costs and higher benefits than conservative management [22]. The incremental cost per quality-adjusted life year gained for CPAP was below GBP 20,000 (approx. USD 30,000). A cost-effectiveness study of a sleep clinic population study provided estimates (from a payer perspective) ranging from USD 2,000 to 11,000 per quality-adjusted life year over 5 years for treating moderate-to-severe OSA [23, 24]. These values have been considered as a very good deal for payers when compared to the use of blood-pressure-lowering drugs in hypertensive patients or comprehensive diabetes care [23, 25].

The incidence of OSA has been much less studied than its prevalence. A longitudinal cohort study of US communities (2,968 men and women, mean age ± SD 62.1 ± 9.9 years) [26] assessed SDB at 2 time points that were 5 years apart. Over the 5-year period, the overall incidence of moderate-to-severe OSA, defined by an AHI >15, was 11.1% in men and 4.9% in women [26]. These sex differences in the incidence of OSA remained significant after adjusting for confounding variables. Weight change was a critical factor for the progression of the disease; however, OSA progressed over time, even in those with stable weight.

Table 2. Definition of OSA according to the International Classification of Sleep Disorders, 2nd edition [1]

A, B and D or C and D satisfy the criteria

(A) At least 1 of the following applies:
- (1) the patient complains of unintentional sleep episodes during wakefulness, excessive sleepiness, unrefreshing sleep, fatigue or insomnia
- (2) the patient wakes with breath holding, gasping or choking
- (3) the bed partner reports loud snoring, breathing interruption or both during the patient's sleep

(B) Polysomnographic recording shows the following:
- (1) 5 or more scorable respiratory events[1] per hour of sleep
- (2) evidence of respiratory effort during all or a portion of each respiratory event[2]

OR

(C) Polysomnographic recording shows the following:
- (1) 15 or more scorable respiratory events[1] per hour of sleep
- (2) evidence of respiratory effort during all or a portion of each respiratory event[2]

(D) The disorder is not more accurately explained by another current sleep disorder, medical or neurological disorder, medication use, or substance use disorder

Reprinted with permission.

[1] Apneas, hypopneas or RERAs.

[2] In the case of a RERA, this is best seen with the use of esophageal manometry.

Table 3. Example of community-based population studies for the prevalence of polysomnographically defined OSA

Reference, year of publication	Country and race	OSA definition	Age range years	Prevalence, %	
				men	women
Young et al. [5], 1993	USA (Caucasian)	AHI ≥5 + ES	30–60	4	2
Bixler et al. [11], 2001	USA (Caucasian)	AHI ≥10 + ES	20–100	3.9	1.2
Ip et al. [12], 2001	China (Asiatic)	AHI ≥5 + ES	30–60	4.1	–
Ip et al. [13], 2004	China (Asiatic)	AHI ≥5 + ES	30–60	–	2.1
Kim et al. [14], 2004	Korea (Asiatic)	AHI ≥5 + ES	40–69	4.5	3.2
Reddy et al. [15], 2009	India (Asiatic)	AHI ≥5 + ES	30–65	4	1.5

ES = Excessive sleepiness.

3 Risk Factors for Obstructive Sleep Apnea

3.1 Overweight, Obesity, Metabolic Syndrome and Alterations in Glucose Metabolism

Obesity is the strongest risk factor for OSA [27, 28]. The relationship between metabolic syndrome, insulin resistance and type 2 diabetes mellitus and the risk of developing or aggravating OSA is reviewed in chapter 3 [this vol., pp. 67–137].

3.2 *Age*

The association between age and sleep apnea is complex because the distribution of OSA prevalence by age is multimodal [10, 29–32]. The prevalence of OSA associated with a higher risk of morbidity and mortality increases with age and peaks at approximately 55 years of age [10, 29, 31, 32]. This increase plateaus after 65 years, although the reasons for this phenomenon are unknown [10, 11, 29, 32]. For example, an epidemiological study [29] performed in men revealed that the prevalence of OSA defined by an AHI ≥10 plus clinical findings, e.g. daytime sleepiness, hypertension or another cardiovascular complication, was 1.2% (95% confidence interval, CI, 0.4–3.8), 4.7% (95% CI 3.1–7.1) and 1.7% (95% CI 0.3–9.1) in the groups aged 20–44, 45–64 and ≥65 years, respectively. In contrast, the prevalence of OSA, defined solely by an AHI ≥10, was 3.2% (95% CI 1.6–6.4), 11.8% (95% CI 9.1–15.3) and 23.9% (95% CI 15.7–41.7) in the same age groups, respectively. Similar findings have also been reported in other studies [11, 32].

Sleep apnea in the elderly may be less severe than in middle-aged patients, and may not be associated with the same increase in mortality and morbidity [33]. In the elderly, the prevalence of OSA is approximately 2–3 times that observed in middle-aged patients [11, 29, 34]. A previous study [34] revealed that, in adults aged 65–99 years, the prevalence of OSA (AHI ≥10) was 70% in men and 56% in women. It remains to be clarified whether OSA in the elderly is a different condition from that observed in middle-aged patients [33].

3.3 *Gender*

OSA is more common in men than in women [35]. In the general population, the male-to-female ratio for OSA prevalence ranges between 2:1 and 4:1 (table 3). The development of OSA is affected by gender differences including overweight and obesity, upper airway dimensions and collapsibility [see chapter 3, this vol., pp. 67–137], and hormonal factors. A relatively high progesterone/estrogen ratio and low testosterone levels may help protect women against OSA, as suggested by studies of the relationship between OSA and menopause, testosterone administration and polycystic ovary syndrome.

3.3.1 Menopause, a Risk Factor for Obstructive Sleep Apnea

OSA is more common among postmenopausal women than among premenopausal women [11, 36, 37]. PSG on 1,000 women and 741 men, recruited by telephone interview, indicated that the prevalence of SDB (AHI ≥10 and daytime symptoms) was 1.2% in women and 3.9% in men ($p = 0.0006$) [11]. The prevalence of SDB in premenopausal women was 0.6%, whereas the prevalence in postmenopausal women without hormone replacement therapy was 2.7% ($p = 0.02$). In the Wisconsin Cohort, the odds ratio compared to premenopausal women with an AHI >15 increases from 1.1 during the perimenopause to 3.5 in the postmenopause [37]. The risk for SDB was also found to increase throughout the menopausal transition, independently of confounding factors.

Studies of the effects of hormone replacement therapy on OSA prevalence have provided some evidence for the role of estrogen and progesterone levels in this condition. Several studies, with a small number of subjects, reported that hormone replacement therapy may improve sleep apnea [38–40]. Data collected from the Sleep Heart Health Study (n = 2,852) indicated a 40–50% reduction in the prevalence of sleep apnea (AHI ≥15) in postmenopausal women receiving hormone replacement therapy when compared with women not receiving such medication (age, BMI and other relevant possible confounders were controlled in this study) [36].

Overall, these studies suggest that the menopause is a significant risk factor for SDB. Perimenopausal and postmenopausal women have been suggested to be evaluated for OSA in the presence of symptoms such as snoring, excessive sleepiness or unrefreshing sleep (although unrefreshing sleep and insomnia are common in perimenopausal women, independently of OSA) [37].

3.3.2 Testosterone Levels and the Risk of Obstructive Sleep Apnea

Several studies have shown that the intramuscular administration of testosterone may predispose to OSA [41–43]. Testosterone may also modulate the neural control of breathing [44]; indeed, testosterone administration in premenopausal women has been shown to increase central chemoreflex responsiveness to CO_2 during wakefulness [45] and the apneic threshold during nonrapid eye movement sleep, facilitating the occurrence of central apneas and breathing instability during sleep [46].

3.3.3 Polycystic Ovary Syndrome and the Risk of Obstructive Sleep Apnea

Polycystic ovary syndrome is characterized by chronic hyperandrogenism, oligomenorrhea, oligoanovulation, central obesity, insulin resistance, dyslipidemia, disordered gonadotropin secretion and polycystic ovaries [47]. The prevalence of OSA has been reported to be as high as 60–70% in women with polycystic ovary syndrome [48–50]. Although controversial [49, 51], this could be potentially related to the high androgen levels observed in this condition [48, 50].

3.4 *Craniofacial Anatomy*

Abnormalities of the bony and soft tissue structures in the upper airway may compromise the pharyngeal airspace and increase the risk of obstructive respiratory events during sleep (they may act through changes in upper airway compliance rather than a direct impingement on airway caliber). Abnormalities in the bony structures of the upper airway include the reduction of the mandibular body size, inferior position of the hyoid bone and retroposition of the maxilla [52, 53]. A meta-analysis of studies investigating craniofacial risk factors showed that mandibular body length had the strongest association with an increased risk of OSA [52]. Abnormalities of the soft tissues of the upper airway include tonsillar hypertrophy, submucosal edema and excess fat deposited along the lateral pharyngeal walls [53, 54]. However, many OSA patients do not demonstrate anatomical abnormalities in their upper airway, while subjects with a narrow upper airway due to anatomical abnormalities do not have OSA [55, 56].

3.5 *Smoking and Alcohol Consumption*

The daily exposure to passive smoking of subjects who have never smoked has been associated with a 1.6-fold increased risk of being a habitual snorer (95% CI 1.2–2.1), after adjusting for age and BMI [57]. In epidemiological studies, current smoking has been associated with a higher prevalence of snoring [57–62] and OSA [62–64]. For example, in the Wisconsin Sleep Cohort Study, current smokers had a 4.4 times increased risk of moderate or worse OSA than individuals who had never smoked [64]. Upper airway inflammation [65, 66] and overnight withdrawal from nicotine [64] have been hypothesized to contribute to the effects of tobacco consumption on OSA. By contrast, analysis of data from the Sleep Heart Health Study revealed an inverse association between current smoking and OSA [67]; after adjusting for confounding factors including age and BMI, current smokers had significantly fewer respiratory disturbance events than did nonsmokers (although the pack-year exposure did not differ across RDI quartiles). These discrepancies remain unexplained, and there is a need to clarify the link between tobacco consumption and OSA.

Alcohol consumption before bedtime has also been shown to increase the number and duration of hypopnea and apnea events [68, 69], but this is a controversial finding [70, 71]. These potential effects on the AHI levels have been hypothesized to be the result of alcohol-induced oropharyngeal muscle hypotonia [72–74]. Population-based, cross-sectional studies have reported a significant association between chronic alcohol consumption and snoring or OSA [63, 75, 76], whereas other cross-sectional [77–79] or longitudinal [80] studies did not. A population-based cross-sectional study in women revealed a significant relationship between alcohol dependence, defined by the CAGE alcohol-screening questionnaire [81], and snoring frequency only in women with a BMI <20 [82]. It was speculated that alcohol-induced hypotonia may be more important in women with a BMI <20 than in overweight/obese women. Overall, these discrepant findings may be related to methodological biases including the methods of assessment for snoring and OSA that differ between studies, e.g. the use of a questionnaire, type 3 monitoring and PSG, and the lack of a reliable metric to assess alcohol consumption in epidemiological studies. Whether acute alcohol ingestion requires higher CPAP levels to prevent apnea and hypopnea remains unresolved [83, 84].

3.6 *Familial and Genetic Predisposition*

First-degree relatives of OSA patients have an approximately 2-fold greater risk for OSA than those without OSA, and familial susceptibility to OSA increases directly with the number of affected relatives [85–87]. A familial basis for OSA has been reported in a nonobese population [88], and obesity was found to explain only 40% of the genetic variance in the severity of OSA in an obese cohort [89]. The Cleveland

Family Study demonstrated that up to 35% of the variance in the severity of OSA, assessed by measuring the AHI, can be attributed, independently of the BMI, to genetic factors with possible racial differences in the mode of inheritance [90].

Genetic determinants of craniofacial morphology, obesity and control of breathing have been implicated as the genetic underpinnings of OSA [91, 92]. Obesity is the greatest risk factor for OSA, but genes involved in the development of OSA, obesity and regional fat distribution appear to be different [92]. Questions about family history of OSA may help to identify patients with the condition [9].

4 Obstructive Sleep Apnea Symptoms and Signs

4.1 *Daytime Symptoms*

4.1.1 Excessive Sleepiness

The American Academy of Sleep Medicine (AASM) Standards of Practice Committee defines excessive sleepiness as 'sleepiness that occurs in a situation when an individual would usually be expected to be awake and alert' [93].

4.1.1.1 Measurements of Subjective Sleepiness: The Patient's Perception of Sleepiness and Sleep Propensity. The state of acute sleepiness, i.e. an individual's level of sleepiness at a particular time, can be assessed with various rating scales, including visual analog scales [94], the Karolinska Sleepiness Scale [95] and the Stanford Sleepiness Scale [96]. These measures are useful to assess current sleepiness and for research purposes, e.g. to assess the effect of a drug on the circadian variation of sleepiness [97]. The Karolinska Sleepiness Scale measures the perception of the need for sleep and the feelings and symptoms associated with a drowsy state [95]. The Stanford Sleepiness Scale was one of the first self-rating scales used to assess various degrees of alertness/sleepiness [96]. It can show slight differences between groups of subjects assessed in clinical studies, but the scores of patients and normal subjects may not always be significantly different [98, 99]. The Epworth Sleepiness Scale is a measure of sleep propensity, e.g. the tendency to nod off [100]. It has been shown to be well correlated with a patient's own perception of sleepiness, but to have a weak or absent correlation with objective measures of sleepiness [101, 102]. Although the reliability and validity of the Epworth Sleepiness Scale has been questioned [103], it is a widely used tool.

Subjective sleepiness has many facets, and there can be discordance in the findings among the different types of measures of subjective sleepiness in a single patient or group of patients [104]. It is of note that all of the rating scales mentioned above are simple methods to assess sleepiness, but they suffer from the risk of unintended bias or purposeful falsification [97, 105].

4.1.1.2 Measurements of Objective Sleepiness and Wakefulness. The gold standard measures of objective and subjective sleepiness are the Multiple Sleep Latency Test (MSLT) and the Maintenance of Wakefulness Test (MWT), respectively [106]. The

MSLT is a validated and objective measure of the ability or tendency to fall asleep under standardized conditions and in the absence of external alerting factors, i.e. patients are instructed not to resist the onset of sleep [93, 107]. The MSLT begins at 1.5–3 h after the termination of a nocturnal PSG. It assesses, on 4 or 5 occasions (nap sessions) separated by 2-hour intervals, the sleep latency and the stage of sleep achieved at the onset of sleep. According to the AASM Standards of Practice Committee [93], 'the MSLT is not routinely indicated in the initial evaluation and diagnosis of OSA or in the assessment of change following treatment with nasal CPAP'. As the co-occurrence of OSA and narcolepsy is well documented [108], the MSLT may be indicated when a patient with OSA is suspected of having narcolepsy (particularly after a therapeutic trial of CPAP has failed to improve sleepiness or other symptoms suggest narcolepsy).

The MWT is a validated and objective measure of the ability to stay awake for a defined period of time [93, 107]. Patients are seated in bed and are instructed to remain awake for as long as possible. The MWT may be used, e.g. in truck drivers, to assess the effect of CPAP administration on the ability of OSA patients to stay awake [107]. A mean sleep latency of less than 15–20 min on the 40-min MWT is considered to be abnormal [107]. Staying awake on all trials of a 40-min MWT provides the strongest objective data available supporting an individual's ability to stay awake [93]. However, completely normal values do not necessarily ensure safety as there is little evidence linking mean sleep latency on the MWT with the risk of accidents in real-life circumstances. Therefore, the AASM Standards of Practice Committee emphasizes that clinical judgment (taking into account medical history, sleep habits, side effects of medication, compliance with treatment etc.) should always prevail in the assessment of patients for sleep impairment and the risk of accidents, i.e. the clinician's decision should not rely solely on mean sleep latency test results [93].

Significant but modest correlations have been reported between the MSLT and MWT [109]. This may be related to the fact that these tests measure different factors, i.e. wakefulness and sleepiness, respectively. Most often, the MWT and MSLT show an improvement with the effective treatment of OSA, but in contrast to the MWT, the MSLT does not usually normalize after treatment [110].

Other tests have been proposed to objectively assess vigilance, such as the Oxford Sleep Resistance Test [111, 112] and the Psychomotor Vigilance Task [113, 114].

4.1.2 Excessive Sleepiness in the General Population and in Patients with Obstructive Sleep Apnea

In the general population, the prevalence of excessive sleepiness is approximately 5–10%. In a Finnish population study, 11.0% of women and 6.7% of men reported excessive sleepiness every day or almost every day [115]. Similar prevalence rates were reported for excessive sleepiness in a general population sample (8.7%, with an equal prevalence for men and women; n = 16,583, ranging in age from 20 to 100 years) [116].

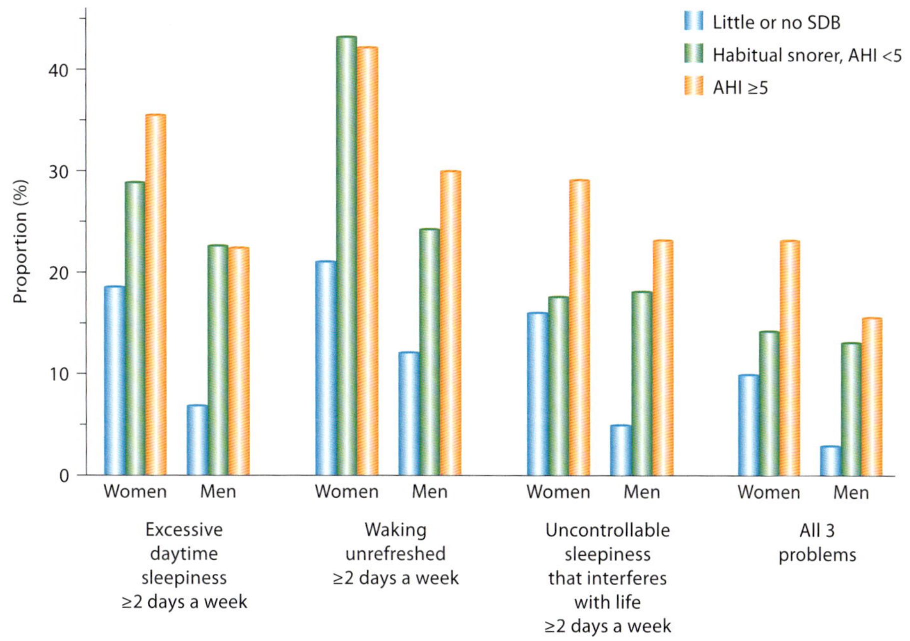

Fig. 2. Proportion of men and women reporting hypersomnolence, according to the category of SDB. Compared with subjects with little or no SDB, habitual snorers and subjects with an AHI ≥5 were significantly ($p < 0.001$) more likely to have hypersomnolence (the prevalence of hypersomnolence was higher among women than men, $p < 0.01$). Note that most subjects with an AHI ≥5 were not hypersomnolent and that hypersomnolence was significantly prevalent in subjects with little or no SDB, e.g. approximately 20% of women with little or no SDB reported excessive sleepiness ≥2 days a week. Data from the Wisconsin Sleep Cohort Study (n = 602, age range 30–60 years). After Young et al. [5], with permission. © 1993 Massachusetts Medical Society.

In patients with OSA, excessive sleepiness is a cardinal symptom; however, many apneic subjects demonstrate minimal evidence of this symptom (fig. 2) [5, 99]. Excessive sleepiness is frequently underestimated or denied by patients with OSA (fig. 3) [117] because they may fail to view sleepiness as a reportable problem since they have adapted to this condition over time. Numerous studies have demonstrated that, compared with sham CPAP or oral placebo, effective CPAP treatment improves excessive sleepiness [118–122].

Excessive sleepiness may be due to factors independent of OSA including OSA comorbidities (obesity, depression and diabetes mellitus), sleep disorders other than OSA (sleep deprivation) or side effects due to medication [116, 123, 124]. The simultaneous assessment of potential risk factors associated with excessive sleepiness in a general population sample (n = 16,583, ranging in age from 20 to 100 years) revealed that depression was the most significant risk factor for excessive sleepiness,

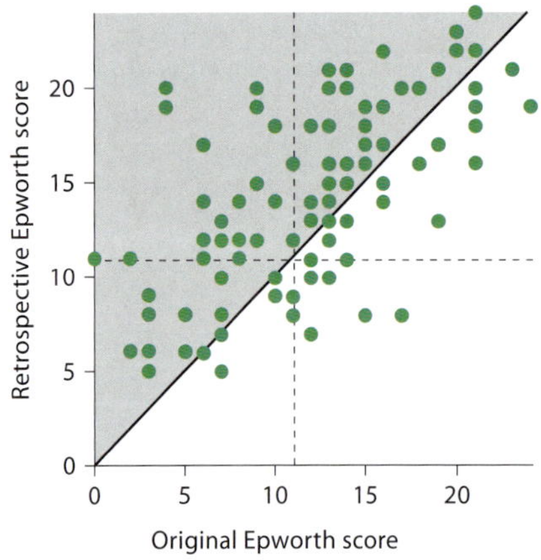

Fig. 3. Original and retrospective Epworth ratings for pretreatment sleepiness in patients with OSA. To assess the underreporting of excessive sleepiness, patients (n = 99) repeated their ratings of the pretreatment Epworth sleepiness scale: first, before diagnosis of OSA (i.e. at presentation: original Epworth score) and after starting treatment with CPAP therapy (retrospective Epworth score). The diagonal line is the line of identity. Patients above the line of identity underrated the Epworth score (gray area), and patients below the line of identity overrated the Epworth score. More patients originally underrated the Epworth score (67%) than overrated it (29%, $p < 0.001$). Patients with an originally 'normal' and retrospectively 'sleepy' Epworth score (upper left quadrant, n = 24) comprised 24% of all patients. After Engleman et al. [117], with permission.

followed by BMI, age, typical sleep duration, diabetes, smoking and finally sleep apnea [116]. It is suggested that patients with excessive sleepiness should be thoroughly assessed for depression, obesity and diabetes, independently of whether SDB is present.

In sum, the majority of patients with OSA does not complain about or may deny excessive sleepiness, and excessive sleepiness, the cardinal sign of OSA, may be due to conditions other than OSA in these individuals.

4.1.3 Fatigue

Fatigue and sleepiness are two separate entities, but these two terms have been frequently interchanged in the literature, and patients themselves may have difficulties in discriminating between them [97, 125]. Several definitions of fatigue have been proposed that describe self-reported patient perceptions and the consequences of fatigue on performance, e.g. physical or mental performance, or the ability to function at normal capacity [97]. Fatigue has been defined as an overwhelming sense of tiredness, lack of energy and a feeling of exhaustion associated with impaired physical and/or cognitive functioning that needs to be distinguished from symptoms of depression, which include a lack of self-esteem, sadness, and despair or hopelessness

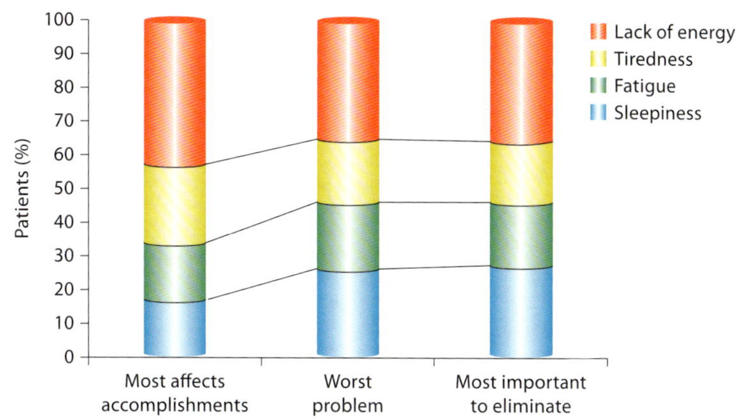

Fig. 4. Frequency of lack of energy, tiredness, fatigue and sleepiness in 117 men and 73 women with OSA. Lack of energy, tiredness and fatigue were reported to be a problem more often or almost always by the majority of the patients (62, 61 and 57%, respectively) than sleepiness (47%). Lack of energy was considered as the major problem by the majority of patients. Specifically, 44% of patients said that lack of energy most affected their ability to accomplish what they wanted, 36% considered lack of energy to be their worst problem, and 36% said that this problem was the one they were most eager to have cured. In comparison, only 16% of patients said sleepiness most affected their accomplishments, 25% said sleepiness was their worst problem, and 27% said that sleepiness was the one problem that they were most eager to have cured. After Chervin [129], with permission.

[97]. Fatigue in patients with OSA has been measured with tools such as the Fatigue Severity Scale [126], visual analog scales [104] and questionnaires such as the fatigue-inertia subscale of the Profile of Mood States [127]. Fatigue is widely reported in patients with OSA, e.g. up to 40% of OSA patients recruited by advertising or word-of-mouth referral [128]. Complaints of fatigue, tiredness and lack of energy have been reported to be more frequent and more distressing to OSA patients than excessive sleepiness (fig. 4) [129]. Increased fatigue levels have been associated with the increased severity of depressive symptoms in OSA patients [130].

4.2 Sleep-Related Symptoms

4.2.1 Snoring, Witnessed Apneas and Nocturnal Choking

The prevalence of habitual snoring in the general population ranges from 15 to 47% in men and from 6 to 33% in women [80, 131, 132]. Snoring is a predominant symptom of OSA that frequently depends on the patient's sleeping position. Snoring is frequently underestimated or denied by patients and is typically reported by their bed partners; approximately 75% of patients who deny snoring are proven to be snorers when measured objectively [133]. Snoring is a cause of poor sleep quality for the patient's partner or a family nuisance [134]. It has been reported to be independently

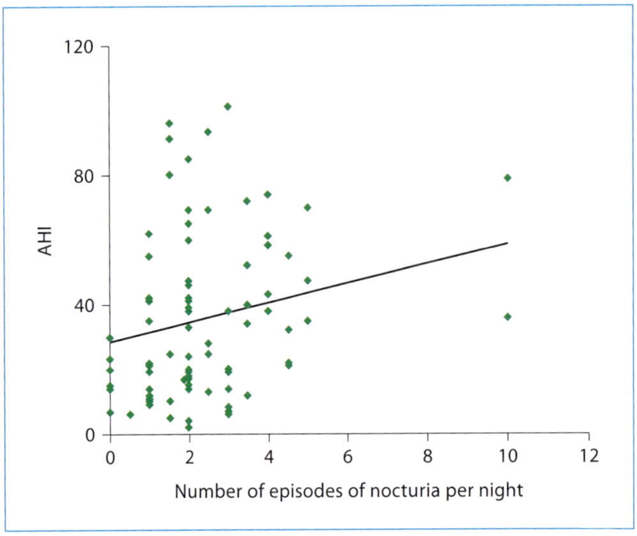

Fig. 5. Correlation between the number of episodes of nocturia per night with the AHI ($r = 0.25$, $p < 0.01$) in patients with OSA ($n = 97$). After Margel et al. [146], with permission.

associated with excessive sleepiness [135], cognitive decline [136], poor academic performance in medical students [137], and a higher risk of cardiovascular (e.g. hypertension and stroke) disease [138, 139] and type 2 diabetes [140].

Witnessed apneas and nocturnal choking are related to apneic events and are typically reported by bed partners. They have also been reported in up to 6% of the normal nonapneic population [141].

4.2.2 Nocturia

Nocturia is defined by the International Continence Society as 'waking once or more at night to urinate' (each void is preceded by and followed by sleep) [142]. The prevalence of nocturia has been reported to be greater in OSA patients than in non-OSA control subjects [143–145]. Nocturia, defined as ≥2 urinations at night, has been reported to be as high as 50% in patients with SDB [144]. The number of voids at night has been found to correlate with the severity of OSA as assessed using the AHI (fig. 5) [146].

Mechanisms that lead to nocturia in OSA patients may include increased atrial natriuretic peptide levels [145, 147, 148]. Obstructive respiratory events combined with sustained ventilatory effort in OSA generate a negative intrathoracic pressure, causing the heart to receive a false signal of volume overload. The hormonal response to this signal includes an increase in atrial natriuretic peptide secretion and, hence, increased urine production. CPAP treatment eliminates the negative intrathoracic pressure and may reduce the secretion of atrial natriuretic peptide, resolving the nocturia [143, 144, 146–149]. Nocturia in OSA patients may also be due to an increased

Table 4. Psychiatric comorbidities in Veterans Health Administration beneficiaries, with and without sleep apnea

Comorbidity	Sleep apnea group (n = 122,052) %	Non-sleep-apnea group (n = 3,525,276) %	Odds ratio	95% CI	χ^2 p value
Depression	21.75	9.43	2.67	2.63–2.71	<0.0001
Anxiety	16.67	8.39	2.18	2.15–2.22	<0.0001
Posttraumatic stress disorder	11.85	4.74	2.70	2.65–2.74	<0.0001
Psychosis	5.13	3.75	1.40	1.35–1.43	<0.0001
Bipolar disorders	4.06	1.88	2.20	2.15–2.27	<0.0001
Dementia	2.13	1.81	1.18	1.13–1.23	<0.0001

After Sharafkhaneh et al. [155], with permission.

awareness of bladder fullness secondary to arousal [150] and/or transmission to the bladder of positive intra-abdominal pressure associated with recurrent obstructive respiratory events [151].

4.3 *Sequelae*

Sequelae are prevalent in patients with OSA and may influence the clinician's diagnostic process to identify OSA.

4.3.1 Psychological Changes and Psychiatric Symptoms

Psychiatric symptoms or disorders associated with OSA [152] include depression [153–156], anxiety [157], hypochondriasis, conversion-hysteria symptoms [158], delirium [159], posttraumatic stress disorder [160] and homicidal behavior [161]. Examination of the Veterans Health Administration database, which contains health care data for more than 4 million veterans, has shown that the prevalence of comorbid psychiatric conditions is significantly higher in individuals with diagnosed sleep apnea than in individuals free from this diagnosis (after controlling for age, sex, ethnicity and other medical conditions) (table 4) [155]. In this study population, up to 20% of the subjects presenting with sleep apnea had depression and vice versa [155], and similar findings have been reported by others [153]. Other authors have observed elevated rates of OSA in patients with depression [162] and in those with chronic schizophrenia [163].

Depressive symptoms are observed in up to 50% of patients with OSA [153–156]. They appear to be more common and more severe in women with OSA than in men [156]. Symptoms of depression and anxiety, although prevalent in OSA, correlate poorly or not at all with OSA severity as assessed using the AHI [156, 164, 165]. These symptoms have been considered to be similar to those associated with chronic general medical conditions [154, 155, 166, 167] and are characterized by elevated somatic and cognitive symptoms of depression without affective symptoms, thus differing from the affective mood changes observed in more typical forms of depression. Some authors have reported that CPAP may improve depressive symptoms [120, 166, 168, 169], but this has yet to be confirmed [170–172].

Mood changes associated with OSA could be secondary to neural injury [165, 173, 174], to consequences of OSA such as excessive sleepiness [175] and impaired quality of life [175], and to conditions associated with OSA such as metabolic syndrome and cardiovascular diseases, which are risk factors for depression [154].

In sum, whether depression is independently associated with OSA remains to be elucidated. OSA should be suspected in depressed patients in the presence of typical OSA symptoms or symptoms such as irritability, tiredness, disrupted sleep, difficulties with concentration and accomplishing tasks, generally decreased social, familial or professional performance [166], important sleep/wake complaints [176], depression that is resistant to treatment [177, 178], risk factors such as metabolic syndrome or cardiovascular diseases [167, 179, 180], and simultaneous antihypertensive and antidepressant medications [181]. Depression should be suspected in OSA patients with insomnia [155], excessive somnolence and fatigue [130], or 'apparently mild' depressive symptoms that are not significantly improved by CPAP therapy [116, 182].

4.3.2 Health-Related Quality of Life

Quality of life is an abstract, multidimensional and subjective concept that can be defined as the level of the patient's overall sense of well-being [183]. Health-related quality of life is the measure of the impact of a disease on the patient's quality of life. It is assessed by measuring the impact of the disease on social, psychological and physical dimensions in their life, the burden of symptoms and the perception of their overall well-being [183]. Several tools, including generic and disease-specific quality of life measures, have been used to assess the impact of the condition and the outcome of treatment in SDB. The choice between these tools depends on the reason for their use. The use of a generic, e.g. the SF-36, and a disease-specific questionnaire to assess health-related quality of life in OSA patients has been recommended [183, 184].

Clinic- and population-based studies have shown that patients with OSA have a significantly impaired quality of life [183, 185, 186]. Similarly to the symptoms associated with OSA, quality of life scores are weakly or not at all related to objective measures of OSA severity, such as the AHI and nocturnal hypoxemia [187, 188]. Several studies, including a randomized, double-blind, controlled, parallel trial of therapeutic versus subtherapeutic CPAP, have shown that CPAP improves quality of life scores [119, 134, 189–191]. A meta-analysis of studies published between 1966 and 2007 comparing values of CPAP with controls indicated that CPAP does not improve the general quality of life scores, but does improve physical domains and vitality [192]. It was suggested that study design and quality of life questionnaire tools are important to capture and evaluate information efficiently and that generic quality of life instruments may not be adequate to detect important changes in quality of life in patients with OSA. According to the Cochrane database review [193], quality of life is significantly improved by CPAP administration when compared with a placebo pill or sham CPAP. Improvement in health status assessed by the Nottingham Health Profile or the SF-36 may be related to a feeling of increased well-being following the treatment of sleepiness [193]. It has been suggested that nasal CPAP improves the health-related quality of life by alleviating depression [168]. It is not clear whether the impaired health-related quality of life is directly related to OSA or to factors associated with the syndrome, such as obesity, sleepiness and depression [188].

4.3.3 Performance Alterations

A wide range of performance alterations have been associated with OSA, including social and familial dysfunction (fig. 6a, b), impaired work performance [194], and increased risk of vehicle and industrial accidents [195].

4.3.3.1 Alterations in Cognitive Function. Cognitive function deficit is a key factor that may contribute to performance alterations in patients with OSA [196]. Cognitive function can be broadly divided into 3 functional areas: attention, memory and learning abilities, and executive performance [99]. A meta-analysis indicated that vigilance, motor coordination and executive functions ranged from moderately to markedly impaired in adults with untreated sleep apnea, whereas intelligence and verbal and visual perceptual abilities were not affected [197]. Mild sleep apnea is usually associated with small cognitive impairments, whereas moderate or severe OSA may be associated with moderate-to-large cognitive performance deficits [99, 198–200]. Neuropsychological performance alterations were negatively correlated with AHI, independently of age, sex and educational status [201]. It was estimated that an AHI of 15 is equivalent to the decrement in psychomotor efficiency associated with 5 additional years of age, or to 50% of the decrement associated with hypnosedative use [201]. Furthermore, age and depression may aggravate the adverse effects of OSA on cognitive functions. The combined effects of age and OSA were demonstrated to produce significant impairments in behavioral performance and cerebral responses beyond that of either variable alone [202]. Similarly, using imaging techniques, neural injury was shown to differ between OSA patients with and without depressive symptoms [203]. These studies may underscore the importance of the early detection of OSA.

The neuropsychological impairments in OSA have been related to functional alterations in the prefrontal, anterior cingulate, hippocampal and parietal areas of the brain (for a review on this subject, see Desseilles et al. [204] and Lim and Veasey [205]). It

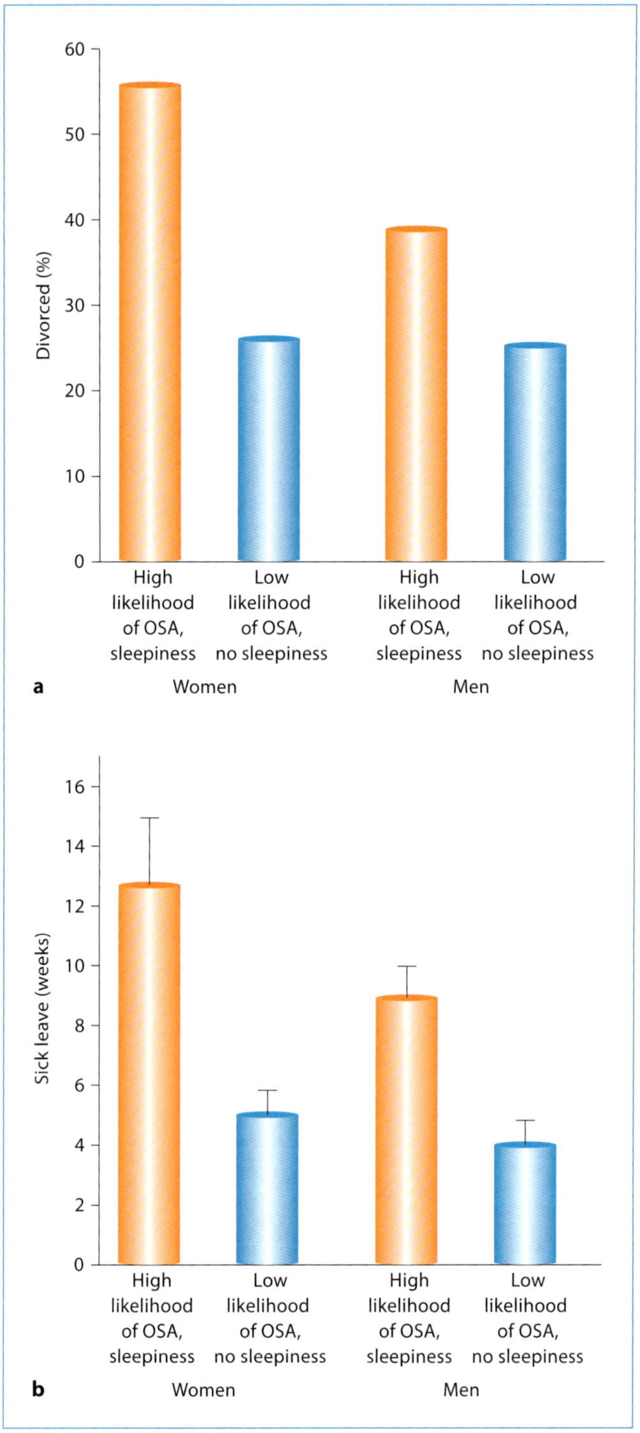

Fig. 6. Impact of self-reported sleep-related breathing disturbances on divorce and sick leave rates. **a** Percentage of women and men divorced at least once in subjects with a high likelihood of OSA plus frequent sleepiness (n = 155 women and 338 men) compared with subjects having a low likelihood of OSA and no reported sleepiness (n = 481 women and 216 men). Odds ratio (women): 4.6, 95% CI: 3.4–6.3; odds ratio (men): 1.9, 95% CI: 1.4–2.5. The multivariate analysis revealed that a high likelihood of OSA or sleepiness or both were independent predictors of the divorce rate. **b** Amount of sick leave in the previous 12 months in subjects with a high likelihood of OSA plus frequent sleepiness (n = 155 women and 338 men) compared with subjects having a low likelihood of OSA and no reported sleepiness (n = 481 women and 216 men). Multivariate analysis revealed that a high likelihood of OSA or sleepiness or both was an independent predictor for the amount of sick leave (women, $p < 0.0001$; men, $p = 0.002$). After Grunstein et al. [267], with permission.

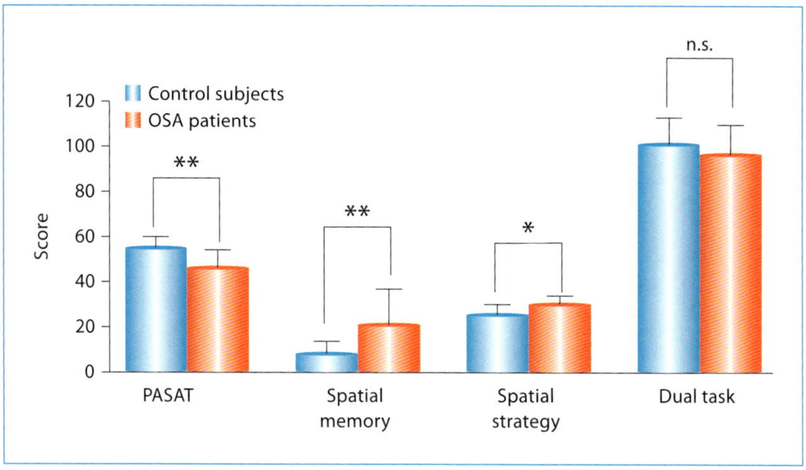

Fig. 7. Comparison of performance in working memory tasks between 25 patients with OSA and 25 matched control subjects. The working memory assessment was based on the evaluation of the maintenance and processing of information using the Paced Auditory Serial Addition Test (PASAT), the Self-Ordered Spatial Memory Task to assess spatial memory and spatial strategy, and tests requiring simultaneous work on 2 types of information (auditory short-term memory plus tracking tasks). OSA patients obtained significantly lower scores than controls for the PASAT. They obtained significantly higher scores than controls for spatial memory and strategy tests (spatial memory and spatial strategy with low scores indicate an efficient strategy). However, dual-task performance did not differ significantly between OSA patients and controls. ** $p < 0.001$; * $p < 0.05$; n.s. = not significant. After Naegele et al. [214], with permission; see also for an extensive description of each of these tests.

is controversial whether OSA patients present with a loss of gray matter in regions involved in various cognitive functions [206–209]. An overrecruitment of brain regions to compensate for cognitive deficits (cognitive reserve) may mask the cognitive decline associated with OSA [210, 211]. Not all cognitive function alterations are reversed after CPAP administration, and they may represent neuronal damage [212].

4.3.3.2 *Memory Impairment.* Memory is currently considered as a collection of mental abilities including episodic memory, semantic memory, procedural memory and working memory (for a review on this subject, see Budson et al. [213]). Several memory systems, but not all [214], have been reported to be impaired in patients with OSA, including verbal and visual episodic memory [215–217], procedural memory [217, 218] and working memory (fig. 7) [199, 219, 220], although the latter is not consistently affected [216, 221]. Memory has been shown to improve, at least partially, with effective treatment of OSA [215, 216, 219, 220, 222]. Sleep fragmentation and intermittent nocturnal hypoxia are likely to contribute to memory dysfunction [99].

4.3.3.3 *Motor Vehicle Accidents.* Two research groups have extensively reviewed studies of the link between OSA and the risk for motor vehicle accidents in commercial and noncommercial drivers [223, 224]. They found that OSA patients had an up to approximately 5 times greater risk for motor vehicle accidents than non-OSA individuals [223, 224]. Factors that have been associated with this increased risk include the BMI; however, OSA severity and excessive sleepiness were not consistently linked with this increased risk [223, 224]. Alcohol may increase the risk of traffic accidents in OSA patients compared with non-OSA subjects [225]. Following CPAP therapy, the driving performance of OSA patients improves when tested by simulators [226], and the risk of motor vehicle accidents appears to return to normal [227–230].

5 Characteristic Clinical Features of Obstructive Sleep Apnea in Patients with Metabolic or Cardiovascular Disorders

The characteristic clinical features of OSA in patients with metabolic or cardiovascular disorders are reviewed in chapters 3 and 6, respectively [this vol., pp. 67–137 and 197–265]. Briefly, OSA is highly prevalent in patients with metabolic disorders, e.g. type 2 diabetes, but it may not be predicted using clinical data [231]. The International Diabetes Federation recently published clinical practice recommendations suggesting that OSA patients should be routinely screened for markers of metabolic disturbance, including fasting glucose. Similarly, it recommended that the possibility of OSA should be considered in the assessment of all patients with type 2 diabetes.

The failure to recognize OSA in patients with cardiovascular diseases is related to several causes (table 5), including the lack of sleep medicine training in health professional education, restricted patient access to appropriate investigations, and the poor specificity and predictive value of OSA signs and symptoms [232]. OSA patients with chronic heart failure, stroke or coronary artery disease may be less sleepy and less obese than OSA patients without these conditions [see chapter 6, this vol., pp. 197–265]; therefore, the absence of subjective sleepiness or obesity is not a reliable measure to rule out OSA in these patients.

6 A Brief Presentation of the Strategies and Tests to Identify Obstructive Sleep Apnea and Treatment Options According to the American Academy of Sleep Medicine Guidelines

6.1 Guidelines

The AASM guidelines for the evaluation of adult patients with OSA are based on consensus, i.e. 'developed to address important areas of clinical practice that had not been the subject of a previous AASM practice parameter, or where the available empirical data were limited or inconclusive' [4]. The diagnostic process is described as starting in 1 of 3 clinical settings: the evaluation of a patient's complaint, routine health

Table 5. Potential reasons that sleep issues have not been embraced by the cardiology community

Concern	Response	Potential solution
Clinician factors		
Lack of awareness by physicians	Traditionally, no teaching in medical school and residency	Enhanced medical education
Lack of classic symptoms such as sleepiness in chronic heart failure [268]	Routine, thorough questioning in medical history	High index of suspicion
Concerns about the confounding of OSA by covariates, such as obesity, in prior studies [269]	Large, rigorous studies have now shown the independent effects of OSA [270]	Interventional studies help to show that treatment of sleep apnea per se is important [271]
Lack of mechanistic research, particularly for sleep deprivation	Data are evolving; field is young	Further research
Lack of definitive multicenter, randomized, controlled studies	Ethical barriers to withholding therapy in symptomatic OSA patients Poor adherence and potential lack of efficacy in asymptomatic OSA patients	Further research Develop better treatments Large-scale studies
Patient factors		
Lack of awareness by patients	Traditional lack of importance placed on sleep duration and symptoms of sleep disorders	Public education Lay press
Reluctance to undergo diagnostic testing	A sleep study is innocuous compared to many diagnostic tests in cardiology	Patient education Development of newer technologies to diagnose sleep disorders in the home
Reluctance to use CPAP or other positive airway pressure devices	Some patients feel much better Develop better technologies Adherence is comparable to other chronic medical therapies [272]	Develop better technologies Provide more definitive data
	Bed partner is often happy with the alleviation of snoring	Patient education
	Newer technologies with blowers, masks and humidifiers are available	Intensive support [273]

After Malhotra et al. [232], with permission.

maintenance evaluation and evaluation of patients at high risk for OSA (fig. 8) [4]. The presence of OSA symptoms leads to a comprehensive sleep evaluation to categorize patients according to their risk for OSA. This evaluation includes the assessment of symptoms and secondary conditions that may occur as a result of OSA and a physical evaluation.

- A patient presenting with any of the symptoms, signs and sequelae detailed above in this chapter may be suspected of having OSA [4]; however, signs and symptoms in isolation are of little utility to identify OSA [32, 233–236]. Anamnesis of the patient's partner may provide useful information about cognitive function and symptoms that OSA patients may often underreport or deny, e.g. snoring and excessive somnolence [185, 237, 238]. It is of note that the clinical impression of sleep experts has been reported to be accurate in only 52–60 and 65–70% of cases in 2 respective studies [233, 239].
- Questionnaires such as the Wisconsin questionnaire, the sleep disorder questionnaire, the self-report questionnaire, the multivariate apnea prediction index and the Berlin questionnaire have been used to identify OSA [240–242]. The Berlin questionnaire is among the most widely used [242], and it has been considered to be useful in specific populations such as preoperative patients [243] and patients at risk of the recurrence of atrial fibrillation after catheter ablation [244]. However, it has a low specificity (65%) in patients with resistant hypertension [245] and a low sensitivity and specificity (62 and 43%, respectively) in a sleep clinic population [246]. Overall, the Berlin questionnaire, which was developed and initially validated in primary care centers, may have limited diagnostic utility in populations other than that in which it was initially validated. A modified version of the Berlin questionnaire administered to patients' bed partners has also been shown to have a low specificity (54%) [247].
- Prediction models mainly consisting of a combination of weighted clinical characteristics have been developed from patient population studies in order to help identify patients with [242, 248] or without OSA [249]. Most of these prediction models include features such as body habitus measurements and bed partners' reports of snoring, apneas and gasping respiration. Although the sensitivity of some prediction models may be high, their specificity is often low. According to the AASM guidelines, no clinical model is recommended to predict the severity of OSA [4, 250, 251].
- The AASM consensus-derived features [4] that may suggest the presence of OSA include increased neck circumference (>43 cm in men and >41 cm in women), BMI ≥30, a modified Mallampati score of 3 or 4, and the presence of retrognathia, lateral peritonsillar narrowing, macroglossia, tonsillar hypertrophy, elongated/enlarged uvula, high arched/narrow hard palate, nasal abnormalities (polyps, deviation, valve abnormalities and turbinate hypertrophy) and/or overjet.

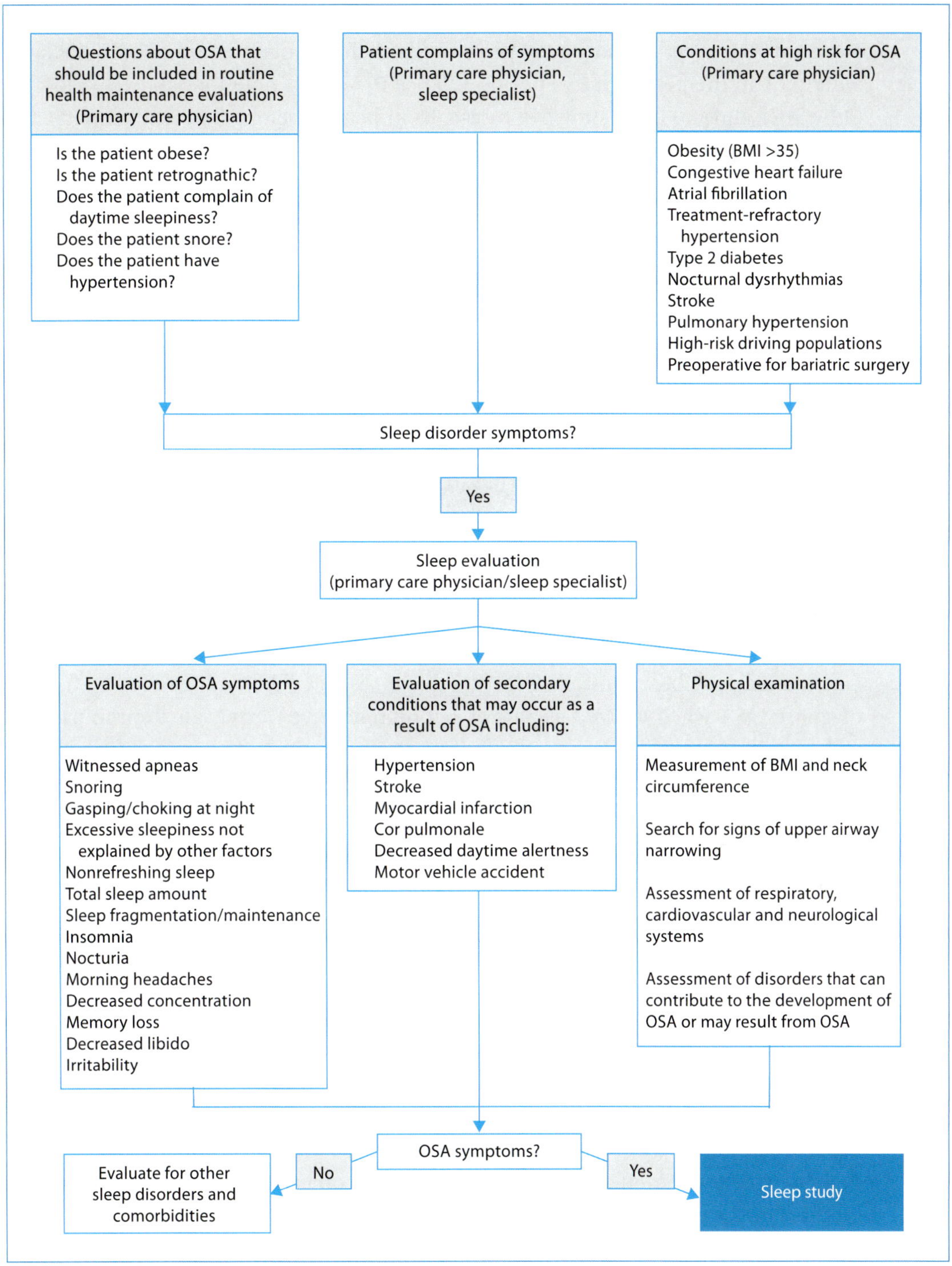

Fig. 8. Consensus-based recommendations for the diagnosis of OSA in adults, after the Adult OSA Task Force of the AASM (see text) [4], with permission.

Patients with a high risk for OSA should undergo a sleep study to confirm its presence [4]; indeed, adverse respiratory and cardiovascular outcomes are associated with OSA in the perioperative period [252, 253]. It is of note that an evaluation for OSA, including a sleep study, is routinely indicated before bariatric surgery and upper airway surgery for snoring or OSA [250]. For patients who are not at a high risk for OSA, the diagnostic strategy and timing for the patient depend on the risk of OSA and the presence of daytime impairment or associated morbidity [4].

6.2 *Diagnostic Tests*

The Standards of Practice Committee of the American Sleep Disorders Association (the previous name of the AASM) developed definitions and delineated levels of equipment type for monitoring that can lead to the diagnosis of OSA [254]. Type 1 monitoring, the gold standard diagnostic test for OSA, is a full, attended PSG in a laboratory setting [255]. Type 2 monitoring is a full, unattended PSG. Type 3 monitoring is performed using limited channel devices (usually with 4–7 channels). Type 4 monitoring is performed using 1 or 2 channels, usually with oximetry as one of the parameters.

The AASM developed guidelines for the indications of PSG and for the use of unattended portable monitors in the diagnosis of OSA in adult patients [250, 251]. PSG is routinely indicated for the diagnosis of sleep-related breathing disorders [250]. Unattended portable monitoring for the diagnosis of OSA in adults may be used to diagnose OSA when utilized as part of a comprehensive sleep evaluation in patients with a high pretest likelihood of moderate-to-severe OSA (the probability of OSA before a diagnostic test result is known; table 6) [251]. It should record, at a minimum, airflow and respiratory effort with biosensors conventionally used for in-laboratory PSG. Patients not considered appropriate for portable monitoring should undergo in-laboratory PSG [4]. However, no definitive resolution exists for the application of these guidelines in specific populations, e.g. sleep clinic screening in high-risk groups such as chronic heart failure patients and preoperative patients.

6.3 *Treatment Options*

OSA is a chronic disorder that requires long-term, multidisciplinary management. Education of the patient is administered (table 7), and treatment outcomes are evaluated (table 8) before initiating the treatment for OSA and at a follow-up visit [4]. Treatment options including medical, behavioral and surgical therapies are briefly described here. The effects of treatment on outcomes assessing OSA pathogenic mechanisms and cardiovascular and metabolic changes associated with OSA are reported in the relevant chapters of this book.

6.3.1 Positive Airway Pressure Administration

Positive airway pressure is the gold standard treatment for OSA. It is the most effective currently available treatment for OSA. It is administered to patients via a nasal or

Table 6. Clinical guidelines for the use of unattended portable monitors in the diagnosis of OSA in adult patients

Unattended portable monitoring for the diagnosis of OSA:
• *is not appropriate* for the diagnosis of OSA in patients – with significant comorbid medical conditions that may degrade the accuracy of portable monitoring, including, but not limited to, moderate-to-severe pulmonary disease, neuromuscular disease or congestive heart failure – suspected of having comorbid sleep disorders
• *is not appropriate* for general screening[1] of asymptomatic populations
• *may be used* as an alternative to PSG for the diagnosis of OSA in patients with a high pretest probability of moderate-to-severe OSA; negative or technically inadequate portable monitoring tests in patients with a high pretest probability of moderate-to-severe OSA should prompt in-laboratory PSG
• *may be indicated* for the diagnosis of OSA in patients for whom in-laboratory PSG is not possible by virtue of immobility, safety or critical illness
• *may be indicated* to monitor the response to non-CPAP treatments for sleep apnea

After Collop et al. [251], with permission.
[1] Screening is a strategy used in a population to detect a disease in subjects without signs or symptoms of that disease.

Table 7. Components of patient education programs, after the AASM clinical guidelines for the evaluation, management and long-term care of OSA in adults [4]

- Findings of study, severity of disease
- Pathophysiology of OSA
- Explanation of the natural course of the disease and associated disorders
- Risk factor identification, explanation of exacerbating factors and risk factor modification
- Genetic counseling when indicated
- Treatment options
- What to expect from the treatment
- Outline the patient's role in the treatment, address their concerns and set goals
- Consequences of untreated disease
- Drowsy driving/sleepiness counseling
- Patient quality assessment and other feedback regarding evaluation

Reprinted with permission.

facial mask and prevents upper airway obstruction during sleep by acting as a pneumatic splint of the upper airway. It can cure abnormal breathing during sleep and improve sleep quality, sleepiness and quality of life [256]. It should be offered as an option to all patients (AASM consensus) [4], is the treatment of choice for moderate-

Table 8. General OSA outcome assessment, after the AASM clinical guidelines for the evaluation, management and long-term care of OSA in adults [4]

- Resolution of sleepiness
- OSA-specific quality of life measures
- Patient and spousal satisfaction
- Adherence to therapy
- Avoidance of factors that worsen the disease
- Obtaining an adequate amount of sleep
- Practicing proper sleep hygiene
- Weight loss for overweight/obese patients

Reprinted with permission.

to-severe OSA and may be proposed to patients with mild OSA [4, 256]. The relatively poor adherence to positive airway pressure treatment (30–60%) is a critical problem as it reduces its efficacy [257]. Various strategies have been proposed to improve treatment adherence including education, support, cognitive behavioral approaches, humidification of the inspired air, appropriate selection of the mask, addition of a pressure ramp, use of partial pressure reduction during expiration (pressure relief), and changes from CPAP to bilevel or autotitrating modes of positive airway pressure administration [2, 4, 257].

6.3.2 Oral Appliances

Oral appliances are efficacious therapeutic options for OSA [258]. Most are custom made by a dentist experienced in the use of this device for OSA patients. Mandibular repositioning devices, also termed mandibular repositioning appliances, mandibular advancement devices, mandibular advancement appliances or mandibular advancement splints, tend to prevent upper airway collapse by protruding the mandible [258] and are the most frequently used types of oral appliance for the treatment of OSA. Tongue-retaining devices maintain the tongue in a protruded position during sleep [258]. Overall, the administration of positive airway pressure is more efficacious than oral appliances. According to the AASM [4, 259], oral appliances are indicated in patients with severe OSA only as a second-line therapy after an initial trial with positive airway pressure treatment. They are indicated in patients with mild-to-moderate OSA who prefer an oral appliance to positive airway pressure therapy, who are not appropriate candidates for positive airway pressure therapy, or who fail positive airway pressure therapy or behavioral measures.

6.3.3 Weight Loss

Obesity is the strongest risk factor for OSA, and weight loss is associated with a decrease in OSA severity [see chapter 3, this vol., pp. 67–137] [260–262]. A population-based longitudinal study showed that after adjusting for sex, age and cigarette smoking, for each 1% decrease or increase in body weight, an approximately 3% decrease or increase in the AHI is expected, respectively [10, 30]. Prospective, randomized, controlled trials have confirmed the efficacy of weight loss in reducing the severity of OSA, not only in mild, but also in moderate-to-severe OSA [261–263]. Although the results of dietary changes are encouraging for the improvement of OSA, weight loss and the mean reduction in the AHI are greater after bariatric surgery than after dieting [10, 264, 265]. Exercise, avoidance of alcohol and sedatives at bedtime, and positional therapy are also behavioral treatments for OSA [4]. A backpack or a tennis ball may be second-line treatments to keep patients in a non-supine position who have a higher index of sleep apnea in a supine position than in other positions.

6.3.4 Surgery

The consensus-derived AASM guidelines consider that surgery may be a treatment option for OSA in some patients [4]. Its indication depends on the severity of OSA, patients' eligibility for surgery, general sleep evaluation, presence of medical, psychological or social comorbidities, and the determination of patients to undergo this therapy [4]. Surgical options (table 9), their likelihood of success, the objectives, risks and benefits of the procedure, and alternative treatments should be presented to patients. It is beyond the scope of this chapter to review the specifics of surgery for OSA. The consensus-derived AASM guidelines [4] state that:

1 surgery may be considered as a second-line treatment for OSA when the outcome of positive airway pressure therapy is inadequate, such as when the patient is intolerant of positive airway pressure or when positive airway pressure therapy cannot eliminate OSA;
2 surgery may be considered as a second-line treatment for OSA when there is an inadequate treatment outcome with an oral appliance, when the patient is intolerant of the oral appliance, or when oral appliance therapy provides an unacceptable improvement in the clinical outcome of OSA;
3 surgery may be considered as an adjunct therapy when obstructive anatomy or functional deficiencies compromise other therapies or to improve the patient's tolerance of other OSA treatments [4];
4 surgery may be considered as a primary treatment in patients with mild OSA who have severe obstructing anatomy that is surgically correctible, e.g. tonsillar hypertrophy obstructing the pharyngeal airway;
5 maxillary and mandibular advancement can improve PSG parameters comparable to positive airway pressure in the majority of patients [4]; most other sleep apnea surgeries are rarely curative for OSA but may improve the clinical outcome;
6 laser-assisted uvulopalatoplasty is not recommended for the treatment of OSA [266].

Table 9. Potential surgical procedures for OSA by site, after the AASM clinical guidelines for the evaluation, management and long-term care of OSA in adults [4]

Nasal procedures	• Septoplasty • Functional rhinoplasty • Nasal valve surgery • Turbinate reduction • Nasal polypectomy • Endoscopic procedures
Oral, oropharyngeal, and nasopharyngeal procedures	• Uvulopalatopharyngoplasty and variations • Palatal advancement pharyngoplasty • Tonsillectomy and/or adenoidectomy • Excision of tori mandibulares • Palatal implants
Hypopharyngeal procedures	• Tongue reduction ◦ Partial glossectomy ◦ Tongue ablation ◦ Lingual tonsillectomy • Tongue advancement/stabilization ◦ Genioglossus advancement ◦ Hyoid suspension ◦ Mandibular advancement ◦ Tongue suspension
Laryngeal procedures	• Epiglottoplasty • Hyoid suspension
Global airway procedures	• Maxillomandibular advancement • Bariatric surgery

Tracheostomy is currently a rarely performed upper airway bypass procedure. It can eliminate OSA but it does not appropriately treat central hypoventilation syndrome. Reprinted with permission.

7 Conclusion

OSA is a disease with serious consequences, not only for the patients, but also for their immediate family and wider society. Clinical assessment alone lacks accuracy, and objective testing is therefore needed to make the diagnosis. The AASM guidelines help clinicians in the diagnosis and therapeutic strategy for the management of OSA. There is a need for simplified validated procedures to identify OSA. There is also a need for guidelines, involving the collaboration of scientific societies concerned with the disease, to address the management of OSA in specific subpopulations at high risk for OSA such as cardiac patients who may present with OSA without the cardinal signs of the disease, i.e. snoring, excessive sleepiness and obesity.

8 References

1 American Academy of Sleep Medicine: International Classification of Sleep Disorders: Diagnostic and Coding Manual, ed 2. Westchester, American Academy of Sleep Medicine, 2005, pp 35–77.

2 Kushida CA, Chediak A, Berry RB, Brown LK, Gozal D, Iber C, Parthasarathy S, Quan SF, Rowley JA: Clinical guidelines for the manual titration of positive airway pressure in patients with obstructive sleep apnea. J Clin Sleep Med 2008;4:157–171.

3 Bao G, Guilleminault C: Upper airway resistance syndrome – one decade later. Curr Opin Pulm Med 2004;10:461–467.

4 Epstein LJ, Kristo D, Strollo PJ Jr, Friedman N, Malhotra A, Patil SP, Ramar K, Rogers R, Schwab RJ, Weaver EM, Weinstein MD: Clinical guideline for the evaluation, management and long-term care of obstructive sleep apnea in adults. J Clin Sleep Med 2009;5:263–276.

5 Young T, Palta M, Dempsey J, Skatrud J, Weber S, Badr S. The occurrence of sleep-disordered breathing among middle-aged adults. N Engl J Med 1993;328:1230–1235.

6 Gottlieb DJ, Whitney CW, Bonekat WH, Iber C, James GD, Lebowitz M, Nieto FJ, Rosenberg CE: Relation of sleepiness to respiratory disturbance index: the Sleep Heart Health Study. Am J Respir Crit Care Med 1999;159:502–507.

7 Redline S, Yenokyan G, Gottlieb DJ, Shahar E, O'Connor GT, Resnick HE, Diener-West M, Sanders MH, Wolf PA, Geraghty EM, Ali T, Lebowitz M, Punjabi NM: Obstructive sleep apnea-hypopnea and incident stroke: the Sleep Heart Health Study. Am J Respir Crit Care Med 2010;182:269–277.

8 Mokhlesi B: Obesity hypoventilation syndrome: a state-of-the-art review. Respir Care 2010;55:1347–1362, discussion 1363–1365.

9 Punjabi NM: The epidemiology of adult obstructive sleep apnea. Proc Am Thorac Soc 2008;5:136–143.

10 Young T, Peppard PE, Gottlieb DJ: Epidemiology of obstructive sleep apnea: a population health perspective. Am J Respir Crit Care Med 2002;165:1217–1239.

11 Bixler EO, Vgontzas AN, Lin HM, Ten Have T, Rein J, Vela-Bueno A, Kales A: Prevalence of sleep-disordered breathing in women: effects of gender. Am J Respir Crit Care Med 2001;163:608–613.

12 Ip MS, Lam B, Lauder IJ, Tsang KW, Chung KF, Mok YW, Lam WK: A community study of sleep-disordered breathing in middle-aged Chinese men in Hong Kong. Chest 2001;119:62–69.

13 Ip MS, Lam B, Tang LC, Lauder IJ, Ip TY, Lam WK: A community study of sleep-disordered breathing in middle-aged Chinese women in Hong Kong: prevalence and gender differences. Chest 2004;125: 127–134.

14 Kim J, In K, Kim J, You S, Kang K, Shim J, Lee S, Lee J, Lee S, Park C, Shin C: Prevalence of sleep-disordered breathing in middle-aged Korean men and women. Am J Respir Crit Care Med 2004;170:1108–1113.

15 Reddy EV, Kadhiravan T, Mishra HK, Sreenivas V, Handa KK, Sinha S, Sharma SK: Prevalence and risk factors of obstructive sleep apnea among middle-aged urban Indians: a community-based study. Sleep Med 2009;10:913–918.

16 Young T, Evans L, Finn L, Palta M: Estimation of the clinically diagnosed proportion of sleep apnea syndrome in middle-aged men and women. Sleep 1997;20:705–706.

17 Rosen RC, Zozula R, Jahn EG, Carson JL: Low rates of recognition of sleep disorders in primary care: comparison of a community-based versus clinical academic setting. Sleep Med 2001;2:47–55.

18 Kapur V, Blough DK, Sandblom RE, Hert R, de Maine JB, Sullivan SD, Psaty BM: The medical cost of undiagnosed sleep apnea. Sleep 1999;22:749–755.

19 Mar J, Rueda JR, Duran-Cantolla J, Schechter C, Chilcott J: The cost-effectiveness of nCPAP treatment in patients with moderate-to-severe obstructive sleep apnoea. Eur Respir J 2003;21:515–522.

20 Ayas NT, FitzGerald JM, Fleetham JA, White DP, Schulzer M, Ryan CF, Ghaeli R, Mercer GW, Cooper P, Tan MC, Marra CA: Cost-effectiveness of continuous positive airway pressure therapy for moderate to severe obstructive sleep apnea/hypopnea. Arch Intern Med 2006;166:977–984.

21 Deutsch PA, Simmons MS, Wallace JM: Cost-effectiveness of split-night polysomnography and home studies in the evaluation of obstructive sleep apnea syndrome. J Clin Sleep Med 2006;2:145–153.

22 McDaid C, Griffin S, Weatherly H, Duree K, van der Burgt M, van Hout S, Akers J, Davies RJ, Sculpher M, Westwood M: Continuous positive airway pressure devices for the treatment of obstructive sleep apnoea-hypopnoea syndrome: a systematic review and economic analysis. Health Technol Assess 2009;13:iii–iv, xi–xiv, 1–119, 143–274.

23 Kapur VK, Alfonso-Cristancho R: Just a good deal or truly a steal? Medical cost savings and the impact on the cost-effectiveness of treating sleep apnea. Sleep 2009;32:135–136.

24 Kapur VK: Obstructive sleep apnea: diagnosis, epidemiology, and economics. Respir Care 2010;55: 1155–1167.

25 Neumann PJ, Levine BS: Do HEDIS measures reflect cost-effective practices? Am J Prev Med 2002;23:276–289.

26 Newman AB, Foster G, Givelber R, Nieto FJ, Redline S, Young T: Progression and regression of sleep-disordered breathing with changes in weight: the Sleep Heart Health Study. Arch Intern Med 2005; 165:2408–2413.

27 Young T, Peppard PE, Taheri S: Excess weight and sleep-disordered breathing. J Appl Physiol 2005;99: 1592–1599.

28 Schwartz AR, Patil SP, Laffan AM, Polotsky V, Schneider H, Smith PL: Obesity and obstructive sleep apnea: pathogenic mechanisms and therapeutic approaches. Proc Am Thorac Soc 2008;5:185–192.

29 Bixler EO, Vgontzas AN, Ten Have T, Tyson K, Kales A: Effects of age on sleep apnea in men. 1. Prevalence and severity. Am J Respir Crit Care Med 1998;157:144–148.

30 Peppard PE, Young T, Palta M, Dempsey J, Skatrud J: Longitudinal study of moderate weight change and sleep-disordered breathing. JAMA 2000;284: 3015–3021.

31 Durán J, Esnaola S, Rubio R, Iztueta A: Obstructive sleep apnea-hypopnea and related clinical features in a population-based sample of subjects aged 30 to 70 years. Am J Respir Crit Care Med 2001;163:685–689.

32 Young T, Shahar E, Nieto FJ, Redline S, Newman AB, Gottlieb DJ, Walsleben JA, Finn L, Enright P, Samet JM: Predictors of sleep-disordered breathing in community-dwelling adults: the Sleep Heart Health Study. Arch Intern Med 2002;162:893–900.

33 Launois SH, Pepin JL, Levy P: Sleep apnea in the elderly: a specific entity? Sleep Med Rev 2007;11:87–97.

34 Ancoli-Israel S, Kripke DF, Klauber MR, Mason WJ, Fell R, Kaplan O: Sleep-disordered breathing in community-dwelling elderly. Sleep 1991;14:486–495.

35 Lin CM, Davidson TM, Ancoli-Israel S: Gender differences in obstructive sleep apnea and treatment implications. Sleep Med Rev 2008;12:481–496.

36 Shahar E, Redline S, Young T, Boland LL, Baldwin CM, Nieto FJ, O'Connor GT, Rapoport DM, Robbins JA. Hormone replacement therapy and sleep-disordered breathing. Am J Respir Crit Care Med 2003; 167:1186–1192.

37 Young T, Finn L, Austin D, Peterson A: Menopausal status and sleep-disordered breathing in the Wisconsin Sleep Cohort Study. Am J Respir Crit Care Med 2003;167:1181–1185.

38 Keefe DL, Watson R, Naftolin F: Hormone replacement therapy may alleviate sleep apnea in menopausal women: a pilot study. Menopause 1999;6: 196–200.

39 Manber R, Kuo TF, Cataldo N, Colrain IM: The effects of hormone replacement therapy on sleep-disordered breathing in postmenopausal women: a pilot study. Sleep 2003;26:163–168.

40 Polo-Kantola P, Rauhala E, Helenius H, Erkkola R, Irjala K, Polo O: Breathing during sleep in menopause: a randomized, controlled, crossover trial with estrogen therapy. Obstet Gynecol 2003;102:68–75.

41 Matsumoto AM, Sandblom RE, Schoene RB, Lee KA, Giblin EC, Pierson DJ, Bremner WJ: Testosterone replacement in hypogonadal men: effects on obstructive sleep apnoea, respiratory drives, and sleep. Clin Endocrinol (Oxf) 1985;22: 713–721.

42 Schneider BK, Pickett CK, Zwillich CW, Weil JV, McDermott MT, Santen RJ, Varano LA, White DP: Influence of testosterone on breathing during sleep. J Appl Physiol 1986;61:618–623.

43 Liu PY, Yee B, Wishart SM, Jimenez M, Jung DG, Grunstein RR, Handelsman DJ: The short-term effects of high-dose testosterone on sleep, breathing, and function in older men. J Clin Endocrinol Metab 2003;88:3605–3613.

44 White DP, Schneider BK, Santen RJ, McDermott M, Pickett CK, Zwillich CW, Weil JV: Influence of testosterone on ventilation and chemosensitivity in male subjects. J Appl Physiol 1985;59:1452–1457.

45 Mateika JH, Diamond MP, Badr MS: Ventilatory sensitivity to carbon dioxide before and after episodic hypoxia in women treated with testosterone. J Appl Physiol 2007;102:1832–1838.

46 Zhou XS, Rowley JA, Demirovic F, Diamond MP, Badr MS: Effect of testosterone on the apneic threshold in women during NREM sleep. J Appl Physiol 2003;94:101–107.

47 Tasali E, Van Cauter E, Ehrmann DA: Polycystic ovary syndrome and obstructive sleep apnea. Sleep Med Clin 2008;3:37–46.

48 Fogel RB, Malhotra A, Pillar G, Pittman SD, Dunaif A, White DP: Increased prevalence of obstructive sleep apnea syndrome in obese women with polycystic ovary syndrome. J Clin Endocrinol Metab 2001;86:1175–1180.

49 Vgontzas AN, Legro RS, Bixler EO, Grayev A, Kales A, Chrousos GP: Polycystic ovary syndrome is associated with obstructive sleep apnea and daytime sleepiness: role of insulin resistance. J Clin Endocrinol Metab 2001;86:517–520.

50 Gopal M, Duntley S, Uhles M, Attarian H: The role of obesity in the increased prevalence of obstructive sleep apnea syndrome in patients with polycystic ovarian syndrome. Sleep Med 2002;3:401–404.

51 Tasali E, Van Cauter E, Ehrmann DA: Relationships between sleep disordered breathing and glucose metabolism in polycystic ovary syndrome. J Clin Endocrinol Metab 2006;91:36–42.

52 Miles PG, Vig PS, Weyant RJ, Forrest TD, Rockette HE Jr: Craniofacial structure and obstructive sleep apnea syndrome – a qualitative analysis and meta-analysis of the literature. Am J Orthod Dentofacial Orthop 1996;109:163–172.

53 Watanabe T, Isono S, Tanaka A, Tanzawa H, Nishino T. Contribution of body habitus and craniofacial characteristics to segmental closing pressures of the passive pharynx in patients with sleep-disordered breathing. Am J Respir Crit Care Med 2002;165:260–265.

54 Schwab RJ, Gupta KB, Gefter WB, Metzger LJ, Hoffman EA, Pack AI: Upper airway and soft tissue anatomy in normal subjects and patients with sleep-disordered breathing: significance of the lateral pharyngeal walls. Am J Respir Crit Care Med 1995;152:1673–1689.

55 Strohl KP: Con: sleep apnea is not an anatomic disorder. Am J Respir Crit Care Med 2003;168:271–272, discussion 272–273.

56 Vgontzas AN: Does obesity play a major role in the pathogenesis of sleep apnoea and its associated manifestations via inflammation, visceral adiposity, and insulin resistance? Arch Physiol Biochem 2008;114:211–223.

57 Franklin KA, Gislason T, Omenaas E, Jogi R, Jensen EJ, Lindberg E, Gunnbjornsdottir M, Nystrom L, Laerum BN, Bjornsson E, Toren K, Janson C: The influence of active and passive smoking on habitual snoring. Am J Respir Crit Care Med 2004;170:799–803.

58 Schmidt-Nowara WW, Coultas DB, Wiggins C, Skipper BE, Samet JM: Snoring in a Hispanic-American population: risk factors and association with hypertension and other morbidity. Arch Intern Med 1990;150:597–601.

59 Jennum P, Sjol A: Epidemiology of snoring and obstructive sleep apnoea in a Danish population, age 30–60. J Sleep Res 1992;1:240–244.

60 Lindberg E, Janson C, Gislason T, Bjornsson E, Hetta J, Boman G: Sleep disturbances in a young adult population: can gender differences be explained by differences in psychological status? Sleep 1997;20:381–387.

61 Hu FB, Willett WC, Colditz GA, Ascherio A, Speizer FE, Rosner B, Hennekens CH, Stampfer MJ: Prospective study of snoring and risk of hypertension in women. Am J Epidemiol 1999;150:806–816.

62 Khoo SM, Tan WC, Ng TP, Ho CH: Risk factors associated with habitual snoring and sleep-disordered breathing in a multi-ethnic Asian population: a population-based study. Respir Med 2004;98:557–566.

63 Stradling JR, Crosby JH. Predictors and prevalence of obstructive sleep apnoea and snoring in 1,001 middle aged men. Thorax 1991;46:85–90.

64 Wetter DW, Young TB, Bidwell TR, Badr MS, Palta M. Smoking as a risk factor for sleep-disordered breathing. Arch Intern Med 1994;154:2219–2224.

65 Kauffmann F, Annesi I, Neukirch F, Oryszczyn MP, Alperovitch A: The relation between snoring and smoking, body mass index, age, alcohol consumption and respiratory symptoms. Eur Respir J 1989;2: 599–603.

66 Young T, Finn L, Palta M: Chronic nasal congestion at night is a risk factor for snoring in a population-based cohort study. Arch Intern Med 2001;161:1514–1519.

67 Newman AB, Nieto FJ, Guidry U, Lind BK, Redline S, Pickering TG, Quan SF: Relation of sleep-disordered breathing to cardiovascular disease risk factors: the Sleep Heart Health Study. Am J Epidemiol 2001;154:50–59.

68 Dolly FR, Block AJ: Increased ventricular ectopy and sleep apnea following ethanol ingestion in COPD patients. Chest 1983;83:469–472.

69 Scanlan MF, Roebuck T, Little PJ, Redman JR, Naughton MT: Effect of moderate alcohol upon obstructive sleep apnoea. Eur Respir J 2000;16:909–913.

70 Scrima L, Hartman PG, Hiller FC: Effect of three alcohol doses on breathing during sleep in 30–49 year old nonobese snorers and nonsnorers. Alcohol Clin Exp Res 1989;13:420–427.

71 Berry RB, Desa MM, Light RW: Effect of ethanol on the efficacy of nasal continuous positive airway pressure as a treatment for obstructive sleep apnea. Chest 1991;99:339–343.

72 Issa FG, Sullivan CE: Alcohol, snoring and sleep apnea. J Neurol Neurosurg Psychiatry 1982;45:353–359.

73 Issa FG, Sullivan CE: Upper airway closing pressures in obstructive sleep apnea. J Appl Physiol 1984;57:520–527.

74 Krol RC, Knuth SL, Bartlett D Jr: Selective reduction of genioglossal muscle activity by alcohol in normal human subjects. Am Rev Respir Dis 1984; 129:247–250.

75 Jennum P, Sjol A: Snoring, sleep apnoea and cardiovascular risk factors: the MONICA II Study. Int J Epidemiol 1993;22:439–444.

76 Peppard PE, Austin D, Brown RL: Association of alcohol consumption and sleep disordered breathing in men and women. J Clin Sleep Med 2007;3:265–270.
77 Bearpark H, Elliott L, Grunstein R, Cullen S, Schneider H, Althaus W, Sullivan C: Snoring and sleep apnea: a population study in Australian men. Am J Respir Crit Care Med 1995;151:1459–1465.
78 Worsnop CJ, Naughton MT, Barter CE, Morgan TO, Anderson AI, Pierce RJ: The prevalence of obstructive sleep apnea in hypertensives. Am J Respir Crit Care Med 1998;157:111–115.
79 Udwadia ZF, Doshi AV, Lonkar SG, Singh CI: Prevalence of sleep-disordered breathing and sleep apnea in middle-aged urban Indian men. Am J Respir Crit Care Med 2004;169:168–173.
80 Lindberg E, Taube A, Janson C, Gislason T, Svardsudd K, Boman G: A 10-year follow-up of snoring in men. Chest 1998;114:1048–1055.
81 Mayfield D, McLeod G, Hall P: The CAGE questionnaire: validation of a new alcoholism screening instrument. Am J Psychiatry 1974;131:1121–1123.
82 Svensson M, Lindberg E, Naessen T, Janson C: Risk factors associated with snoring in women with special emphasis on body mass index: a population-based study. Chest 2006;129:933–941.
83 Mitler MM, Dawson A, Henriksen SJ, Sobers M, Bloom FE: Bedtime ethanol increases resistance of upper airways and produces sleep apneas in asymptomatic snorers. Alcohol Clin Exp Res 1988;12:801–805.
84 Teschler H, Berthon-Jones M, Wessendorf T, Meyer HJ, Konietzko N. Influence of moderate alcohol consumption on obstructive sleep apnoea with and without AutoSet nasal CPAP therapy. Eur Respir J 1996;9:2371–2377.
85 Redline S, Tishler PV, Tosteson TD, Williamson J, Kump K, Browner I, Ferrette V, Krejci P: The familial aggregation of obstructive sleep apnea. Am J Respir Crit Care Med 1995;151:682–687.
86 Redline S, Tishler PV: The genetics of sleep apnea. Sleep Med Rev 2000;4:583–602.
87 Schwab RJ. Genetic determinants of upper airway structures that predispose to obstructive sleep apnea. Respir Physiol Neurobiol 2005;147:289–298.
88 Mathur R, Douglas NJ. Family studies in patients with the sleep apnea-hypopnea syndrome. Ann Intern Med 1995;122:174–178.
89 Patel SR, Larkin EK, Redline S: Shared genetic basis for obstructive sleep apnea and adiposity measures. Int J Obes (Lond) 2008;32:795–800.
90 Buxbaum SG, Elston RC, Tishler PV, Redline S: Genetics of the apnea hypopnea index in Caucasians and African Americans. 1. Segregation analysis. Genet Epidemiol 2002;22:243–253.
91 Casale M, Pappacena M, Rinaldi V, Bressi F, Baptista P, Salvinelli F: Obstructive sleep apnea syndrome: from phenotype to genetic basis. Curr Genomics 2009;10:119–126.
92 Riha RL: Genetic aspects of the obstructive sleep apnoea/hypopnoea syndrome – is there a common link with obesity? Respiration 2009;78:5–17.
93 Littner MR, Kushida C, Wise M, Davila DG, Morgenthaler T, Lee-Chiong T, Hirshkowitz M, Daniel LL, Bailey D, Berry RB, Kapen S, Kramer M: Practice parameters for clinical use of the multiple sleep latency test and the maintenance of wakefulness test. Sleep 2005;28:113–121.
94 Monk TH: A visual analogue scale technique to measure global vigor and affect. Psychiatry Res 1989;27:89–99.
95 Åkerstedt T, Gillberg M: Subjective and objective sleepiness in the active individual. Int J Neurosci 1990;52:29–37.
96 Hoddes E, Zarcone V, Smythe H, Phillips R, Dement WC. Quantification of sleepiness: a new approach. Psychophysiology 1973;10:431–436.
97 Shen J, Barbera J, Shapiro CM: Distinguishing sleepiness and fatigue: focus on definition and measurement. Sleep Med Rev 2006;10:63–76.
98 Roth T, Hartse KM, Zorick F, Conway W: Multiple naps and the evaluation of daytime sleepiness in patients with upper airway sleep apnea. Sleep 1980;3:425–439.
99 Engleman HM, Douglas NJ: Sleep. 4. Sleepiness, cognitive function, and quality of life in obstructive sleep apnoea/hypopnoea syndrome. Thorax 2004;59:618–622.
100 Johns MW: A new method for measuring daytime sleepiness: the Epworth sleepiness scale. Sleep 1991;14:540–545.
101 Chervin RD: The Multiple Sleep Latency Test and Epworth Sleepiness Scale in the assessment of daytime sleepiness. J Sleep Res 2000;9:399–401.
102 Johns MW: Sensitivity and specificity of the Multiple Sleep Latency Test (MSLT), the Maintenance of Wakefulness Test and the Epworth Sleepiness Scale: failure of the MSLT as a gold standard. J Sleep Res 2000;9:5–11.
103 Chervin RD: Epworth Sleepiness Scale? Sleep Med 2003;4:175–176.
104 Sauter C, Asenbaum S, Popovic R, Bauer H, Lamm C, Klosch G, Zeitlhofer J: Excessive daytime sleepiness in patients suffering from different levels of obstructive sleep apnoea syndrome. J Sleep Res 2000;9:293–301.
105 Cluydts R, De Valck E, Verstraeten E, Theys P: Daytime sleepiness and its evaluation. Sleep Med Rev 2002;6:83–96.

106 Sullivan SS, Kushida CA: Multiple sleep latency test and maintenance of wakefulness test. Chest 2008; 134:854–861.
107 Arand D, Bonnet M, Hurwitz T, Mitler M, Rosa R, Sangal RB: The clinical use of the MSLT and MWT. Sleep 2005;28:123–144.
108 Inoue Y, Nanba K, Higami S, Honda Y, Takahashi Y, Arai H: Clinical significance of sleep-related breathing disorder in narcolepsy. Psychiatry Clin Neurosci 2002;56:269–270.
109 Sangal RB, Thomas L, Mitler MM: Maintenance of Wakefulness Test and Multiple Sleep Latency Test: measurement of different abilities in patients with sleep disorders. Chest 1992;101:898–902.
110 Weaver TE: Outcome measurement in sleep medicine practice and research. 1. Assessment of symptoms, subjective and objective daytime sleepiness, health-related quality of life and functional status. Sleep Med Rev 2001;5:103–128.
111 Bennett LS, Stradling JR, Davies RJ: A behavioural test to assess daytime sleepiness in obstructive sleep apnoea. J Sleep Res 1997;6:142–145.
112 Mazza S, Pepin JL, Deschaux C, Naegele B, Levy P: Analysis of error profiles occurring during the OSLER test: a sensitive mean of detecting fluctuations in vigilance in patients with obstructive sleep apnea syndrome. Am J Respir Crit Care Med 2002; 166:474–478.
113 Dinges DF, Pack F, Williams K, Gillen KA, Powell JW, Ott GE, Aptowicz C, Pack AI: Cumulative sleepiness, mood disturbance, and psychomotor vigilance performance decrements during a week of sleep restricted to 4–5 hours per night. Sleep 1997; 20:267–277.
114 Kim H, Dinges DF, Young T: Sleep-disordered breathing and psychomotor vigilance in a community-based sample. Sleep 2007;30:1309–1316.
115 Hublin C, Kaprio J, Partinen M, Heikkila K, Koskenvuo M: Daytime sleepiness in an adult, Finnish population. J Intern Med 1996;239:417–423.
116 Bixler EO, Vgontzas AN, Lin HM, Calhoun SL, Vela-Bueno A, Kales A: Excessive daytime sleepiness in a general population sample: the role of sleep apnea, age, obesity, diabetes, and depression. J Clin Endocrinol Metab 2005;90:4510–4515.
117 Engleman HM, Hirst WS, Douglas NJ: Underreporting of sleepiness and driving impairment in patients with sleep apnoea/hypopnoea syndrome. J Sleep Res 1997;6:272–275.
118 Ballester E, Badia JR, Hernandez L, Carrasco E, de Pablo J, Fornas C, Rodriguez-Roisin R, Montserrat JM: Evidence of the effectiveness of continuous positive airway pressure in the treatment of sleep apnea/hypopnea syndrome. Am J Respir Crit Care Med 1999;159:495–501.
119 Engleman HM, Kingshott RN, Wraith PK, Mackay TW, Deary IJ, Douglas NJ: Randomized placebo-controlled crossover trial of continuous positive airway pressure for mild sleep apnea/hypopnea syndrome. Am J Respir Crit Care Med 1999;159:461–467.
120 Jenkinson C, Davies RJ, Mullins R, Stradling JR: Comparison of therapeutic and subtherapeutic nasal continuous positive airway pressure for obstructive sleep apnoea: a randomised prospective parallel trial. Lancet 1999;353:2100–2105.
121 Faccenda JF, Mackay TW, Boon NA, Douglas NJ: Randomized placebo-controlled trial of continuous positive airway pressure on blood pressure in the sleep apnea-hypopnea syndrome. Am J Respir Crit Care Med 2001;163:344–348.
122 Patel SR, White DP, Malhotra A, Stanchina ML, Ayas NT: Continuous positive airway pressure therapy for treating sleepiness in a diverse population with obstructive sleep apnea: results of a meta-analysis. Arch Intern Med 2003;163:565–571.
123 Resnick HE, Carter EA, Aloia M, Phillips B: Cross-sectional relationship of reported fatigue to obesity, diet, and physical activity: results from the Third National Health and Nutrition Examination Survey. J Clin Sleep Med 2006;2:163–169.
124 Basta M, Lin HM, Pejovic S, Sarrigiannidis A, Bixler E, Vgontzas AN: Lack of regular exercise, depression, and degree of apnea are predictors of excessive daytime sleepiness in patients with sleep apnea: sex differences. J Clin Sleep Med 2008;4:19–25.
125 Neu D, Linkowski P, le Bon O: Clinical complaints of daytime sleepiness and fatigue: how to distinguish and treat them, especially when they become 'excessive' or 'chronic'? Acta Neurol Belg 2010;110: 15–25.
126 Hossain JL, Ahmad P, Reinish LW, Kayumov L, Hossain NK, Shapiro CM: Subjective fatigue and subjective sleepiness: two independent consequences of sleep disorders? J Sleep Res 2005;14:245–253.
127 Bardwell WA, Moore P, Ancoli-Israel S, Dimsdale JE: Fatigue in obstructive sleep apnea: driven by depressive symptoms instead of apnea severity? Am J Psychiatry 2003;160:350–355.
128 Mills PJ, Kim JH, Bardwell W, Hong S, Dimsdale JE: Predictors of fatigue in obstructive sleep apnea. Sleep Breath 2008;12:397–399.
129 Chervin RD: Sleepiness, fatigue, tiredness, and lack of energy in obstructive sleep apnea. Chest 2000; 118:372–379.

130 Jackson ML, Stough C, Howard ME, Spong J, Downey LA, Thompson B: The contribution of fatigue and sleepiness to depression in patients attending the sleep laboratory for evaluation of obstructive sleep apnea. Sleep Breath 2010, E-pub ahead of print.
131 Ohayon MM, Guilleminault C, Priest RG, Caulet M: Snoring and breathing pauses during sleep: telephone interview survey of a United Kingdom population sample. BMJ 1997;314:860–863.
132 Larsson LG, Lindberg A, Franklin KA, Lundback B: Gender differences in symptoms related to sleep apnea in a general population and in relation to referral to sleep clinic. Chest 2003;124:204–211.
133 Hoffstein V, Mateika S, Anderson D: Snoring: is it in the ear of the beholder? Sleep 1994;17:522–526.
134 McArdle N, Kingshott R, Engleman HM, Mackay TW, Douglas NJ: Partners of patients with sleep apnoea/hypopnoea syndrome: effect of CPAP treatment on sleep quality and quality of life. Thorax 2001;56:513–518.
135 Gottlieb DJ, Yao Q, Redline S, Ali T, Mahowald MW: Does snoring predict sleepiness independently of apnea and hypopnea frequency? Am J Respir Crit Care Med 2000;162:1512–1517.
136 Quesnot A, Alperovitch A: Snoring and risk of cognitive decline: a 4-year follow-up study in 1,389 older individuals. J Am Geriatr Soc 1999;47:1159–1160.
137 Ficker JH, Wiest GH, Lehnert G, Meyer M, Hahn EG: Are snoring medical students at risk of failing their exams? Sleep 1999;22:205–209.
138 Davies DP, Rodgers H, Walshaw D, James OF, Gibson GJ: Snoring, daytime sleepiness and stroke: a case-control study of first-ever stroke. J Sleep Res 2003;12:313–318.
139 Thomas GN, Jiang CQ, Lao XQ, McGhee SM, Zhang WS, Schooling CM, Adab P, Lam TH, Cheng KK: Snoring and vascular risk factors and disease in a low-risk Chinese population: the Guangzhou Biobank Cohort Study. Sleep 2006;29:896–900.
140 Al-Delaimy WK, Manson JE, Willett WC, Stampfer MJ, Hu FB: Snoring as a risk factor for type II diabetes mellitus: a prospective study. Am J Epidemiol 2002;155:387–393.
141 Young T, Hutton R, Finn L, Badr S, Palta M: The gender bias in sleep apnea diagnosis: are women missed because they have different symptoms? Arch Intern Med 1996;156:2445–2451.
142 Van Kerrebroeck P, Abrams P, Chaikin D, Donovan J, Fonda D, Jackson S, Jennum P, Johnson T, Lose G, Mattiasson A, Robertson G, Weiss J: The standardisation of terminology in nocturia: report from the Standardisation Sub-committee of the International Continence Society. Neurourol Urodyn 2002;21:179–183.
143 Krieger J, Petiau C, Sforza E, Delanoe C, Hecht MT, Chamouard V: Nocturnal pollakiuria is a symptom of obstructive sleep apnea. Urol Int 1993;50:93–97.
144 Guilleminault C, Lin CM, Goncalves MA, Ramos E: A prospective study of nocturia and the quality of life of elderly patients with obstructive sleep apnea or sleep onset insomnia. J Psychosom Res 2004;56:511–515.
145 Umlauf MG, Chasens ER, Greevy RA, Arnold J, Burgio KL, Pillion DJ: Obstructive sleep apnea, nocturia and polyuria in older adults. Sleep 2004;27:139–144.
146 Margel D, Shochat T, Getzler O, Livne PM, Pillar G: Continuous positive airway pressure reduces nocturia in patients with obstructive sleep apnea. Urology 2006;67:974–977.
147 Krieger J, Laks L, Wilcox I, Grunstein RR, Costas LJ, McDougall JG, Sullivan CE: Atrial natriuretic peptide release during sleep in patients with obstructive sleep apnoea before and during treatment with nasal continuous positive airway pressure. Clin Sci (Lond) 1989;77:407–411.
148 Lin CC, Tsan KW, Lin CY: Plasma levels of atrial natriuretic factor in moderate to severe obstructive sleep apnea syndrome. Sleep 1993;16:37–39.
149 Fitzgerald MP, Mulligan M, Parthasarathy S: Nocturic frequency is related to severity of obstructive sleep apnea, improves with continuous positive airways treatment. Am J Obstet Gynecol 2006;194:1399–1403.
150 Oztura I, Kaynak D, Kaynak HC: Nocturia in sleep-disordered breathing. Sleep Med 2006;7:362–367.
151 Arai H, Furuta H, Kosaka K, Kaneda R, Koshino Y, Sano J, Yokoyama O: Polysomnographic and urodynamic changes in a case of obstructive sleep apnea syndrome with enuresis. Psychiatry Clin Neurosci 1999;53:319–320.
152 Sateia MJ: Update on sleep and psychiatric disorders. Chest 2009;135:1370–1379.
153 Ohayon MM: The effects of breathing-related sleep disorders on mood disturbances in the general population. J Clin Psychiatry 2003;64:1195–1200, quiz 274–276.
154 Schröder CM, O'Hara R: Depression and obstructive sleep apnea (OSA). Ann Gen Psychiatry 2005;4:13.
155 Sharafkhaneh A, Giray N, Richardson P, Young T, Hirshkowitz M: Association of psychiatric disorders and sleep apnea in a large cohort. Sleep 2005;28:1405–1411.
156 McCall WV, Harding D, O'Donovan C: Correlates of depressive symptoms in patients with obstructive sleep apnea. J Clin Sleep Med 2006;2:424–426.
157 Saunamaki T, Jehkonen M: Depression and anxiety in obstructive sleep apnea syndrome: a review. Acta Neurol Scand 2007;116:277–288.

158 Beutler LE, Ware JC, Karacan I, Thornby JI: Differentiating psychological characteristics of patients with sleep apnea and narcolepsy. Sleep 1981;4:39–47.
159 Munoz X, Marti S, Sumalla J, Bosch J, Sampol G: Acute delirium as a manifestation of obstructive sleep apnea syndrome. Am J Respir Crit Care Med 1998;158:1306–1307.
160 Krakow B, Lowry C, Germain A, Gaddy L, Hollifield M, Koss M, Tandberg D, Johnston L, Melendrez D: A retrospective study on improvements in nightmares and post-traumatic stress disorder following treatment for co-morbid sleep-disordered breathing. J Psychosom Res 2000;49:291–298.
161 Mahowald MW, Cramer-Bornemann M, Hannon H, Janjua T, Ullevig C, Patterson A: Did this father's sleep apnea contribute to the inadvertent death of his infant son? Sleep Med 2002;3:369–370.
162 Deldin PJ, Phillips LK, Thomas RJ: A preliminary study of sleep-disordered breathing in major depressive disorder. Sleep Med 2006;7:131–139.
163 Winkelman JW: Schizophrenia, obesity, and obstructive sleep apnea. J Clin Psychiatry 2001;62:8–11.
164 Dominici M, Gomes Mda M: Obstructive sleep apnea (OSA) and depressive symptoms. Arq Neuropsiquiatr 2009;67:35–39.
165 Macey PM, Woo MA, Kumar R, Cross RL, Harper RM: Relationship between obstructive sleep apnea severity and sleep, depression and anxiety symptoms in newly-diagnosed patients. PLoS One 2010; 5:e10211.
166 Millman RP, Fogel BS, McNamara ME, Carlisle CC. Depression as a manifestation of obstructive sleep apnea: reversal with nasal continuous positive airway pressure. J Clin Psychiatry 1989;50:348–351.
167 Aloia MS, Arnedt JT, Smith L, Skrekas J, Stanchina M, Millman RP: Examining the construct of depression in obstructive sleep apnea syndrome. Sleep Med 2005;6:115–121.
168 Kawahara S, Akashiba T, Akahoshi T, Horie T: Nasal CPAP improves the quality of life and lessens the depressive symptoms in patients with obstructive sleep apnea syndrome. Intern Med 2005;44:422–427.
169 Schwartz DJ, Karatinos G: For individuals with obstructive sleep apnea, institution of CPAP therapy is associated with an amelioration of symptoms of depression which is sustained long term. J Clin Sleep Med 2007;3:631–635.
170 Borak J, Cieslicki JK, Koziej M, Matuszewski A, Zielinski J: Effects of CPAP treatment on psychological status in patients with severe obstructive sleep apnoea. J Sleep Res 1996;5:123–127.
171 Yu BH, Ancoli-Israel S, Dimsdale JE: Effect of CPAP treatment on mood states in patients with sleep apnea. J Psychiatr Res 1999;33:427–432.
172 Henke KG, Grady JJ, Kuna ST: Effect of nasal continuous positive airway pressure on neuropsychological function in sleep apnea-hypopnea syndrome: a randomized, placebo-controlled trial. Am J Respir Crit Care Med 2001;163:911–917.
173 Macey PM, Kumar R, Woo MA, Valladares EM, Yan-Go FL, Harper RM: Brain structural changes in obstructive sleep apnea. Sleep 2008;31:967–977.
174 Yaouhi K, Bertran F, Clochon P, Mezenge F, Denise P, Foret J, Eustache F, Desgranges B: A combined neuropsychological and brain imaging study of obstructive sleep apnea. J Sleep Res 2009;18:36–48.
175 Sforza E, de Saint Hilaire Z, Pelissolo A, Rochat T, Ibanez V: Personality, anxiety and mood traits in patients with sleep-related breathing disorders: effect of reduced daytime alertness. Sleep Med 2002;3:139–145.
176 Reynolds CF 3rd, Coble PA, Spiker DG, Neil JF, Holzer BC, Kupfer DJ: Prevalence of sleep apnea and nocturnal myoclonus in major affective disorders: clinical and polysomnographic findings. J Nerv Ment Dis 1982;170:565–567.
177 Fleming JA, Fleetham JA, Taylor DR, Remick RA: A case report of obstructive sleep apnea in a patient with bipolar affective disorder. Can J Psychiatry 1985;30:437–439.
178 Kaplan R: Obstructive sleep apnoea and depression – diagnostic and treatment implications. Aust NZ J Psychiatry 1992;26:586–591.
179 Pillar G, Lavie P: Psychiatric symptoms in sleep apnea syndrome: effects of gender and respiratory disturbance index. Chest 1998;114:697–703.
180 Raikkonen K, Matthews KA, Kuller LH: The relationship between psychological risk attributes and the metabolic syndrome in healthy women: antecedent or consequence? Metabolism 2002;51:1573–1577.
181 Farney RJ, Lugo A, Jensen RL, Walker JM, Cloward TV: Simultaneous use of antidepressant and antihypertensive medications increases likelihood of diagnosis of obstructive sleep apnea syndrome. Chest 2004;125:1279–1285.
182 Bardwell WA, Moore P, Ancoli-Israel S, Dimsdale JE: Does obstructive sleep apnea confound sleep architecture findings in subjects with depressive symptoms? Biol Psychiatry 2000;48:1001–1009.
183 Reimer MA, Flemons WW: Quality of life in sleep disorders. Sleep Med Rev 2003;7:335–349.
184 Flemons WW: Measuring quality of life in patients with sleep apnoea: whose life is it anyway? Thorax 2004;59:457–458.

185 Breugelmans JG, Ford DE, Smith PL, Punjabi NM: Differences in patient and bed partner-assessed quality of life in sleep-disordered breathing. Am J Respir Crit Care Med 2004;170:547–552.
186 Goncalves MA, Paiva T, Ramos E, Guilleminault C: Obstructive sleep apnea syndrome, sleepiness, and quality of life. Chest 2004;125:2091–2096.
187 Bennett LS, Barbour C, Langford B, Stradling JR, Davies RJ: Health status in obstructive sleep apnea: relationship with sleep fragmentation and daytime sleepiness, and effects of continuous positive airway pressure treatment. Am J Respir Crit Care Med 1999;159:1884–1890.
188 Sforza E, Janssens JP, Rochat T, Ibanez V: Determinants of altered quality of life in patients with sleep-related breathing disorders. Eur Respir J 2003;21:682–687.
189 Jenkinson C, Davies RJ, Mullins R, Stradling JR: Long-term benefits in self-reported health status of nasal continuous positive airway pressure therapy for obstructive sleep apnoea. Q J Med 2001;94:95–99.
190 Pichel F, Zamarron C, Magan F, del Campo F, Alvarez-Sala R, Suarez JR: Health-related quality of life in patients with obstructive sleep apnea: effects of long-term positive airway pressure treatment. Respir Med 2004;98:968–976.
191 Siccoli MM, Pepperell JC, Kohler M, Craig SE, Davies RJ, Stradling JR: Effects of continuous positive airway pressure on quality of life in patients with moderate to severe obstructive sleep apnea: data from a randomized controlled trial. Sleep 2008;31:1551–1558.
192 Jing J, Huang T, Cui W, Shen H: Effect on quality of life of continuous positive airway pressure in patients with obstructive sleep apnea syndrome: a meta-analysis. Lung 2008;186:131–144.
193 Giles TL, Lasserson TJ, Smith BH, White J, Wright J, Cates CJ: Continuous positive airways pressure for obstructive sleep apnoea in adults. Cochrane Database Syst Rev 2006;3:CD001106.
194 Omachi TA, Claman DM, Blanc PD, Eisner MD: Obstructive sleep apnea: a risk factor for work disability. Sleep 2009;32:791–798.
195 Rodenstein D: Sleep apnea: traffic and occupational accidents – individual risks, socioeconomic and legal implications. Respiration 2009;78:241–248.
196 Verstraeten E: Neurocognitive effects of obstructive sleep apnea syndrome. Curr Neurol Neurosci Rep 2007;7:161–166.
197 Beebe DW, Groesz L, Wells C, Nichols A, McGee K: The neuropsychological effects of obstructive sleep apnea: a meta-analysis of norm-referenced and case-controlled data. Sleep 2003;26:298–307.
198 Quan SF, Wright R, Baldwin CM, Kaemingk KL, Goodwin JL, Kuo TF, Kaszniak A, Boland LL, Caccappolo E, Bootzin RR: Obstructive sleep apnea-hypopnea and neurocognitive functioning in the Sleep Heart Health Study. Sleep Med 2006;7:498–507.
199 Archbold KH, Borghesani PR, Mahurin RK, Kapur VK, Landis CA: Neural activation patterns during working memory tasks and OSA disease severity: preliminary findings. J Clin Sleep Med 2009;5:21–27.
200 Ayalon L, Ancoli-Israel S, Aka AA, McKenna BS, Drummond SP: Relationship between obstructive sleep apnea severity and brain activation during a sustained attention task. Sleep 2009;32:373–381.
201 Kim HC, Young T, Matthews CG, Weber SM, Woodward AR, Palta M: Sleep-disordered breathing and neuropsychological deficits: a population-based study. Am J Respir Crit Care Med 1997;156: 1813–1819.
202 Ayalon L, Ancoli-Israel S, Drummond SP: Obstructive sleep apnea and age: a double-insult to brain function? Am J Respir Crit Care Med 2010; 182:413–419.
203 Cross RL, Kumar R, Macey PM, Doering LV, Alger JR, Yan-Go FL, Harper RM: Neural alterations and depressive symptoms in obstructive sleep apnea patients. Sleep 2008;31:1103–1109.
204 Desseilles M, Dang-Vu T, Schabus M, Sterpenich V, Maquet P, Schwartz S: Neuroimaging insights into the pathophysiology of sleep disorders. Sleep 2008;31:777–794.
205 Lim DC, Veasey SC: Neural injury in sleep apnea. Curr Neurol Neurosci Rep 2010;10:47–52.
206 Macey PM, Henderson LA, Macey KE, Alger JR, Frysinger RC, Woo MA, Harper RK, Yan-Go FL, Harper RM: Brain morphology associated with obstructive sleep apnea. Am J Respir Crit Care Med 2002;166:1382–1387.
207 Morrell MJ, McRobbie DW, Quest RA, Cummin AR, Ghiassi R, Corfield DR: Changes in brain morphology associated with obstructive sleep apnea. Sleep Med 2003;4:451–454.
208 Gale SD, Hopkins RO: Effects of hypoxia on the brain: neuroimaging and neuropsychological findings following carbon monoxide poisoning and obstructive sleep apnea. J Int Neuropsychol Soc 2004;10:60–71.
209 O'Donoghue FJ, Briellmann RS, Rochford PD, Abbott DF, Pell GS, Chan CHP, Tarquinio N, Jackson GD, Pierce RJ: Cerebral structural changes in severe obstructive sleep apnea. Am J Respir Crit Care Med 2005;171:1185–1190.

210 Alchanatis M, Zias N, Deligiorgis N, Amfilochiou A, Dionellis G, Orphanidou D: Sleep apnea-related cognitive deficits and intelligence: an implication of cognitive reserve theory. J Sleep Res 2005;14:69–75.

211 Castronovo V, Canessa N, Strambi LF, Aloia MS, Consonni M, Marelli S, Iadanza A, Bruschi A, Falini A, Cappa SF: Brain activation changes before and after PAP treatment in obstructive sleep apnea. Sleep 2009;32:1161–1172.

212 Sanchez AI, Martinez P, Miro E, Bardwell WA, Buela-Casal G: CPAP and behavioral therapies in patients with obstructive sleep apnea: effects on daytime sleepiness, mood, and cognitive function. Sleep Med Rev 2009;13:223–233.

213 Budson AE, Price BH: Memory dysfunction. N Engl J Med 2005;352:692–699.

214 Naegele B, Launois SH, Mazza S, Feuerstein C, Pepin JL, Levy P: Which memory processes are affected in patients with obstructive sleep apnea? An evaluation of 3 types of memory. Sleep 2006;29: 533–544.

215 Valencia-Flores M, Bliwise DL, Guilleminault C, Cilveti R, Clerk A: Cognitive function in patients with sleep apnea after acute nocturnal nasal continuous positive airway pressure (CPAP) treatment: sleepiness and hypoxemia effects. J Clin Exp Neuropsychol 1996;18:197–210.

216 Ferini-Strambi L, Baietto C, Di Gioia MR, Castaldi P, Castronovo C, Zucconi M, Cappa SF: Cognitive dysfunction in patients with obstructive sleep apnea (OSA): partial reversibility after continuous positive airway pressure (CPAP). Brain Res Bull 2003;61:87–92.

217 Kloepfer C, Riemann D, Nofzinger EA, Feige B, Unterrainer J, O'Hara R, Sorichter S, Nissen C: Memory before and after sleep in patients with moderate obstructive sleep apnea. J Clin Sleep Med 2009;5:540–548.

218 Rouleau I, Decary A, Chicoine AJ, Montplaisir J: Procedural skill learning in obstructive sleep apnea syndrome. Sleep 2002;25:401–411.

219 Thomas RJ, Rosen BR, Stern CE, Weiss JW, Kwong KK: Functional imaging of working memory in obstructive sleep-disordered breathing. J Appl Physiol 2005;98:2226–2234.

220 Felver-Gant JC, Bruce AS, Zimmerman M, Sweet LH, Millman RP, Aloia MS: Working memory in obstructive sleep apnea: construct validity and treatment effects. J Clin Sleep Med 2007;3:589–594.

221 Lee MM, Strauss ME, Adams N, Redline S: Executive functions in persons with sleep apnea. Sleep Breath 1999;3:13–16.

222 Naegele B, Pepin JL, Levy P, Bonnet C, Pellat J, Feuerstein C: Cognitive executive dysfunction in patients with obstructive sleep apnea syndrome (OSAS) after CPAP treatment. Sleep 1998;21:392–397.

223 Ellen RL, Marshall SC, Palayew M, Molnar FJ, Wilson KG, Man-Son-Hing M: Systematic review of motor vehicle crash risk in persons with sleep apnea. J Clin Sleep Med 2006;2:193–200.

224 Tregear S, Reston J, Schoelles K, Phillips B: Obstructive sleep apnea and risk of motor vehicle crash: systematic review and meta-analysis. J Clin Sleep Med 2009;5:573–581.

225 Vakulin A, Baulk SD, Catcheside PG, Antic NA, van den Heuvel CJ, Dorrian J, McEvoy RD: Effects of alcohol and sleep restriction on simulated driving performance in untreated patients with obstructive sleep apnea. Ann Intern Med 2009;151:447–455.

226 Hack M, Davies RJ, Mullins R, Choi SJ, Ramdassingh-Dow S, Jenkinson C, Stradling JR: Randomised prospective parallel trial of therapeutic versus subtherapeutic nasal continuous positive airway pressure on simulated steering performance in patients with obstructive sleep apnoea. Thorax 2000;55:224–231.

227 Horstmann S, Hess CW, Bassetti C, Gugger M, Mathis J: Sleepiness-related accidents in sleep apnea patients. Sleep 2000;23:383–389.

228 George CF: Reduction in motor vehicle collisions following treatment of sleep apnoea with nasal CPAP. Thorax 2001;56:508–512.

229 Orth M, Duchna HW, Leidag M, Widdig W, Rasche K, Bauer TT, Walther JW, de Zeeuw J, Malin JP, Schultze-Werninghaus G, Kotterba S: Driving simulator and neuropsychological [corrected] testing in OSAS before and under CPAP therapy. Eur Respir J 2005;26:898–903.

230 Mazza S, Pepin JL, Naegele B, Rauch E, Deschaux C, Ficheux P, Levy P: Driving ability in sleep apnoea patients before and after CPAP treatment evaluation on a road safety platform. Eur Respir J 2006;28: 1020–1028.

231 Charles MA, Eschwege E, Basdevant A: Monitoring the obesity epidemic in France: the Obepi surveys 1997–2006. Obesity (Silver Spring) 2008;16:2182–2186.

232 Malhotra A, Loscalzo J: Sleep and cardiovascular disease: an overview. Prog Cardiovasc Dis 2009;51: 279–284.

233 Hoffstein V, Szalai JP: Predictive value of clinical features in diagnosing obstructive sleep apnea. Sleep 1993;16:118–122.

234 Flemons WW, Whitelaw WA, Brant R, Remmers JE. Likelihood ratios for a sleep apnea clinical prediction rule. Am J Respir Crit Care Med 1994;150:1279–1285.

235 Deegan PC, McNicholas WT: Predictive value of clinical features for the obstructive sleep apnoea syndrome. Eur Respir J 1996;9:117–124.

236 Jacobs CK, Coffey J: Clinical inquiries. Sleep apnea in adults: how accurate is clinical prediction? J Fam Pract 2009;58:327–328.

237 Kingshott RN, Sime PJ, Engleman HM, Douglas NJ: Self assessment of daytime sleepiness: patient versus partner. Thorax 1995;50:994–995.

238 Walter TJ, Foldvary N, Mascha E, Dinner D, Golish J: Comparison of Epworth Sleepiness Scale scores by patients with obstructive sleep apnea and their bed partners. Sleep Med 2002;3:29–32.

239 Viner S, Szalai JP, Hoffstein V: Are history and physical examination a good screening test for sleep apnea? Ann Intern Med 1991;115:356–359.

240 Kump K, Whalen C, Tishler PV, Browner I, Ferrette V, Strohl KP, Rosenberg C, Redline S: Assessment of the validity and utility of a sleep-symptom questionnaire. Am J Respir Crit Care Med 1994;150:735–741.

241 Maislin G, Pack AI, Kribbs NB, Smith PL, Schwartz AR, Kline LR, Schwab RJ, Dinges DF: A survey screen for prediction of apnea. Sleep 1995;18:158–166.

242 Netzer NC, Stoohs RA, Netzer CM, Clark K, Strohl KP: Using the Berlin questionnaire to identify patients at risk for the sleep apnea syndrome. Ann Intern Med 1999;131:485–491.

243 Chung F, Ward B, Ho J, Yuan H, Kayumov L, Shapiro C: Preoperative identification of sleep apnea risk in elective surgical patients, using the Berlin questionnaire. J Clin Anesth 2007;19:130–134.

244 Chilukuri K, Dalal D, Marine JE, Scherr D, Henrikson CA, Cheng A, Nazarian S, Spragg D, Berger R, Calkins H: Predictive value of obstructive sleep apnoea assessed by the Berlin Questionnaire for outcomes after the catheter ablation of atrial fibrillation. Europace 2009;11:896–901.

245 Gus M, Goncalves SC, Martinez D, de Abreu Silva EO, Moreira LB, Fuchs SC, Fuchs FD: Risk for obstructive sleep apnea by Berlin questionnaire, but not daytime sleepiness, is associated with resistant hypertension: a case-control study. Am J Hypertens 2008;21:832–835.

246 Ahmadi N, Chung SA, Gibbs A, Shapiro CM: The Berlin questionnaire for sleep apnea in a sleep clinic population: relationship to polysomnographic measurement of respiratory disturbance. Sleep Breath 2008;12:39–45.

247 Sagaspe P, Leger D, Taillard J, Bayon V, Chaumet G, Philip P: Might the Berlin Sleep Questionnaire applied to bed partners be used to screen sleep apneic patients? Sleep Med 2010;11:479–483.

248 Rowley JA, Aboussouan LS, Badr MS: The use of clinical prediction formulas in the evaluation of obstructive sleep apnea. Sleep 2000;23:929–938.

249 Gurubhagavatula I, Maislin G, Pack AI: An algorithm to stratify sleep apnea risk in a sleep disorders clinic population. Am J Respir Crit Care Med 2001;164:1904–1909.

250 Kushida CA, Littner MR, Morgenthaler T, Alessi CA, Bailey D, Coleman J Jr, Friedman L, Hirshkowitz M, Kapen S, Kramer M, Lee-Chiong T, Loube DL, Owens J, Pancer JP, Wise M: Practice parameters for the indications for polysomnography and related procedures: an update for 2005. Sleep 2005;28:499–521.

251 Collop NA, Anderson WM, Boehlecke B, Claman D, Goldberg R, Gottlieb DJ, Hudgel D, Sateia M, Schwab R: Clinical guidelines for the use of unattended portable monitors in the diagnosis of obstructive sleep apnea in adult patients. Portable Monitoring Task Force of the American Academy of Sleep Medicine. J Clin Sleep Med 2007;3:737–747.

252 Adesanya AO, Lee W, Greilich NB, Joshi GP: Perioperative management of obstructive sleep apnea. Chest 2010;138:1489–1498.

253 Stierer TL, Wright C, George A, Thompson RE, Wu CL, Collop N: Risk assessment of obstructive sleep apnea in a population of patients undergoing ambulatory surgery. J Clin Sleep Med 2010;6:467–472.

254 Practice parameters for the use of portable recording in the assessment of obstructive sleep apnea. Standards of Practice Committee of the American Sleep Disorders Association. Sleep 1994;17:372–377.

255 Iber C, Ancoli-Israel S, Chesson A, Quan SF, American Academy of Sleep Medicine: The AASM Manual for the Scoring of Sleep and Associated Events: Rules, Terminology and Technical Specifications, ed 1. Westchester, American Academy of Sleep Medicine, 2007.

256 Kushida CA, Littner MR, Hirshkowitz M, Morgenthaler TI, Alessi CA, Bailey D, Boehlecke B, Brown TM, Coleman J Jr, Friedman L, Kapen S, Kapur VK, Kramer M, Lee-Chiong T, Owens J, Pancer JP, Swick TJ, Wise MS: Practice parameters for the use of continuous and bilevel positive airway pressure devices to treat adult patients with sleep-related breathing disorders. Sleep 2006;29:375–380.

257 Weaver TE, Sawyer AM. Adherence to continuous positive airway pressure treatment for obstructive sleep apnoea: implications for future interventions. Indian J Med Res 2010;131:245–258.

258 Chan AS, Cistulli PA: Oral appliance treatment of obstructive sleep apnea: an update. Curr Opin Pulm Med 2009, E-pub ahead of print.

259 Kushida CA, Morgenthaler TI, Littner MR, Alessi CA, Bailey D, Coleman J Jr, Friedman L, Hirshkowitz M, Kapen S, Kramer M, Lee-Chiong T, Owens J, Pancer JP: Practice parameters for the treatment of snoring and obstructive sleep apnea with oral appliances: an update for 2005. Sleep 2006;29:240–243.
260 Morgenthaler TI, Kapen S, Lee-Chiong T, Alessi C, Boehlecke B, Brown T, Coleman J, Friedman L, Kapur V, Owens J, Pancer J, Swick T: Practice parameters for the medical therapy of obstructive sleep apnea. Sleep 2006;29:1031–1035.
261 Foster GD, Borradaile KE, Sanders MH, Millman R, Zammit G, Newman AB, Wadden TA, Kelley D, Wing RR, Pi-Sunyer FX, Reboussin D, Kuna ST: A randomized study on the effect of weight loss on obstructive sleep apnea among obese patients with type 2 diabetes: the Sleep AHEAD study. Arch Intern Med 2009;169:1619–1626.
262 Tuomilehto HP, Seppa JM, Partinen MM, Peltonen M, Gylling H, Tuomilehto JO, Vanninen EJ, Kokkarinen J, Sahlman JK, Martikainen T, Soini EJ, Randell J, Tukiainen H, Uusitupa M: Lifestyle intervention with weight reduction: first-line treatment in mild obstructive sleep apnea. Am J Respir Crit Care Med 2009;179:320–327.
263 Johansson K, Neovius M, Lagerros YT, Harlid R, Rossner S, Granath F, Hemmingsson E: Effect of a very low energy diet on moderate and severe obstructive sleep apnoea in obese men: a randomised controlled trial. BMJ 2009;339:b4609.
264 Buchwald H, Avidor Y, Braunwald E, Jensen MD, Pories W, Fahrbach K, Schoelles K: Bariatric surgery: a systematic review and meta-analysis. JAMA 2004;292:1724–1737.
265 Greenburg DL, Lettieri CJ, Eliasson AH: Effects of surgical weight loss on measures of obstructive sleep apnea: a meta-analysis. Am J Med 2009;122: 535–542.
266 Littner M, Kushida CA, Hartse K, Anderson WM, Davila D, Johnson SF, Wise MS, Hirshkowitz M, Woodson BT: Practice parameters for the use of laser-assisted uvulopalatoplasty: an update for 2000. Sleep 2001;24:603–619.
267 Grunstein RR, Stenlof K, Hedner JA, Sjostrom L: Impact of self-reported sleep-breathing disturbances on psychosocial performance in the Swedish Obese Subjects (SOS) Study. Sleep 1995;18:635–643.
268 Arzt M, Young T, Finn L, Skatrud JB, Ryan CM, Newton GE, Mak S, Parker JD, Floras JS, Bradley TD: Sleepiness and sleep in patients with both systolic heart failure and obstructive sleep apnea. Arch Intern Med 2006;166:1716–1722.
269 Wright J, Johns R, Watt I, Melville A, Sheldon T: Health effects of obstructive sleep apnoea and the effectiveness of continuous positive airways pressure: a systematic review of the research evidence. BMJ 1997;314:851–860.
270 Peppard PE, Young T, Palta M, Skatrud J: Prospective study of the association between sleep-disordered breathing and hypertension. N Engl J Med 2000;342:1378–1384.
271 Becker HF, Jerrentrup A, Ploch T, Grote L, Penzel T, Sullivan CE, Peter JH: Effect of nasal continuous positive airway pressure treatment on blood pressure in patients with obstructive sleep apnea. Circulation 2003;107:68–73.
272 Kripalani S, Yao X, Haynes RB: Interventions to enhance medication adherence in chronic medical conditions: a systematic review. Arch Intern Med 2007;167:540–550.
273 Hoy CJ, Vennelle M, Kingshott RN, Engleman HM, Douglas NJ. Can intensive support improve continuous positive airway pressure use in patients with the sleep apnea/hypopnea syndrome? Am J Respir Crit Care Med 1999;159:1096–1100.

Inflammation, Oxidative Stress, and Procoagulant and Thrombotic Activity in Adults with Obstructive Sleep Apnea

2

Chapter 2

Inflammation, Oxidative Stress, and Procoagulant and Thrombotic Activity in Adults with Obstructive Sleep Apnea

Abstract

Obstructive sleep apnea (OSA) is currently considered to be an inflammatory disorder. Evidence suggests that the chronic intermittent hypoxia and, possibly, sleep loss and fragmentation associated with OSA increase the levels of various markers of inflammation, oxidative stress, and procoagulant and thrombotic activity. These alterations may contribute to the development of endothelial and metabolic dysfunction, atherosclerosis and cardiovascular disorders associated with OSA. However, these alterations are also associated with OSA comorbidities, making it difficult to discern which effects are attributable to OSA and/or these other conditions. Well-designed longitudinal and interventional studies that take confounding variables into account are needed to demonstrate a causal link between OSA and inflammation, to assess specific mechanisms that could explain these alterations and to address whether they may be improved by continuous positive airway pressure therapy.

Obstructive sleep apnea (OSA) has been associated with increased levels of many of the mediators involved in inflammatory processes, oxidative stress, and procoagulant and thrombotic activity [1, 2]. The release of these mediators is triggered by the chronic intermittent hypoxia and, possibly, sleep loss and fragmentation associated with OSA [3, 4]. Their adverse effects on specific body tissues may lead to the development of the cardiovascular and metabolic disorders associated with OSA [5].

1 Inflammatory Response to Chronic Intermittent Hypoxia

1.1 Intermittent Hypoxia Activates Transcription Factors Involved in Inflammatory Processes

In contrast to sustained hypoxia, intermittent hypoxia is associated with repetitive episodes of reoxygenation. Intermittent and sustained hypoxia may produce their effects by activating distinct transcription factors involved in inflammatory processes [6]. The roles of 2 of these factors have been studied in OSA: nuclear factor κB (NF-κB) and hypoxia-inducible factors (HIFs) [6]. In vitro studies have suggested that NF-κB

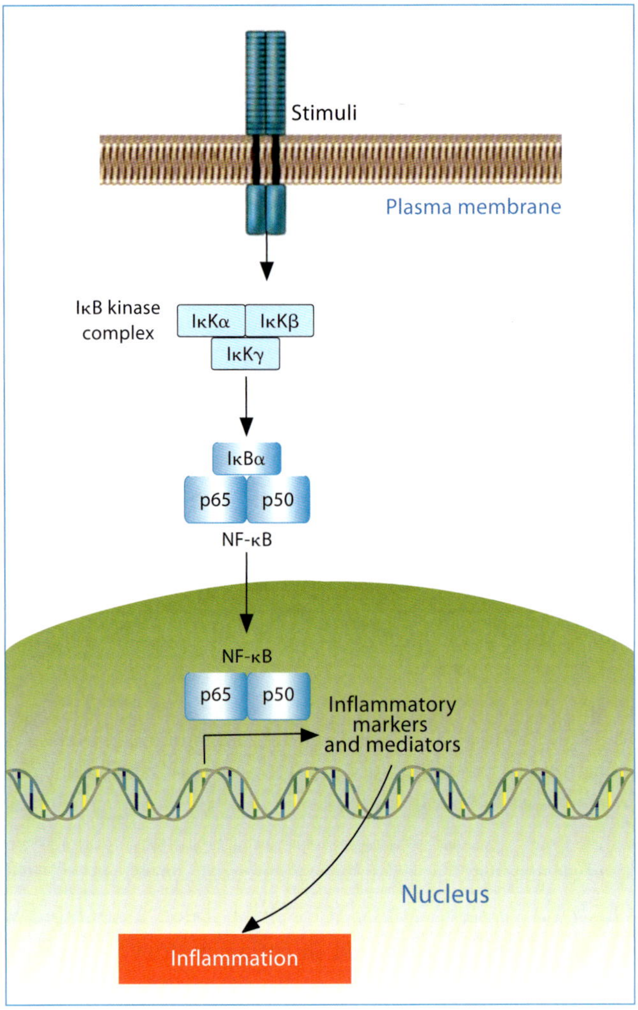

Fig. 1. Simplified scheme of the cytoplasmic activation of NF-κB showing its translocation to the nucleus. In non-stimulated cells, NF-κB remains inactive in the cytoplasm due to its interaction with the NF-κB inhibitor (IκB). In response to multiple stimuli, such as inflammatory cytokines or reactive oxygen species, NF-κB is activated. This activation is achieved by the phosphorylation of IκB by the IκB kinase complex (IκK complex, which contains several subunits including 2 related catalytic subunits, IκKα and IκKβ, and a regulatory subunit, IκKγ), a critical regulatory step in NF-κB function. The phosphorylation of IκB frees NF-κB from its inhibitor, and the freed NF-κB can then translocate to the nucleus where it activates the transcription of a variety of target genes involved in the inflammatory process. After Shoelson et al. [14], with permission.

may be selectively activated by intermittent hypoxia in contrast to HIF-1, which is mainly activated by sustained hypoxia [7, 8]. However, studies using cell culture and animal models have demonstrated that HIFs are activated by frequent and repeated exposure to intermittent hypoxia [9–12]. A potential interaction between NF-κB and HIF-1 further complicates the understanding of the mechanisms for the activation of transcription factors by intermittent hypoxia [6]. How these experimental models are applicable to OSA is, to our knowledge, currently unknown.

1.1.1 The Nuclear Factor κB Pathway

NF-κB is a generic name for a family of dimeric transcription factors composed of several proteins, including p50 and p65 (RelA), RelB, c-Rel, p50 (NF-κB1) and p52 (NF-κB2). The classical NF-κB pathway (fig. 1) is activated by mediators including

Table 1. NF-κB target gene products that are potentially involved in the pathogenesis of atherosclerosis, and/or insulin resistance and type 2 diabetes

Cytokines and chemokines	Transcription factors	Receptors and surface proteins	Others
TNF-α	TNFR p55	p65 RelA	PAI-1
IFN-γ	TNFR p75	NF-κB p50	SAA
Resistin	IFNR subunits	IκKα	Angiotensinogen
IL-1β	IL-1R	IκKβ	CRP
IL-6	IL-6R	IκBα	COX-2
IL-8	CD40 ligand	A20	iNOS
IL-10	E-selectin		VEGF
IL-12	P-selectin		IGFBP
IL-18	ICAM-1		MnSOD
Lymphotoxins	VCAM-1		
TGF-β	CCR-2		
MCP-1	TLR-2		
MIP-α	TLR-4		
MIP-1β	Lox-1		
MIP-2	RAGE		
MIP-3α	RANTES		

TNFR = TNF receptor; IFN = interferon; IFNR = interferon receptor; IL-1R = IL-1 receptor; TGF-β = transforming growth factor β; MCP-1 = monocyte chemoattractant protein 1; MIP = macrophage inflammatory protein; ICAM = intercellular adhesion molecule; VCAM = vascular cell adhesion molecule; CCR = chemokine receptor; TLR = Toll-like receptor; Lox-1 = lectin-like oxidized low-density lipoprotein receptor; RAGE = receptor for advanced glycation end-products; RANTES = a chemokine, 'regulated upon activation, normal T-cell expressed and secreted'; NF-κB is a generic name for a family of dimeric transcription factors composed of several proteins (e.g. p50 and p65) that share a domain responsible for DNA binding and the binding of NF-κB inhibitor (IκB); NF-κB activation is achieved by the phosphorylation of IκB by the IκB kinase complex (IκK complex), which contains several subunits including 2 related catalytic subunits, IκKα and IκKβ; A20 is an inducible zinc finger protein; PAI-1 = plasminogen activator inhibitor 1; SAA = serum amyloid A; CRP = C-reactive protein; COX-2 = cyclooxygenase enzyme 2; iNOS = inducible nitric oxide synthase; VEGF = vascular endothelial growth factor; IGFBP = insulin-like growth factor-binding protein; MnSOD = manganese superoxide dismutase. After Shoelson et al. [14], with permission.

inflammatory cytokines [e.g. tumor necrosis factor (TNF) α and interleukin (IL) 1], chemokines (e.g. IL-8) and possibly reactive oxygen species (ROS). NF-κB mediates the coordinate expression of inflammatory molecules involved in the development of various disorders such as atherosclerosis and insulin resistance/type 2 diabetes (table 1) [13, 14]. The NF-κB nonclassical signaling pathway has a central role in the expression of genes involved in the development and maintenance of secondary lymphoid organs. An endothelial cell in vitro model indicated that intermittent hypoxia may activate NF-κB, at least in part, via the activation of p38 mitogen-

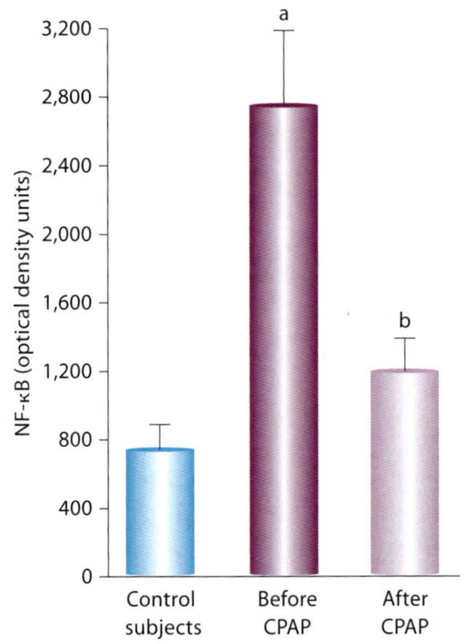

Fig. 2. Increased monocyte NF-κB activity in OSA patients and its reversal with continuous positive airway pressure (CPAP) treatment. NF-κB band intensity from 5 patients quantified using densitometry and expressed as arbitrary optical density units (means ± SEM). [a] $p < 0.05$ compared with controls, [b] $p < 0.05$ compared with pre-CPAP values. After Greenberg et al. [15], with permission.

activated protein kinase; pharmacological inhibition of p38 abolished the activation of NF-κB by intermittent hypoxia, and depletion of p38 significantly reduced intermittent hypoxia-induced NF-κB activity [8].

1.1.1.1 *Activation of the NF-κB Pathway in OSA.* The critical role of inflammation mediated by the activation of the NF-κB pathway in OSA is suggested by:

- higher levels of NF-κB activity in circulating monocytes (fig. 2) [15, 16] and neutrophils [16] from OSA patients than from control subjects;
- increased expression of NF-κB in freshly harvested venous endothelial cells from obese OSA patients compared to obese non-OSA patients [17];
- increased levels of NF-κB target gene products in OSA patients, including the cytokines TNF-α (fig. 3) [7, 18, 19], IL-6 [20], macrophage chemotactic protein 1 [21] and IL-8 [18], and adhesion molecules [22], which have been shown to be reduced by the administration of continuous positive airway pressure (CPAP) [18, 20]. However, the association between IL-6 levels and OSA has yet to be replicated [18]. The increase in TNF-α may be due to a genetic predisposition, e.g. the TNF-α (–308A) allele (consisting of a guanine-to-adenine substitution at position –308 in the promoter region) has been associated with the diagnosis of OSA [23, 24].

1.1.2 The Hypoxia-Inducible Factor Pathway

HIF-1 is the prototypical member of the HIF family [6, 12] and consists of an O_2-regulated α-subunit and a constitutive β-subunit. HIF-1 transcriptional activity is

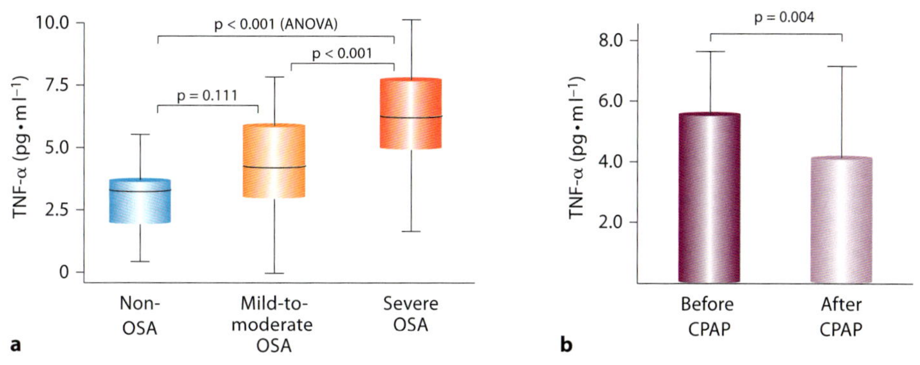

Fig. 3. Serum levels of TNF-α in subjects without OSA, with mild-to-moderate OSA and with severe OSA, and the impact of 6 weeks of continuous positive airway pressure (CPAP) therapy. **a** At baseline, TNF-α levels are significantly different between the 3 groups ($p < 0.001$; groups matched for age, body mass index, smoking status and other relevant variables) and higher in the severe OSA group ($n = 31$) than in the non-OSA ($n = 30$; $p < 0.001$) and mild-to-moderate OSA groups ($n = 35$; $p < 0.001$). TNF-α levels in the mild-to-moderate OSA group were not significantly different from those in the non-OSA group ($p = 0.11$). The boxes represent values within the interquartile range, the whiskers represent the data range, and the line across the boxes represents the median values. **b** Continuous positive airway pressure (CPAP) treatment ($n = 49$) lowered TNF-α levels ($p < 0.004$). After Ryan et al. [18], with permission. © American Thoracic Society.

induced under continuous and chronic intermittent hypoxia. HIF-1 activates the transcription of genes encoding proteins that increase oxygen supply to the cell or adapt the cell metabolism to reduced oxygen delivery. The O_2-regulated α-subunit of HIF-2α creates a heterodimer with HIF-1β to activate target genes, which are similar to those activated by HIF-1 [25], while HIF-3α may inhibit HIF signaling.

The effects of intermittent and sustained hypoxia on HIF-1α accumulation may differ. This has been shown in pheochromocytoma 12 cell cultures, which share many properties with carotid body glomus cells, including O_2-regulated neurotransmitter release and the expression of tyrosine hydroxylase, the rate-limiting enzyme for catecholamine production [6]. In this cell line, intermittent hypoxia induced a higher HIF 1α protein level than sustained hypoxia, for a given intensity and duration [9]. HIF-1α levels remain high during reoxygenation in the intermittent hypoxic situation, whereas they return to control levels within 10 min of reoxygenation following sustained hypoxia [10]. Intermittent hypoxia upregulates HIF-1α protein levels in pheochromocytoma 12 cells and rodents, whereas it downregulates the expression of HIF-2α (fig. 4) [12]. Sustained hypoxia is associated with an increase in the levels and transcriptional activity of HIF-2α and HIF-1 levels [12]. By contrast, chronic intermittent hypoxia is associated with the increased expression of HIF-2α and HIF-3α in the rat carotid body, while sustained hypoxia is associated with an increase in the expression of the HIF-1α subtype [11].

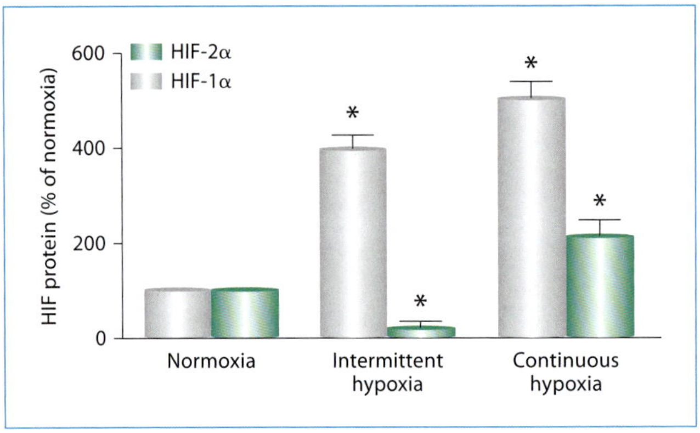

Fig. 4. Intermittent hypoxia results in HIF-2α degradation in the rat pheochromocytoma 12 cell line. Representative HIF-2α and HIF-1α protein levels analyzed by immunoblot in the pheochromocytoma 12 cell line exposed to normoxia, 60 cycles of intermittent hypoxia (each cycle consisted of 30 s of 1.5% O_2 followed by 5 min of 20% O_2) or continuous hypoxia (1.5% O_2 for 4 h). Average data of densitometric analysis of the immunoblots are presented as the mean ± SEM from 4 independent experiments. * $p < 0.05$. After Nanduri et al. [12], with permission.

1.1.2.1 *Activation of the HIF Pathway in OSA.* Two HIF-1-dependent factors have been studied in OSA patients: vascular endothelial growth factor (VEGF; a cytokine regulating angiogenesis) and erythropoietin (a glycoprotein hormone that controls erythropoiesis). Obese OSA patients with cardiovascular comorbidities have increased circulating levels of VEGF that was correlated with OSA severity and reduced by CPAP administration in patients who were compliant with treatment and who had improved nocturnal hypoxia [26]. However, obesity and hypertension are also associated with increased levels of VEGF [27], and this may contribute to the increased VEGF levels observed in OSA patients with these conditions [28]. Increased levels of VEGF have also been reported in otherwise healthy patients with OSA [29], but this remains controversial [28]. It should be noted that VEGF may be activated by $O_2^-\bullet$-independent mechanisms, e.g. via TNF-α (whose levels are increased in OSA), or by angiotensin II and the activation of angiotensin I receptors [18, 30]. It remains to be determined whether the levels of circulating erythropoietin are also increased in OSA. They have been reported to be similar in OSA patients and in normal control subjects [7], whereas nocturnal erythropoietin levels were higher in obese patients with severe OSA than in matched control subjects [31].

1.1.3 Tissue-Specific Effects of Chronic Intermittent Hypoxia

Body tissues respond to intermittent hypoxia in different ways (table 2) [5]. NF-κB may be predominantly activated in endothelial cells and adipose tissue, whereas HIFs may have a predominant role in oxygen-sensing by the carotid bodies [5]. This has been reviewed by Garvey et al. [5].

Table 2. Tissue-specific effects of intermittent hypoxia

Tissue	Mechanism	Effects
Carotid body	Oxygen-sensing by HIF-1α	Enhanced sympathetic activity Increased blood pressure Decreased baroreflex sensitivity
Endothelium	Activation of NF-κB	Inflammatory cytokine production Surface adhesion molecule expression Increased apoptotic endothelial cells? Decreased circulating endothelial progenitor cells?
Adipose tissue	Activation of NF-κB	Dysregulation of adipokine production

After Garvey et al. [5], with permission.

In summary, in OSA, the mechanisms linking chronic intermittent hypoxia, the activation of the HIF and NF-κB pathways, the interactions between them, and the tissue-specific adverse effects of intermittent hypoxia remain largely unknown [5, 6].

1.2 *Oxidative and Nitrosative Stress*

Intermittent hypoxia is associated with recurrent episodes of reoxygenation, as occurs in ischemia-reperfusion injury, and with the increased production of ROS and reactive nitrogen species (RNS) [1, 2, 32, 33]; therefore, OSA is potentially an oxidative stress condition [2, 32]. ROS possibly activate transcription factors including NF-κB and increase the expression of proinflammatory mediators, e.g. TNF-α, IL-6 and adhesion molecules (see above). These mediators may activate inflammatory cells (such as monocytes and lymphocytes) or endothelial cells that contribute to the endothelial dysfunction, atherosclerosis and cardiovascular disorders associated with OSA. However, although in vitro and animal studies provide evidence for oxidative stress, data from clinical studies in OSA patients are contradictory. This may be related to bias, including the presence of confounders and the unreliable methods used to measure oxidative stress [1].

1.2.1 Sources and Cellular Effects of Reactive Oxidative and Nitrosative Species

ROS and RNS play key roles in vascular physiology and pathology [34]. The most important species are peroxide (H_2O_2), superoxide anion ($O_2^{-}\bullet$), nitric oxide (NO), and peroxynitrite ($ONOO^-$; fig. 5) [35]. These highly reactive molecules originate in structural cells, e.g. endothelial cells and vascular smooth muscle cells, and in inflammatory and immune cells, e.g. granulocytes and monocytes. They all may generate oxidants within the vessel wall. The major cardiovascular sources of ROS include the enzymes nicotinamide adenine dinucleotide (phosphate) [NAD(P)H] oxidase, xanthine oxidoreductase, NO synthase, mitochondrial cytochromes and hemoglobin.

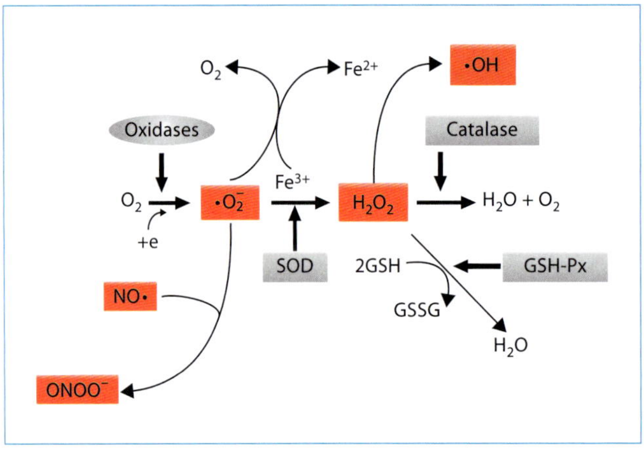

Fig. 5. Vascular ROS. Highlighted in red are some of the most important ROS in vascular cells. Oxidases convert oxygen to superoxide anion (O_2^-•), which is then dismutated to peroxide (H_2O_2) by superoxide dismutase (SOD). H_2O_2 can be converted to H_2O by catalase or glutathione peroxidase (GSH-Px) or to hydroxyl radical (•OH) after reaction with Fe^{2+}. O_2^-• reacts rapidly with nitric oxide (NO•) to form peroxynitrite ($ONOO^-$). GSSG = Oxidized glutathione; GSH = reduced glutathione. After Griendling and FitzGerald [35], with permission.

ROS and RNS are involved in cellular signaling pathways and transcriptional regulation, with specific roles in the modulation of cellular events (termed the redox signaling function of ROS and RNS) [36]. In the physiological state, they contribute to the maintenance of cellular homeostasis. They serve as a secondary messenger system that transmits information via the modulation of intracellular signaling molecules [34], e.g. ROS generated by NAD(P)H oxidase activate other enzymatic or transcription factor pathways. NO can bind to the transition metal center of proteins such as guanylate cyclase, whose activation is largely responsible for NO-induced vasodilation, the inhibition of platelet aggregation and the proliferation of smooth muscle cells. However, the majority of NO action is mediated by S-nitrosylation (the covalent attachment of NO to cysteine thiol) [37].

Excess ROS and RNS cause radical-induced oxidation and damage, resulting in cell dysfunction, necrosis and/or apoptosis [36]. The interplay between ROS and RNS contributes to vascular inflammation and endothelial dysfunction, and is involved in the development and progression of atherosclerosis and cardiovascular diseases [34]. Their excess production may also cause direct oxidative and nitrosative injury to lipids, deoxyribonucleic acid (DNA) and proteins. Excess ROS and RNS contribute to diminish NO bioactivity and thereby damage cellular function (NO contributes to cytotoxicity, mainly by reacting with O_2^-• to produce $ONOO^-$; fig. 6) [34, 38]. This may be a potential mechanism that leads to the endothelial dysfunction associated with OSA, as evidenced by the reduced NO-dependent vasodilation responses of OSA patients [39]. In contrast, the increased availability of NO may reduce oxidative stress

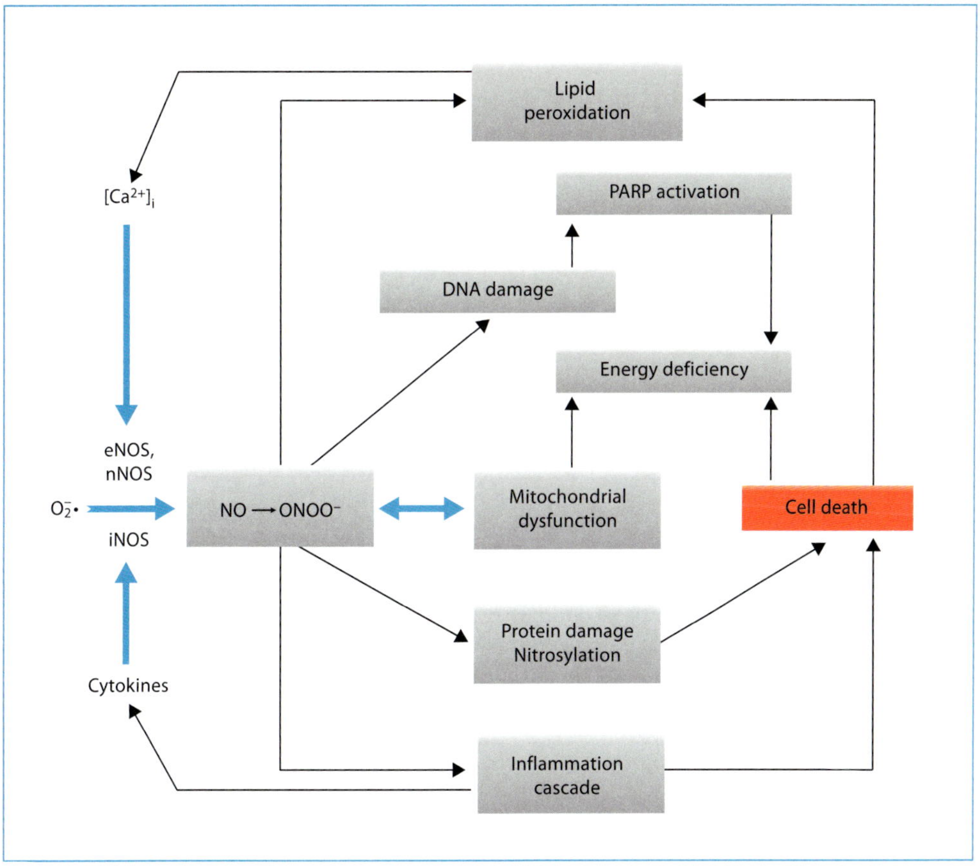

Fig. 6. Detrimental peroxide-dependent mechanisms. Superoxide ($O_2^{-}\cdot$) anions react with nitric oxide (NO•) to produce peroxynitrite ($ONOO^-$). The protonation of $ONOO^-$ generates peroxynitrous acid (ONOOH). $ONOO^-$ and ONOOH are powerful oxidants and nitrating/nitrosating agents that can initiate lipid peroxidation cascades, damage DNA and proteins, inactivate mitochondrial respiratory complexes and deplete cellular thiols. The accumulation of these effects can lead to cell death and energy deficiency. Some of these mechanisms, including lipid peroxidation [45, 47–49], DNA oxidation [54] and cell apoptosis [121], have been reported in OSA. eNOS = Endothelial NO synthase; nNOS = neuronal NO synthase; iNOS = inducible NO synthase; PARP = polyadenosine diphosphate ribosyl polymerase (all of these enzymes are involved in a number of cellular processes, mainly DNA repair and programmed cell death). $[Ca^{2+}]_i$ = Intracellular Ca^{2+}. After Manukhina et al. [38], with permission.

and protect the endothelium and endothelial repair mechanisms, e.g. the recruitment and proliferation of endothelial progenitor cells [40].

1.2.2 Oxidative and Nitrosative Stress in Obstructive Sleep Apnea

Several mechanisms may be responsible for the increased production of ROS and RNS in OSA, including the recurrent hypoxia and reoxygenation cycles [41–43] and the increase in inflammatory responses, sympathetic activity and catecholamine-induced ROS production seen in the disease [42].

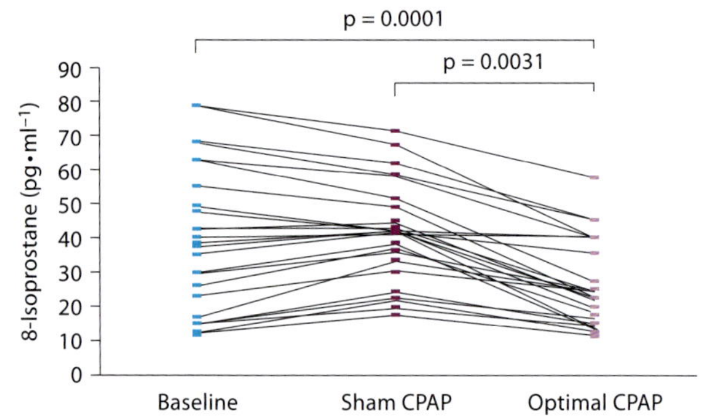

Fig. 7. Individual plasma 8-isoprostane concentrations at baseline, after sham CPAP and after optimal CPAP in OSA patients. After Alonso-Fernandez et al. [44], with permission.

Oxidative stress in OSA has been assessed by measuring lipid peroxidation using malondialdehyde, thiobarbituric-acid-reactive substances and oxidized low-density lipoprotein levels in urine, plasma, exhaled condensate or sputum samples. The negative findings of studies assessing oxidative stress in OSA patients may be related to biases including the use of unreliable dosage methods, as reviewed by Arnardottir et al. [1]. The proposed gold standard method for assessing oxidative stress in OSA is the measurement of 8-isoprostane levels, a marker of lipid peroxidation, by gas chromatography/negative ion chemical ionization mass spectrometry in urine samples taken after the sleep period or in plasma during sleep [1].

Several studies have reported increased lipid peroxidation in OSA patients. Plasma 8-isoprostane concentrations were examined in a prospective randomized, placebo-controlled study of newly diagnosed middle-aged males with OSA and no other known comorbidity (n = 31) and healthy control subjects (n = 15) of the same age, gender and body mass index (BMI) [44]. OSA patients were randomized to sham CPAP and effective CPAP application for 12 weeks. The concentrations of 8-isoprostane were significantly higher in OSA patients than in healthy subjects and were significantly lowered after CPAP therapy, but not after sham CPAP (fig. 7) [44]. Increased 8-isoprostane levels have also been observed in urine [45] (fig. 8) and exhaled breath condensates [46, 47] from overweight or obese OSA patients compared to control subjects; these levels were lowered by CPAP administration [45, 47]. Furthermore, increased levels of lipid peroxidation (assessed by measuring the plasma levels of thiobarbituric-acid-reactive substances) [48, 49] were observed in overweight OSA patients with a history of smoking compared to control subjects [49]; peroxidation was lowered by CPAP treatment [48, 49]. Higher levels of oxidized low-density lipoproteins have been found in otherwise healthy OSA patients than in non-OSA subjects, and these levels were reduced after the administration of CPAP for 3 months [50]. Finally, higher plasma levels of malondialdehyde have been found in obese OSA

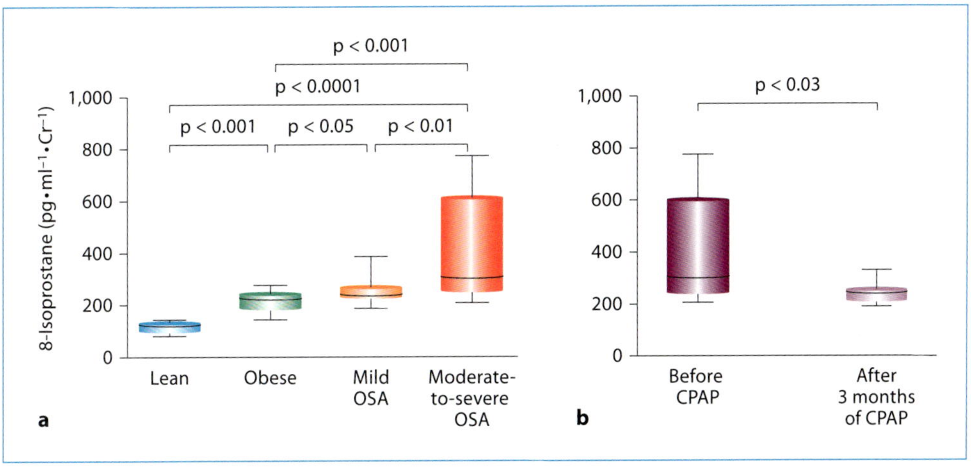

Fig. 8. Lipid peroxidation in OSA patients: effect of CPAP therapy. **a** Overnight urinary excretion of 8-isoprostane in lean subjects without OSA (n = 12), obese subjects without OSA (n = 18), obese patients with mild OSA (n = 20) and obese patients with moderate-to-severe OSA (n = 20). **b** Effect of CPAP on overnight urinary excretion of 8-isoprostane in patients with moderate-to-severe OSA (n = 20) after treatment with nasal CPAP for 3 months. Participants were free of diseases other than OSA and obesity. The boundaries of each box represent the interquartile range (25th–75th percentiles), the horizontal line inside the box represents the median, and the error bars outside the box represent the 95% confidence intervals. After Minoguchi et al. [45], with permission.

patients than in non-OSA control subjects, and these levels were also reduced after the administration of CPAP for 3 months [51].

The increased production of ROS by monocytes and neutrophils has been observed in overweight or obese OSA patients compared to control subjects with normal or nearly normal BMI, and this increased production was lowered by CPAP therapy [41, 42]. In these studies, the OSA patients and control subjects were smokers [42] or had cardiovascular comorbidities [41]. Increased levels of oxidative stress have been observed in freshly harvested venous endothelial cells [52] and in microvascular walls obtained by forearm subcutaneous biopsy [53] from OSA patients compared to control subjects [see chapter 4, this vol., pp. 139–169].

Abnormal levels of additional oxidative stress markers have also been observed in OSA patients, including increases in the levels of: (1) DNA oxidation [54]; (2) urinary uric acid (the purine catabolic end-product of xanthine oxidoreductase) in OSA patients compared to control subjects, which decreased with CPAP treatment [55]; (3) plasma homocysteine in OSA patients with cardiovascular diseases [56] or with a much higher BMI than control subjects [57]. Homocysteine levels decreased after long-term CPAP treatment in 12 OSA patients suffering from various cardiovascular diseases or diabetes [58]. In addition, decreased antioxidant capacity has been observed in obese or nearly obese patients with severe OSA [59, 60], which returned to the levels observed in control subjects after CPAP therapy [60]; these patients were smokers [59,

60] or had hypertension [60]. Furthermore, changes in the structure of serum albumin and the impairment of its antioxidant properties, which were improved following CPAP therapy, have been reported in OSA patients [61]. Finally, an improvement in vascular reactivity has been observed in OSA patients after treatment with vitamin C (an antioxidant) [62] or allopurinol (a xanthine oxidase inhibitor) [63].

However, other studies have failed to find a significant difference in oxidative stress markers between OSA patients and control subjects. A study of otherwise healthy male patients with moderate-to-severe OSA (n = 41) and closely matched OSA-free control subjects (n = 35) measured the baseline plasma indices of oxidative stress and lipid peroxidation before sleep, after 4 h of untreated OSA and in the morning after 4 h of effective CPAP treatment [64]. The baseline measures were not significantly different between OSA patients and control subjects, and neither untreated OSA, CPAP treatment nor normal sleep affected the levels of any of the oxidative stress measures. In addition, there was no association between the severity of OSA and any of the measures of oxidative stress. There was no significant difference in the levels of thiobarbituric-acid-reactive substances between obese patients with severe OSA and lean control subjects without symptoms suggesting OSA [65]. Similar 3-nitrotyrosine plasma levels were observed before and after sleep in 10 men with untreated moderate-to-severe OSA, who were free of other diseases and medication, and in 10 healthy male control subjects with a similar age and BMI [66]. Neither normal nor apneic sleep significantly modified the circulating levels of free 3-nitrotyrosine, which were similar before and after sleep in normal and apneic subjects. Three studies have failed to find a significant difference in homocysteine levels [60, 67, 68]. Two of these studies assessed patients free from OSA comorbidities, and the OSA patients and healthy control subjects were carefully matched for confounding variables such as BMI and age [67, 68].

2 Inflammatory Response to Sleep Loss and Fragmentation

The sleep of OSA patients is characterized by increased fragmentation and reduced slow wave and rapid eye movement sleep. Poor sleep and short sleep are considered to be risk factors for adverse cardiovascular and metabolic events, including the development of hypertension, alterations in glucose metabolism and obesity [3, 69]. Chronic inflammation could be an intermediate mechanism linking the sleep loss and fragmentation associated with OSA and the later development of cardiovascular disorders. However, this still remains to be demonstrated, and it is important to distinguish sleep deprivation per se from sleep fragmentation that is secondary to sleep apnea because the former can occur without the coexistence of sleep apnea. Experimental and clinical studies have reported an association between sleep deprivation and increased circulating levels of inflammatory mediators, including soluble intercellular adhesion molecule 1 and E-selectin, IL-1β, IL-6, TNF-α and IL-17 [69–

71]. Acute total and short-term partial sleep deprivation is associated with an increase in the concentration of high-sensitivity C-reactive protein (CRP) [70, 72]. Conversely, analysis of the data from the Wisconsin Sleep Cohort Study indicated that there is no association between CRP levels and sleep duration [73].

3 Hypercoagulability and Thrombosis

Increased procoagulant and thrombotic activity is associated with endothelial dysfunction and the development of atherosclerosis [74]. It is unclear whether OSA is an independent risk factor for an increased coagulation state because comorbidities such as metabolic syndrome may also alter coagulation and thrombosis in OSA patients.

Several alterations in coagulation homeostasis have been reported in OSA. The levels of type 1 plasminogen activator inhibitor (PAI) 1 (a factor derived from adipose tissue, and of which increased levels indicate decreased fibrinolytic activity) are higher in OSA patients with cardiovascular comorbidities than in controls [75, 76]. These increased levels were lowered after 2 weeks of CPAP therapy in a small number of patients (n = 18) [77]; however, PAI-1 levels have been noted to be similar in OSA patients and healthy controls after adjustment for blood pressure and BMI [78]. Similarly, in patients with OSA and metabolic syndrome, the metabolic syndrome may be of more importance in determining PAI-1 levels than OSA; indeed, in the absence of metabolic syndrome, the apnea-hypopnea index (AHI) accounted for only approximately 10% of the variance in PAI-1 levels [75]. The levels of PAI-1 in the adults from the Cleveland Family Study (n = 537) [79] were increased by 12% in the morning (95% confidence interval, CI, 5–20%; $p < 0.001$) and 11% in the evening (95% CI 2–20%; $p = 0.01$) per 5-unit AHI increase, until an AHI of 15, when no further increase in PAI-1 was demonstrated. Similarly, levels of fibrinogen were increased in the morning by an average of 8.4 $mg \cdot dl^{-1}$ (95% CI 3.12–13.65; $p = 0.002$) per 5-unit AHI increase, until an AHI of 15. It is suggested that even mild OSA levels may increase prothrombotic processes. Plasma fibrinogen levels in OSA patients with cardiovascular comorbidities were found to be similar [80] or higher than those of non-OSA control patients [81]. CPAP treatment was shown to lower [82] or not to lower [83] plasma fibrinogen levels. Excessive platelet activity was observed in OSA patients with cardiovascular or metabolic comorbidities [83–85], and this activity was [84, 85] or was not [83] reduced by CPAP therapy. It is also unclear as to whether the levels of P-selectin, a marker of platelet activation, do [86] or do not [83] correlate with OSA severity. Increased levels of activated coagulation factor VII were found in overweight or obese OSA patients with hypertension, and these were lowered by CPAP therapy [87]. In addition, compared to unmatched controls at baseline, higher levels of the activated coagulation factors XIIa and VIIa, and the thrombin-antithrombin ratio have been recorded; however, these levels did not fall after 1 month of CPAP treatment [83]. Studies of D-dimer levels in OSA patients have also produced inconsistent findings [77, 79, 88–90].

Several hypotheses have been proposed to explain the presence of a hypercoagulative state in OSA patients [91]: increased $O_2^-\bullet$ release by neutrophils may enhance thrombus formation and limit the levels of bioavailable NO [42]; increased circulating catecholamine levels may activate platelet adrenergic receptors and enhance aggregation; poor sleep quality, which has been associated with increased levels of von Willebrand factor (a mediator of platelet adhesion), soluble tissue factor antigen (an initiator of the coagulation cascade) [89] and plasma D-dimer [92, 93]. The mechanisms linking OSA and the presence of a hypercoagulative state remain to be explained.

4 Systemic Inflammation

Low-grade inflammation may contribute to the development of the cardiovascular and metabolic diseases associated with OSA. The presence of a low-grade inflammatory state is also recognized as a critical process in adipose tissue dysfunction in obesity [94]. This makes it difficult to characterize the relationship between OSA and inflammation as obesity is a confounding factor of OSA [94, 95].

Systemic inflammation is associated with the increased activation of immune and inflammatory cells. In OSA patients, the increased activation of cells such as circulating monocytes [15, 16], neutrophils [16, 42] and platelets [83, 86] has been observed. CD4+ and CD8+ T cells of OSA patients undergo phenotypic and functional changes and acquire cytotoxic activity; CD8+ T cells become particularly cytotoxic against endothelial cells. These cellular changes are improved or reversed by treatment with CPAP [41, 96, 97].

Leukotrienes (LTs) and CRP are markers of low-grade inflammation that have been evaluated in OSA. LTB_4, a potent chemoattractant, and cysteinyl LTs (C, D_4, E_4) have been linked to the genesis and progression of atherosclerosis and, potentially, to the development of cardiovascular disorders [98]. The majority of studies on the relationship between LTs and OSA have been performed in children [99–105], and these studies suggested that children with OSA may have higher LT levels than children without OSA. Only a few studies have assessed the role of LTs in adults with OSA [95, 106, 107]. Nonobese adults with OSA ($n = 40$) had higher urinary LTE_4 levels than non-OSA control subjects matched for age, sex and BMI ($n = 25$) [95]. Urinary LTE_4 levels correlated with the percentage of time spent with a mean oxygen saturation level <90% ($r = 0.0312$; $p = 0.017$), and urinary LTE_4 levels increased as a function of BMI ($r = 0.445$; $p = 0.0002$) in a larger cohort of adults with OSA ($n = 72$). Compared with baseline, CPAP administration reduced urinary LTE_4 levels by 22% ($p = 0.006$) only in nonobese OSA patients. It is suggested that urinary LTE_4 levels are increased in OSA, in relation to obesity and, to a lesser extent, to the severity of hypoxia. LTB_4 production by polymorphonuclear leukocytes was also increased in nonobese OSA patients compared with age- and BMI-matched control subjects [106]. LTB_4 levels correlated with the mean and minimal arterial oxygen saturation, and CPAP administration significantly reduced the production of LTB_4 by 50%. Finally, higher levels of LTB_4 were observed in the exhaled breath condensates of OSA patients than in obese subjects ($p < 0.01$), which correlated with the AHI ($r = 0.35$, $p < 0.05$). Overall, LTs are potential mediators of the development of the cardiovascular disorders associated with OSA. Research on this topic is, however, at its very beginning.

CRP is an acute-phase reactant synthesized by the liver, which is mainly regulated by IL-6 (adipose tissue is a potent source of IL-6) [108]. Increased CRP levels have been particularly studied as they are considered to be a risk factor for cardiovascular disease; however, their importance has been questioned [109]. Studies with large numbers of participants have suggested that the increase in CRP levels may be related to confounding variables, especially obesity [110]. Studies assessing the relationship between OSA and CRP have provided conflicting results: some have shown that CRP is independently associated with the severity of sleep apnea [20, 111], whereas others did not find this to be the case [57, 68, 80, 112, 113]. For example, high-sensitivity CRP serum levels were measured in BMI-matched subjects without OSA, with mild-to-moderate OSA, and with severe OSA and in non-BMI-matched obese subjects with severe OSA [68]. All participants were free of other disease and were similar in age, smoking habits and cholesterol levels. CRP levels were similar in the 3 BMI-matched groups ($p = 0.7$), but they were significantly higher in the 4th group (which consisted of more obese patients) compared to the other groups ($p < 0.05$). However, there was no independent association between CRP levels and OSA in 907 adult participants of the Wisconsin Sleep Cohort Study [73]. The effect of CPAP therapy on CRP levels is also controversial [20, 112]. In a comparison of CRP, IL-6 and TNF-α circulating levels during and after 1 week of CPAP withdrawal, CPAP withdrawal was associated with the return of OSA and a marked increase in sympathetic activity without a concomitant elevation of these inflammatory markers [114]. However, the pretreatment levels were not reported; thus, a methodological bias was introduced that prevents an unequivocal conclusion being drawn as to the effect of CPAP on these inflammatory markers [115]. The effect of therapeutic ($n = 51$) and subtherapeutic ($n = 49$) CPAP therapy on inflammatory markers, including highly sensitive CRP, IL-6, γ-interferon and anti-inflammatory adiponectin, was also assessed in moderate-to-severe OSA patients at baseline and after 4 weeks of follow-up [116]. The marker levels were not significantly changed after 4 weeks of therapeutic CPAP compared to subtherapeutic CPAP therapy; therefore, it is suggested that 4 weeks of CPAP treatment had no beneficial effect on these blood markers of inflammation in patients with moderate-to-severe OSA.

5 Conclusions and Future Perspectives

The inflammatory process associated with OSA may contribute to the development and aggravation of endothelial dysfunction and insulin resistance. These may, in turn,

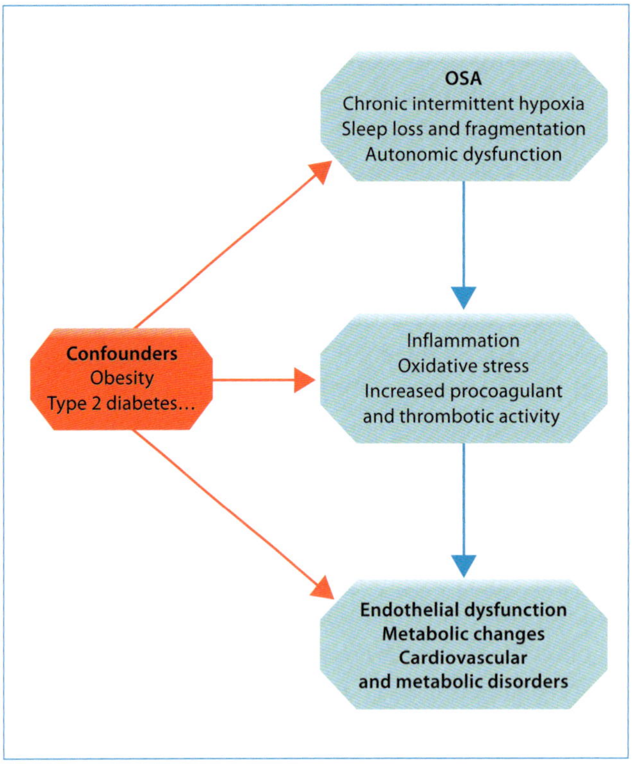

Fig. 9. Key points: the potential relationship between OSA, inflammation, oxidative stress, coagulation and thrombotic activity, and the risk for cardiovascular disorders associated with OSA. OSA is considered as an inflammatory disorder. Increased inflammation processes, oxidative stress, and coagulation and thrombosis activity may elicit endothelial dysfunction which, in turn, may increase the risk of atherosclerosis and cardiovascular disorders. However, OSA comorbidities are confounders that are able to produce similar cardiovascular damage. They may also, in themselves, be risk factors for the development and aggravation of OSA. This makes it difficult to discern whether it is the OSA or the confounders that are the root cause of the cardiovascular and metabolic complications associated with OSA.

be involved in the development of atherosclerosis and other cardiovascular disorders associated with OSA (fig. 9) [117]. Cell studies have been used to identify transcription factors and biochemical pathways linking intermittent hypoxia and inflammatory processes [7, 8, 12], while animal studies have been used to assess the link between these mechanisms and the development of atherosclerosis and cardiovascular and metabolic disorders associated with OSA [for reviews on this subject, see 118–120].

The presence of confounding variables, e.g. obesity, smoking habits, medication and cardiovascular diseases, makes it difficult to determine whether OSA is an independent risk factor for these intermediate mechanisms. There is a need for: (1) prospective studies of well-matched patients and control subjects that pay particular attention to matching the OSA comorbidities; (2) the identification of early inflammatory markers for cardiovascular risk associated with OSA; (3) the identification of OSA subpopulations at risk for cardiovascular diseases, and the assessment of early markers of inflammation in these subpopulations, where genetic studies may help to identify these subpopulations; (4) the assessment of the effects of CPAP administration on inflammatory mechanisms associated with OSA.

6 References

1 Arnardottir ES, Mackiewicz M, Gislason T, Teff KL, Pack AI: Molecular signatures of obstructive sleep apnea in adults: a review and perspective. Sleep 2009;32:447–470.

2 Lavie L, Lavie P: Molecular mechanisms of cardiovascular disease in OSAHS: the oxidative stress link. Eur Respir J 2009;33:1467–1484.

3 Spiegel K, Tasali E, Leproult R, Van Cauter E: Effects of poor and short sleep on glucose metabolism and obesity risk. Nat Rev Endocrinol 2009;5:253–261.

4 Ye J: Emerging role of adipose tissue hypoxia in obesity and insulin resistance. Int J Obes (Lond) 2009;33:54–66.

5 Garvey JF, Taylor CT, McNicholas WT: Cardiovascular disease in obstructive sleep apnoea syndrome: the role of intermittent hypoxia and inflammation. Eur Respir J 2009;33:1195–1205.

6 Nanduri J, Yuan G, Kumar GK, Semenza GL, Prabhakar NR: Transcriptional responses to intermittent hypoxia. Respir Physiol Neurobiol 2008;164: 277–281.

7 Ryan S, Taylor CT, McNicholas WT: Selective activation of inflammatory pathways by intermittent hypoxia in obstructive sleep apnea syndrome. Circulation 2005;112:2660–2667.

8 Ryan S, McNicholas WT, Taylor CT: A critical role for p38 map kinase in NF-kappaB signaling during intermittent hypoxia/reoxygenation. Biochem Biophys Res Commun 2007;355:728–733.

9 Yuan G, Nanduri J, Bhasker CR, Semenza GL, Prabhakar NR: Ca^{2+}/calmodulin kinase-dependent activation of hypoxia inducible factor 1 transcriptional activity in cells subjected to intermittent hypoxia. J Biol Chem 2005;280:4321–4328.

10 Yuan G, Nanduri J, Khan S, Semenza GL, Prabhakar NR: Induction of HIF-1alpha expression by intermittent hypoxia: involvement of NADPH oxidase, Ca^{2+} signaling, prolyl hydroxylases, and mTOR. J Cell Physiol 2008;217:674–685.

11 Lam SY, Tipoe GL, Liong EC, Fung ML: Differential expressions and roles of hypoxia-inducible factor-1alpha, -2alpha and -3alpha in the rat carotid body during chronic and intermittent hypoxia. Histol Histopathol 2008;23:271–280.

12 Nanduri J, Wang N, Yuan G, Khan SA, Souvannakitti D, Peng YJ, Kumar GK, Garcia JA, Prabhakar NR: Intermittent hypoxia degrades HIF-2alpha via calpains resulting in oxidative stress: implications for recurrent apnea-induced morbidities. Proc Natl Acad Sci USA 2009;106:1199–1204.

13 Monaco C, Paleolog E: Nuclear factor kappaB: a potential therapeutic target in atherosclerosis and thrombosis. Cardiovasc Res 2004;61:671–682.

14 Shoelson SE, Lee J, Goldfine AB: Inflammation and insulin resistance. J Clin Invest 2006;116:1793–1801.

15 Greenberg H, Ye X, Wilson D, Htoo AK, Hendersen T, Liu SF: Chronic intermittent hypoxia activates nuclear factor-kappaB in cardiovascular tissues in vivo. Biochem Biophys Res Commun 2006;343: 591–596.

16 Htoo AK, Greenberg H, Tongia S, Chen G, Henderson T, Wilson D, Liu SF: Activation of nuclear factor kappaB in obstructive sleep apnea: a pathway leading to systemic inflammation. Sleep Breath 2006;10:43–50.

17 Jelic S, Lederer DJ, Adams T, Padeletti M, Colombo PC, Factor PH, Le Jemtel TH: Vascular inflammation in obesity and sleep apnea. Circulation 2010; 121:1014–1021.

18 Ryan S, Taylor CT, McNicholas WT: Predictors of elevated nuclear factor-kappaB-dependent genes in obstructive sleep apnea syndrome. Am J Respir Crit Care Med 2006;174:824–830.

19 Sahlman J, Miettinen K, Peuhkurinen K, Seppa J, Peltonen M, Herder C, Punnonen K, Vanninen E, Gylling H, Partinen M, Uusitupa M, Tuomilehto H: The activation of the inflammatory cytokines in overweight patients with mild obstructive sleep apnoea. J Sleep Res 2010;19:341–348.

20 Yokoe T, Minoguchi K, Matsuo H, Oda N, Minoguchi H, Yoshino G, Hirano T, Adachi M: Elevated levels of C-reactive protein and interleukin-6 in patients with obstructive sleep apnea syndrome are decreased by nasal continuous positive airway pressure. Circulation 2003;107:1129–1134.

21 Kim J, Lee CH, Park CS, Kim BG, Kim SW, Cho JH: Plasma levels of MCP-1 and adiponectin in obstructive sleep apnea syndrome. Arch Otolaryngol Head Neck Surg 2010;136:896–899.
22 Ohga E, Nagase T, Tomita T, Teramoto S, Matsuse T, Katayama H, Ouchi Y: Increased levels of circulating ICAM-1, VCAM-1 and L-selectin in obstructive sleep apnea syndrome. J Appl Physiol 1999;87:10–14.
23 Riha RL, Brander P, Vennelle M, McArdle N, Kerr SM, Anderson NH, Douglas NJ: Tumour necrosis factor-alpha (–308) gene polymorphism in obstructive sleep apnoea-hypopnoea syndrome. Eur Respir J 2005;26:673–678.
24 Bhushan B, Guleria R, Misra A, Luthra K, Vikram NK: TNF-alpha gene polymorphism and TNF-alpha levels in obese Asian Indians with obstructive sleep apnea. Respir Med 2009;103:386–392.
25 Elvidge GP, Glenny L, Appelhoff RJ, Ratcliffe PJ, Ragoussis J, Gleadle JM: Concordant regulation of gene expression by hypoxia and 2-oxoglutarate-dependent dioxygenase inhibition: the role of HIF-1alpha, HIF-2alpha, and other pathways. J Biol Chem 2006;281:15215–15226.
26 Lavie L, Kraiczi H, Hefetz A, Ghandour H, Perelman A, Hedner J, Lavie P: Plasma vascular endothelial growth factor in sleep apnea syndrome: effects of nasal continuous positive air pressure treatment. Am J Respir Crit Care Med 2002;165:1624–1628.
27 Garcia de la Torre N, Rubio MA, Bordiu E, Cabrerizo L, Aparicio E, Hernandez C, Sanchez-Pernaute A, Diez-Valladares L, Torres AJ, Puente M, Charro AL: Effects of weight loss after bariatric surgery for morbid obesity on vascular endothelial growth factor-A, adipocytokines, and insulin. J Clin Endocrinol Metab 2008;93:4276–4281.
28 Valipour A, Litschauer B, Mittermayer F, Rauscher H, Burghuber OC, Wolzt M: Circulating plasma levels of vascular endothelial growth factor in patients with sleep disordered breathing. Respir Med 2004;98:1180–1186.
29 De la Pena M, Barcelo A, Barbe F, Pierola J, Pons J, Rimbau E, Ayllon O, Agusti AG: Endothelial function and circulating endothelial progenitor cells in patients with sleep apnea syndrome. Respiration 2008;76:28–32.
30 Takahashi S, Nakamura Y, Nishijima T, Sakurai S, Inoue H: Essential roles of angiotensin II in vascular endothelial growth factor expression in sleep apnea syndrome. Respir Med 2005;99:1125–1131.
31 Winnicki M, Shamsuzzaman A, Lanfranchi P, Accurso V, Olson E, Davison D, Somers VK: Erythropoietin and obstructive sleep apnea. Am J Hypertens 2004;17:783–786.
32 Lavie L: Oxidative stress – a unifying paradigm in obstructive sleep apnea and comorbidities. Prog Cardiovasc Dis 2009;51:303–312.
33 Pialoux V, Hanly PJ, Foster GE, Brugniaux JV, Beaudin AE, Hartmann SE, Pun M, Duggan CT, Poulin MJ: Effects of exposure to intermittent hypoxia on oxidative stress and acute hypoxic ventilatory response in humans. Am J Respir Crit Care Med 2009;180:1002–1009.
34 Stocker R, Keaney JF Jr: Role of oxidative modifications in atherosclerosis. Physiol Rev 2004;84:1381–1478.
35 Griendling KK, FitzGerald GA: Oxidative stress and cardiovascular injury. I. Basic mechanisms and in vivo monitoring of ROS. Circulation 2003;108:1912–1916.
36 Seddon M, Looi YH, Shah AM: Oxidative stress and redox signalling in cardiac hypertrophy and heart failure. Heart 2007;93:903–907.
37 Gaston B, Singel D, Doctor A, Stamler JS: S-nitrosothiol signaling in respiratory biology. Am J Respir Crit Care Med 2006;173:1186–1193.
38 Manukhina EB, Downey HF, Mallet RT: Role of nitric oxide in cardiovascular adaptation to intermittent hypoxia. Exp Biol Med (Maywood) 2006;231:343–365.
39 Gozal D, Kheirandish-Gozal L: Cardiovascular morbidity in obstructive sleep apnea: oxidative stress, inflammation, and much more. Am J Respir Crit Care Med 2008;177:369–375.
40 Thum T, Fraccarollo D, Thum S, Schultheiss M, Daiber A, Wenzel P, Munzel T, Ertl G, Bauersachs J: Differential effects of organic nitrates on endothelial progenitor cells are determined by oxidative stress. Arterioscler Thromb Vasc Biol 2007;27:748–754.
41 Dyugovskaya L, Lavie P, Lavie L: Increased adhesion molecules expression and production of reactive oxygen species in leukocytes of sleep apnea patients. Am J Respir Crit Care Med 2002;165:934–939.
42 Schulz R, Mahmoudi S, Hattar K, Sibelius U, Olschewski H, Mayer K, Seeger W, Grimminger F: Enhanced release of superoxide from polymorphonuclear neutrophils in obstructive sleep apnea: impact of continuous positive airway pressure therapy. Am J Respir Crit Care Med 2000;162:566–570.
43 Lavie L: Obstructive sleep apnoea syndrome – an oxidative stress disorder. Sleep Med Rev 2003;7:35–51.
44 Alonso-Fernandez A, Garcia-Rio F, Arias MA, Hernanz A, de la Pena M, Pierola J, Barcelo A, Lopez-Collazo E, Agusti A: Effects of CPAP on oxidative stress and nitrate efficiency in sleep apnoea: a randomised trial. Thorax 2009;64:581–586.

45 Minoguchi K, Yokoe T, Tanaka A, Ohta S, Hirano T, Yoshino G, O'Donnell CP, Adachi M: Association between lipid peroxidation and inflammation in obstructive sleep apnoea. Eur Respir J 2006;28: 378–385.
46 Carpagnano GE, Kharitonov SA, Resta O, Foschino-Barbaro MP, Gramiccioni E, Barnes PJ: Increased 8-isoprostane and interleukin-6 in breath condensate of obstructive sleep apnea patients. Chest 2002; 122:1162–1167.
47 Carpagnano GE, Kharitonov SA, Resta O, Foschino-Barbaro MP, Gramiccioni E, Barnes PJ: 8-Isoprostane, a marker of oxidative stress, is increased in exhaled breath condensate of patients with obstructive sleep apnea after night and is reduced by continuous positive airway pressure therapy. Chest 2003;124:1386–1392.
48 Barcelo A, Miralles C, Barbe F, Vila M, Pons S, Agusti AG: Abnormal lipid peroxidation in patients with sleep apnoea. Eur Respir J 2000;16:644–647.
49 Lavie L, Vishnevsky A, Lavie P: Evidence for lipid peroxidation in obstructive sleep apnea. Sleep 2004; 27:123–128.
50 Kizawa T, Nakamura Y, Takahashi S, Sakurai S, Yamauchi K, Inoue H: Pathogenic role of angiotensin II and oxidised LDL in obstructive sleep apnoea. Eur Respir J 2009;34:1390–1398.
51 Jurado-Gamez B, Fernandez-Marin MC, Gomez-Chaparro JL, Munoz-Cabrera L, Lopez-Barea J, Perez-Jimenez F, Lopez-Miranda J: Relationship of oxidative stress and endothelial dysfunction in sleep apnoea. Eur Respir J 2011;37:873–879.
52 Jelic S, Padeletti M, Kawut SM, Higgins C, Canfield SM, Onat D, Colombo PC, Basner RC, Factor P, Le Jemtel TH: Inflammation, oxidative stress, and repair capacity of the vascular endothelium in obstructive sleep apnea. Circulation 2008;117: 2270–2278.
53 Patt BT, Jarjoura D, Haddad DN, Sen CK, Roy S, Flavahan NA, Khayat RN: Endothelial dysfunction in the microcirculation of patients with obstructive sleep apnea. Am J Respir Crit Care Med 2010;182: 1540–1545.
54 Yamauchi M, Nakano H, Maekawa J, Okamoto Y, Ohnishi Y, Suzuki T, Kimura H: Oxidative stress in obstructive sleep apnea. Chest 2005;127:1674–1679.
55 Sahebjani H: Changes in urinary uric acid excretion in obstructive sleep apnea before and after therapy with nasal continuous positive airway pressure. Chest 1998;113:1604–1608.
56 Lavie L, Perelman A, Lavie P: Plasma homocysteine levels in obstructive sleep apnea: association with cardiovascular morbidity. Chest 2001;120:900–908.
57 Can M, Acikgoz S, Mungan G, Bayraktaroglu T, Kocak E, Guven B, Demirtas S: Serum cardiovascular risk factors in obstructive sleep apnea. Chest 2006;129:233–237.
58 Jordan W, Berger C, Cohrs S, Rodenbeck A, Mayer G, Niedmann PD, von Ahsen N, Ruther E, Kornhuber J, Bleich S: CPAP-therapy effectively lowers serum homocysteine in obstructive sleep apnea syndrome. J Neural Transm 2004;111: 683–689.
59 Christou K, Moulas AN, Pastaka C, Gourgoulianis KI: Antioxidant capacity in obstructive sleep apnea patients. Sleep Med 2003;4:225–228.
60 Barcelo A, Barbe F, de la Pena M, Vila M, Perez G, Pierola J, Duran J, Agusti AG: Antioxidant status in patients with sleep apnoea and impact of continuous positive airway pressure treatment. Eur Respir J 2006;27:756–760.
61 Faure P, Tamisier R, Baguet JP, Favier A, Halimi S, Levy P, Pepin JL: Impairment of serum albumin antioxidant properties in obstructive sleep apnoea syndrome. Eur Respir J 2008;31:1046–1053.
62 Grebe M, Eisele HJ, Weissmann N, Schaefer C, Tillmanns H, Seeger W, Schulz R: Antioxidant vitamin C improves endothelial function in obstructive sleep apnea. Am J Respir Crit Care Med 2006;173: 897–901.
63 El Solh AA, Saliba R, Bosinski T, Grant BJ, Berbary E, Miller N: Allopurinol improves endothelial function in sleep apnoea: a randomised controlled study. Eur Respir J 2006;27:997–1002.
64 Svatikova A, Wolk R, Lerman LO, Juncos LA, Greene EL, McConnell JP, Somers VK: Oxidative stress in obstructive sleep apnoea. Eur Heart J 2005; 26:2435–2439.
65 Alzoghaibi MA, Bahammam AS: Lipid peroxides, superoxide dismutase and circulating IL-8 and GCP-2 in patients with severe obstructive sleep apnea: a pilot study. Sleep Breath 2005;9:119–126.
66 Svatikova A, Wolk R, Wang HH, Otto ME, Bybee KA, Singh RJ, Somers VK: Circulating free nitrotyrosine in obstructive sleep apnea. Am J Physiol Regul Integr Comp Physiol 2004;287:R284–R287.
67 Svatikova A, Wolk R, Magera MJ, Shamsuzzaman AS, Phillips BG, Somers VK: Plasma homocysteine in obstructive sleep apnoea. Eur Heart J 2004;25: 1325–1329.
68 Ryan S, Nolan GM, Hannigan E, Cunningham S, Taylor C, McNicholas WT: Cardiovascular risk markers in obstructive sleep apnoea syndrome and correlation with obesity. Thorax 2007;62:509–514.
69 Mullington JM, Haack M, Toth M, Serrador JM, Meier-Ewert HK: Cardiovascular, inflammatory, and metabolic consequences of sleep deprivation. Prog Cardiovasc Dis 2009;51:294–302.

70 Van Leeuwen WM, Lehto M, Karisola P, Lindholm H, Luukkonen R, Sallinen M, Harma M, Porkka-Heiskanen T, Alenius H: Sleep restriction increases the risk of developing cardiovascular diseases by augmenting proinflammatory responses through IL-17 and CRP. PLoS One 2009;4:e4589.
71 Sauvet F, Leftheriotis G, Gomez-Merino D, Langrume C, Drogou C, Van Beers P, Bourrilhon C, Florence G, Chennaoui M: Effect of acute sleep deprivation on vascular function in healthy subjects. J Appl Physiol 2010;108:68–75.
72 Meier-Ewert HK, Ridker PM, Rifai N, Regan MM, Price NJ, Dinges DF, Mullington JM: Effect of sleep loss on C-reactive protein, an inflammatory marker of cardiovascular risk. J Am Coll Cardiol 2004;43:678–683.
73 Taheri S, Austin D, Lin L, Nieto FJ, Young T, Mignot E: Correlates of serum C-reactive protein (CRP) – no association with sleep duration or sleep disordered breathing. Sleep 2007;30:991–996.
74 Croce K, Libby P: Intertwining of thrombosis and inflammation in atherosclerosis. Curr Opin Hematol 2007;14:55–61.
75 Von Kanel R, Loredo JS, Ancoli-Israel S, Mills PJ, Dimsdale JE: Elevated plasminogen activator inhibitor 1 in sleep apnea and its relation to the metabolic syndrome: an investigation in 2 different study samples. Metabolism 2007;56:969–976.
76 Zamarron C, Ricoy J, Riveiro A, Gude F: Plasminogen activator inhibitor-1 in obstructive sleep apnea patients with and without hypertension. Lung 2008;186:151–156.
77 Von Kanel R, Loredo JS, Ancoli-Israel S, Dimsdale JE: Association between sleep apnea severity and blood coagulability: treatment effects of nasal continuous positive airway pressure. Sleep Breath 2006;10:139–146.
78 Rangemark C, Hedner JA, Carlson JT, Gleerup G, Winther K: Platelet function and fibrinolytic activity in hypertensive and normotensive sleep apnea patients. Sleep 1995;18:188–194.
79 Mehra R, Xu F, Babineau DC, Tracy RP, Jenny NS, Patel SR, Redline S: Sleep-disordered breathing and prothrombotic biomarkers: cross-sectional results of the Cleveland Family Study. Am J Respir Crit Care Med 2010;182:826–833.
80 Saletu M, Nosiska D, Kapfhammer G, Lalouschek W, Saletu B, Benesch T, Zeitlhofer J: Structural and serum surrogate markers of cerebrovascular disease in obstructive sleep apnea (OSA): association of mild OSA with early atherosclerosis. J Neurol 2006;253:746–752.
81 Steiner S, Jax T, Evers S, Hennersdorf M, Schwalen A, Strauer BE: Altered blood rheology in obstructive sleep apnea as a mediator of cardiovascular risk. Cardiology 2005;104:92–96.
82 Chin K, Ohi M, Kita H, Noguchi T, Otsuka N, Tsuboi T, Mishima M, Kuno K: Effects of NCPAP therapy on fibrinogen levels in obstructive sleep apnea syndrome. Am J Respir Crit Care Med 1996;153:1972–1976.
83 Robinson GV, Pepperell JC, Segal HC, Davies RJ, Stradling JR: Circulating cardiovascular risk factors in obstructive sleep apnoea: data from randomised controlled trials. Thorax 2004;59:777–782.
84 Akinnusi ME, Paasch LL, Szarpa KR, Wallace PK, El Solh AA: Impact of nasal continuous positive airway pressure therapy on markers of platelet activation in patients with obstructive sleep apnea. Respiration 2009;77:25–31.
85 Oga T, Chin K, Tabuchi A, Kawato M, Morimoto T, Takahashi K, Handa T, Taniguchi R, Kondo H, Mishima M, Kita T, Horiuchi H: Effects of obstructive sleep apnea with intermittent hypoxia on platelet aggregability. J Atheroscler Thromb 2009;16:862–869.
86 O'Brien LM, Serpero LD, Tauman R, Gozal D: Plasma adhesion molecules in children with sleep-disordered breathing. Chest 2006;129:947–953.
87 Chin K, Kita H, Noguchi T, Otsuka N, Tsuboi T, Nakamura T, Shimizu K, Mishima M, Ohi M: Improvement of factor VII clotting activity following long-term NCPAP treatment in obstructive sleep apnoea syndrome. Q J Med 1998;91:627–633.
88 Shitrit D, Peled N, Shitrit AB, Meidan S, Bendayan D, Sahar G, Kramer MR: An association between oxygen desaturation and D-dimer in patients with obstructive sleep apnea syndrome. Thromb Haemost 2005;94:544–547.
89 Von Kanel R, Loredo JS, Ancoli-Israel S, Mills PJ, Natarajan L, Dimsdale JE: Association between polysomnographic measures of disrupted sleep and prothrombotic factors. Chest 2007;131:733–739.
90 Von Kanel R, Natarajan L, Ancoli-Israel S, Mills PJ, Loredo JS, Dimsdale JE: Day/night rhythm of hemostatic factors in obstructive sleep apnea. Sleep 2010;33:371–377.
91 Quan SF, Gersh BJ: Cardiovascular consequences of sleep-disordered breathing: past, present and future: report of a workshop from the National Center on Sleep Disorders Research and the National Heart, Lung, and Blood Institute. Circulation 2004;109:951–957.
92 Mausbach BT, Ancoli-Israel S, von Kanel R, Patterson TL, Aschbacher K, Mills PJ, Ziegler MG, Dimsdale JE, Calleran S, Grant I: Sleep disturbance, norepinephrine, and D-dimer are all related in elderly caregivers of people with Alzheimer disease. Sleep 2006;29:1347–1352.

93 Von Kanel R, Dimsdale JE, Ancoli-Israel S, Mills PJ, Patterson TL, McKibbin CL, Archuleta C, Grant I: Poor sleep is associated with higher plasma proinflammatory cytokine interleukin-6 and procoagulant marker fibrin D-dimer in older caregivers of people with Alzheimer's disease. J Am Geriatr Soc 2006;54:431–437.
94 Gonzalez-Periz A, Claria J: Resolution of adipose tissue inflammation. Sci World J 2010;10:832–856.
95 Stanke-Labesque F, Back M, Lefebvre B, Tamisier R, Baguet JP, Arnol N, Levy P, Pepin JL: Increased urinary leukotriene E_4 excretion in obstructive sleep apnea: effects of obesity and hypoxia. J Allergy Clin Immunol 2009;124:364–370.
96 Dyugovskaya L, Lavie P, Lavie L: Phenotypic and functional characterization of blood gammadelta T cells in sleep apnea. Am J Respir Crit Care Med 2003;168:242–249.
97 Dyugovskaya L, Lavie P, Hirsh M, Lavie L: Activated CD8+ T-lymphocytes in obstructive sleep apnoea. Eur Respir J 2005;25:820–828.
98 Riccioni G, Back M, Capra V: Leukotrienes and atherosclerosis. Curr Drug Targets 2010;11:882–887.
99 Goldbart AD, Goldman JL, Li RC, Brittian KR, Tauman R, Gozal D: Differential expression of cysteinyl leukotriene receptors 1 and 2 in tonsils of children with obstructive sleep apnea syndrome or recurrent infection. Chest 2004;126:13–18.
100 Goldbart AD, Goldman JL, Veling MC, Gozal D: Leukotriene modifier therapy for mild sleep-disordered breathing in children. Am J Respir Crit Care Med 2005;172:364–370.
101 Goldbart AD, Krishna J, Li RC, Serpero LD, Gozal D: Inflammatory mediators in exhaled breath condensate of children with obstructive sleep apnea syndrome. Chest 2006;130:143–148.
102 Kheirandish L, Goldbart AD, Gozal D: Intranasal steroids and oral leukotriene modifier therapy in residual sleep-disordered breathing after tonsillectomy and adenoidectomy in children. Pediatrics 2006;117:e61–e66.
103 Berlucchi M, Salsi D, Valetti L, Parrinello G, Nicolai P: The role of mometasone furoate aqueous nasal spray in the treatment of adenoidal hypertrophy in the pediatric age group: preliminary results of a prospective, randomized study. Pediatrics 2007;119: e1392–e1397.
104 Kaditis AG, Ioannou MG, Chaidas K, Alexopoulos EI, Apostolidou M, Apostolidis T, Koukoulis G, Gourgoulianis K: Cysteinyl leukotriene receptors are expressed by tonsillar T cells of children with obstructive sleep apnea. Chest 2008;134:324–331.
105 Kaditis AG, Alexopoulos E, Chaidas K, Ntamagka G, Karathanasi A, Tsilioni I, Kiropoulos TS, Zintzaras E, Gourgoulianis K: Urine concentrations of cysteinyl leukotrienes in children with obstructive sleep-disordered breathing. Chest 2009;135: 1496–1501.
106 Lefebvre B, Pepin JL, Baguet JP, Tamisier R, Roustit M, Riedweg K, Bessard G, Levy P, Stanke-Labesque F: Leukotriene B_4: early mediator of atherosclerosis in obstructive sleep apnoea? Eur Respir J 2008;32: 113–120.
107 Petrosyan M, Perraki E, Simoes D, Koutsourelakis I, Vagiakis E, Roussos C, Gratziou C: Exhaled breath markers in patients with obstructive sleep apnoea. Sleep Breath 2008;12:207–215.
108 Blake GJ, Ridker PM: C-reactive protein and other inflammatory risk markers in acute coronary syndromes. J Am Coll Cardiol 2003;41:37S–42S.
109 Danesh J, Wheeler JG, Hirschfield GM, Eda S, Eiriksdottir G, Rumley A, Lowe GD, Pepys MB, Gudnason V: C-reactive protein and other circulating markers of inflammation in the prediction of coronary heart disease. N Engl J Med 2004;350: 1387–1397.
110 Khera A, de Lemos JA, Peshock RM, Lo HS, Stanek HG, Murphy SA, Wians FH Jr, Grundy SM, McGuire DK: Relationship between C-reactive protein and subclinical atherosclerosis: the Dallas Heart Study. Circulation 2006;113:38–43.
111 Lui MM, Lam JC, Mak HK, Xu A, Ooi C, Lam DC, Mak JC, Khong PL, Ip MS: C-reactive protein is associated with obstructive sleep apnea independent of visceral obesity. Chest 2009;135:950–956.
112 Akashiba T, Akahoshi T, Kawahara S, Majima T, Horie T: Effects of long-term nasal continuous positive airway pressure on C-reactive protein in patients with obstructive sleep apnea syndrome. Intern Med 2005;44:899–900.
113 Sharma SK, Mishra HK, Sharma H, Goel A, Sreenivas V, Gulati V, Tahir M: Obesity, and not obstructive sleep apnea, is responsible for increased serum hs-CRP levels in patients with sleep-disordered breathing in Delhi. Sleep Med 2008;9: 149–156.
114 Phillips CL, Yang Q, Williams A, Roth M, Yee BJ, Hedner JA, Berend N, Grunstein RR: The effect of short-term withdrawal from continuous positive airway pressure therapy on sympathetic activity and markers of vascular inflammation in subjects with obstructive sleep apnoea. J Sleep Res 2007;16: 217–225.
115 Atkeson A, Yeh SY, Malhotra A, Jelic S: Endothelial function in obstructive sleep apnea. Prog Cardiovasc Dis 2009;51:351–362.

116 Kohler M, Ayers L, Pepperell JC, Packwood KL, Ferry B, Crosthwaite N, Craig S, Siccoli MM, Davies RJ, Stradling JR: Effects of continuous positive airway pressure on systemic inflammation in patients with moderate to severe obstructive sleep apnoea: a randomised controlled trial. Thorax 2009;64:67–73.
117 Bradley TD, Floras JS: Obstructive sleep apnoea and its cardiovascular consequences. Lancet 2009;373: 82–93.
118 Dematteis M, Godin-Ribuot D, Arnaud C, Ribuot C, Stanke-Labesque F, Pepin JL, Levy P: Cardiovascular consequences of sleep-disordered breathing: contribution of animal models to understanding the human disease. ILAR J 2009;50: 262–281.
119 Jun J, Polotsky VY: Metabolic consequences of sleep-disordered breathing. ILAR J 2009;50: 289–306.
120 Kanagy NL: Vascular effects of intermittent hypoxia. ILAR J 2009;50:282–288.
121 Ayers L, Ferry B, Craig S, Nicoll D, Stradling JR, Kohler M: Circulating cell-derived microparticles in patients with minimally symptomatic obstructive sleep apnoea. Eur Respir J 2009;33:574–580.

Metabolic Disorders Associated with Obstructive Sleep Apnea in Adults

3

Chapter 3

Metabolic Disorders Associated with Obstructive Sleep Apnea in Adults

Abstract

The relationship between metabolic disorders and obstructive sleep apnea (OSA) is multidirectional. Obesity is recognized as the strongest risk factor for OSA. It is unknown whether metabolic syndrome and insulin resistance/type 2 diabetes mellitus contribute to the development or aggravation of OSA, although this is likely. Conversely, OSA may be a risk factor for metabolic disorders. Strong evidence suggests that OSA may increase the risk of developing insulin resistance, glucose intolerance and type 2 diabetes mellitus. OSA has also been associated with the development and/or aggravation of obesity, dyslipidemia, metabolic syndrome and nonalcoholic fatty liver disease – a liver manifestation of metabolic syndrome. In addition, metabolic disorders are confounding factors in OSA. Metabolic disorders and OSA share common intermediate pathogenic pathways, including alterations in autonomic nervous system regulation, increased inflammatory activity, and alterations in adipokine levels and endothelial dysfunction, which may be involved in the interplay between these conditions. Overall, this complexity makes it especially difficult to reveal and understand the links between OSA and metabolic and cardiovascular disorders. The International Diabetes Federation has recently published clinical practice recommendations suggesting that OSA patients should be routinely screened for markers of metabolic disturbance and cardiovascular risk, such as waist circumference, blood pressure, and fasting lipid and glucose levels. It also recommends that the possibility of OSA should be considered in the assessment of all patients with type 2 diabetes mellitus and metabolic syndrome.

1 Obesity and Obstructive Sleep Apnea

Obesity is known to be a cause of obstructive sleep apnea (OSA). It is also a confounding factor in the disease; in addition, obesity is likely to be a consequence of OSA. This complexity makes it especially difficult to interpret the relationship between the two conditions and between OSA and other cardiovascular and metabolic disorders. Extensive reviews devoted to this topic have recently been published [1–6].

1.1 Obesity Is the Major Risk Factor for Obstructive Sleep Apnea

1.1.1 Definition of Obesity

Obesity is defined as 'abnormal or excessive fat accumulation that may impair health' [7, 8]. The body mass index (BMI) is a simple index of weight to height that is commonly used to classify overweight and obesity in adult populations and individuals

Table 1. The international classification of adult underweight, overweight and obesity according to the BMI

Classification	BMI principal cutoff points
Underweight	<18.50
Severe thinness	<16.00
Moderate thinness	16.00–16.99
Mild thinness	17.00–18.49
Normal range	18.50–24.99
Overweight	≥25.00
Pre-obese	25.00–29.99
Obese	≥30.00
Obese class I	30.00–34.99
Obese class II	35.00–39.99
Obese class III	≥40.00

There has been a growing debate on whether there is a need to develop different BMI cutoff points for different ethnic groups, due to increasing evidence that the associations between BMI, percentage of body fat and body fat distribution differ between populations. It has been suggested that health risks could increase below the cutoff point of 25 that defines overweight in the current WHO classification system. The WHO Expert Consultation has recommended that countries should use all principal and secondary cutoff points for reporting purposes, in order to facilitate international comparisons [349]. WHO = World Health Organization. Adapted from the WHO [7], with permission.

(table 1) [7], and is defined as the weight in kilograms divided by the square of the height in meters. BMI classification is the same for both sexes and for all ages of adults; however, it should only be considered as a rough guide because it may not correspond to the same degree of fatness in different individuals [7].

Obesity is a worldwide epidemic affecting approximately 6% of the population [7–9]. By 2015, the World Health Organization (WHO) predicts that approximately 10% of the global population will be obese. A mailed questionnaire survey in France, which was performed in 1997, 2000, 2003 and 2006, sampled 20,000 representative French households by the method of quotas (the Obepi study) and showed that the prevalence of adult obesity increased progressively from 8.6% (95% confidence interval, CI, 8.2–8.8) in 1997 to 13.1% (12.7–13.5) in 2006 [10]. This increase was detected in all ages, socioeconomic strata and regions. Although the prevalence of obesity increased in parallel in men and women from 1997 to 2003, the rate of increase was lower in men between 2003 and 2006. In the USA, data from the National Health and Nutrition Examination Survey, a nationally representative sample of the US population, revealed that the prevalence of overweight or obese adults (age >20 years) was 66.6%, and the prevalence of obese adults was 32.2% in 2003–2004 [11]. In 2007–2008, these figures were 68 and 33.8%, respectively [12]. Over a 10-year period (1999–2008), obesity showed no significant trend among women, whereas there was

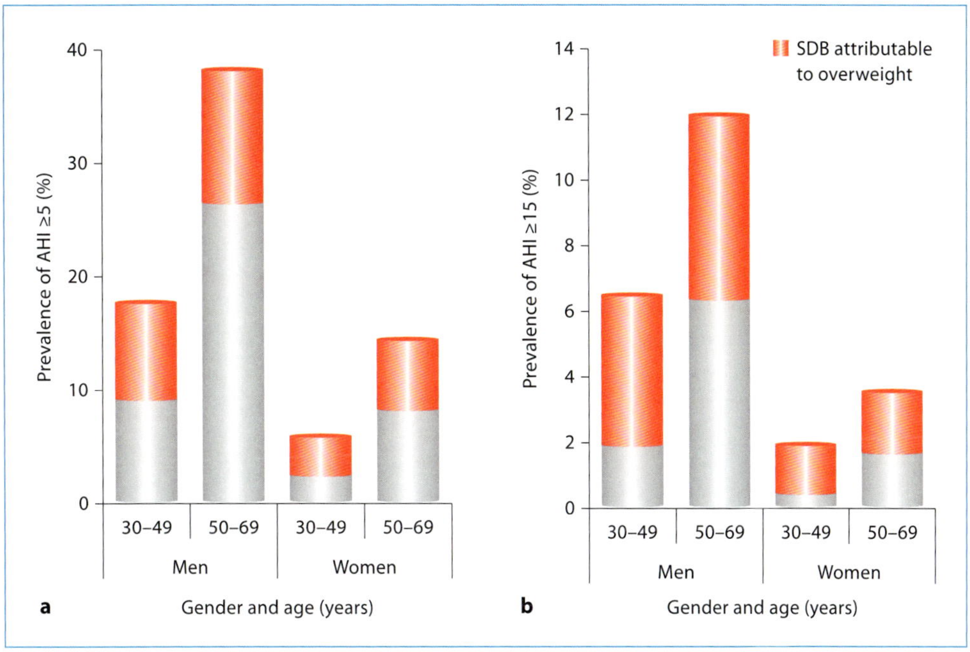

Fig. 1. Estimated prevalence of mild or worse (AHI ≥5; **a**) and moderate or worse sleep-disordered breathing (SDB; AHI ≥15; **b**) and the prevalence of SDB attributable to excess weight (BMI ≥25) by sex and age. After Young et al. [18], with permission.

a significant linear trend in men (the 3 most recent data points, however, did not differ significantly from each other) [12]. This suggests that the previously observed increase in the prevalence of obesity does not appear to have proceeded at the same rate over the past 10 years, particularly for women and possibly for men.

1.1.2 Clinical and Population Studies of the Relationship between Obesity and the Risk for Obstructive Sleep Apnea

The prevalence of OSA is highly associated with overweight and obesity in cross-sectional clinic-based studies and population-based studies [3, 4, 13–17]. The prevalence of obesity in OSA patients is 50–70%, while the prevalence of OSA in obese subjects is approximately 40%, and it can be up to 90% in severely obese subjects [3, 4]. In a random sample of middle-aged state employees taken from the Wisconsin Sleep Cohort Study, an increase of 1 standard deviation (SD) in weight or BMI was associated with a 2- or 4-fold increased risk of prevalent sleep apnea, respectively [13]. When the data from this study were reanalyzed, about 17% of adults aged from 30 to 69 years had mild or worse OSA (apnea-hypopnea index, AHI ≥5 events • h^{-1}); of these adults, 41% had OSA attributable to a BMI ≥25 [18]. In addition, approximately 5.7% of adults in the same age bracket had moderate or worse OSA (AHI ≥15), and 58% of these adults had OSA attributable to excess weight (fig. 1). From these

Table 2. Conditional logistic regression coefficients and odds ratios for the development of moderate-to-severe OSA for selected categories of weight gain

Percent gain in weight (versus no gain)	Regression coefficient	Estimated odds ratio for moderate-to-severe OSA	95% CI
5	0.9 (0.3)	2.5	1.5–4.1*
10	1.8 (0.5)	6.0	2.2–17.0*
20	3.6 (1.1)	36.6	4.6 to >50*

Moderate-to-severe OSA = AHI ≥15. Odds ratio adjusted for the change in the number of cigarette packs • $week^{-1}$. Standard errors given in parentheses. * $p < 0.001$ for all. After Peppard et al. [15], with permission.

data, it was predicted that the prevalence of OSA would almost certainly increase, along with the proportion of OSA attributable to obesity, if the expanding epidemic of obesity currently observed in the USA continues.

1.1.3 Impact of Treatment for Obesity on Obstructive Sleep Apnea Severity

Population studies of weight gain or loss support the causal association between excess weight and OSA [18, 19]. Weight gain increases the risk of developing OSA and aggravates existing OSA [15, 19]. A population-based longitudinal study showed that after adjusting for sex, age and cigarette smoking, for each 1% decrease or increase in body weight, an approximately 3% decrease or increase in the AHI is expected, respectively (table 2) [15, 20]. Weight loss is an effective means of reducing OSA severity in overweight patients [19–25].

Prospective, randomized controlled trials have confirmed the efficacy of weight reduction in reducing OSA severity, not only in mild but also in moderate-to-severe OSA [23–25]. In a comparison of the effects of a very low calorie diet with supervised lifestyle counseling versus routine lifestyle counseling in a randomized, controlled parallel-group study with a 1-year follow-up of patients with mild OSA (BMI 28–40), lifestyle intervention was associated with a greater reduction in BMI (mean ± SD –3.5 ± 2.1 vs. –0.8 ± 2.0, respectively) and a higher proportion of objectively cured patients (n = 35) compared with the control group (n = 37, AHI <5; 63 vs. 35%, p = 0.033) [25]. These authors also reported that these changes were sustained at 2 years after the termination of supervised lifestyle counseling (during the 2nd year, no dietary counseling was offered) [26]. The reduction in the AHI was significantly greater in the intervention group (p = 0.049), and the intervention lowered the risk of OSA at the follow-up; the adjusted odds ratio (OR) for OSA was 0.35 (95% CI 0.12–0.97; p = 0.045). A parallel, randomized controlled study was used to assess the impact of a very low energy diet for 7 weeks, followed by a 2-week gradual introduction of normal food in obese men with moderate-to-severe OSA [24]. The control group adhered to their usual diet during the 9 weeks, and both groups had a mean AHI (±SD) of 37 ± 15 at baseline. At week 9, the mean body weight was 20 kg (95% CI 18–21) lower in the intervention group than in the control group, while the mean AHI in the intervention group was 23 events$\cdot h^{-1}$ (95% CI 15–30) lower than in the control group. In the intervention group, 17% of the patients were disease free (AHI <5), with 50% having mild disease (AHI 5–14.9), whereas the AHI of the control group patients, except for 1, remained at 15 or higher. The greatest effect was observed in patients with severe OSA. A 1-year study assessed 264 obese patients with type 2 diabetes (mean BMI ± SD 36.7 ± 5.7) and a mean AHI (±SD) of 23.2 ± 16.5 [23]. The participants were randomly assigned to either a behavioral weight loss program specifically developed for obese patients with type 2 diabetes (intervention group) or to 3 group sessions related to effective diabetes management (control group). At 1 year, more than 3 times as many participants in the intervention group had total remission of their OSA than in the control group. The prevalence of severe OSA in the intervention group was 50% less than that observed in the control group.

Although the results of dietary changes are encouraging for the improvement of OSA, weight loss and the mean reduction in the AHI are greater after bariatric surgery than after dieting [20, 27]. A meta-analysis of the effect of bariatric surgery on OSA demonstrated a critical improvement of OSA in the majority of patients after bariatric surgery [27]. A total of 136 studies were included in this meta-analysis with a total of 22,094 patients: mean age, 39 years (range 16–64 years); 19% were men and 72.6% were women, although sex was not reported for 1,537 patients (8%) [27]. The baseline BMI for 16,944 patients was 46.9 (range 32.3–68.8). The mean percentage of excess weight loss was 61.2% (95% CI 58.1–64.4) for all patients. OSA was resolved in 85.7% of patients and was resolved or improved in 83.6% of patients. Another meta-analysis of 12 studies with 342 patients to identify the effects of surgical weight loss on the AHI demonstrated that the pooled mean BMI was reduced from 55.3 (95% CI 53.5–57.1) to 37.7 (95% CI 36.6–38.9) [28]. The random-effects pooled baseline AHI was also reduced from 54.7 (95% CI 49.0–60.3) to 15.8 (95% CI 12.6–19.0). Thirty-eight percent of patients were cured from OSA (AHI <5), whereas the remaining patients had a mean residual AHI of 16. Overall, these findings suggest that although bariatric surgery significantly reduces the severity of OSA, it does not cure OSA in all patients [27–29].

1.1.4 Gender Differences in Body Mass Index and the Risk for Obstructive Sleep Apnea

OSA is more common in men than in women [30]. In the general population, the male-to-female ratio for OSA prevalence ranges between 2:1 and 4:1 [13, 20, 31]. The predominance of males with OSA may be related to differences in the gender distribution of adipose tissue. Men tend to have a greater degree of visceral obesity, with the main fat deposit located around the abdomen and the upper body, whereas women tend to have the main fat deposit located around the lower body, i.e. around

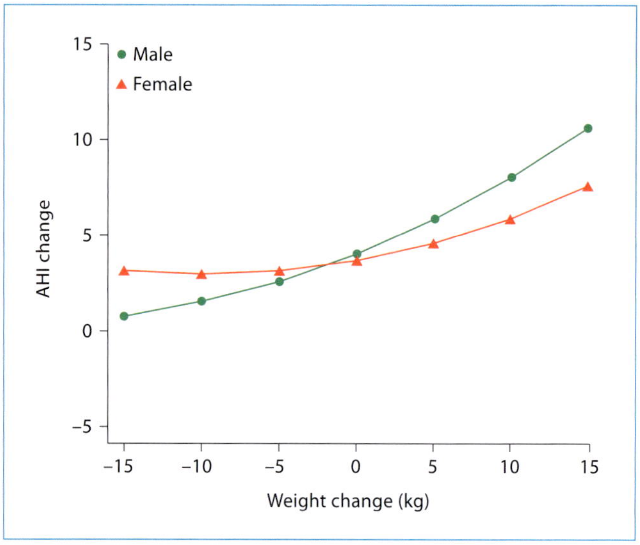

Fig. 2. Change in the AHI by change in weight. After Newman et al. [19], with permission. © 2005 American Medical Association.

the hips and thighs [32]. This gender difference in excess fat deposit location may explain why, for a given degree of upper-body obesity, men have more severe sleep apnea than women.

The effect of weight change on the progression of OSA has been studied in male and female participants in the Sleep Heart Health Study, a longitudinal study of 2,968 men and women (mean age 62 years) assessed 5 years apart [19]. Modest changes in weight were related to an increase or decrease in OSA severity, and this association was stronger in men than in women (fig. 2).

1.2 Visceral Obesity

Visceral obesity (also known as 'central' or 'android' or 'apple shape' obesity) is characterized by the deposition of adipose tissue around the trunk and the accumulation of fat in the abdominal area, including internal fat around the visceral organs (fig. 3). Several studies have used imaging techniques to examine the relationship between intra-abdominal adipose tissue and OSA [33–37]. When the relationship between abdominal visceral fat (measured at the level of the umbilicus using computed tomographic sections) and OSA (AHI >5) was evaluated in obese subjects (n = 37), the visceral adipose tissue area and its ratio to the total adipose tissue area were significantly greater in OSA patients than in non-OSA patients [33]. These 2 parameters were closely correlated with an increase in the apnea index. Computed tomographic scans were used to measure total, subcutaneous and visceral abdominal fat in groups of male obese patients with OSA and in age- and BMI-matched nonapneic controls [34]. OSA patients had a significantly greater amount of visceral fat than the obese controls ($p < 0.05$), and the severity of OSA, assessed using the AHI and minimum

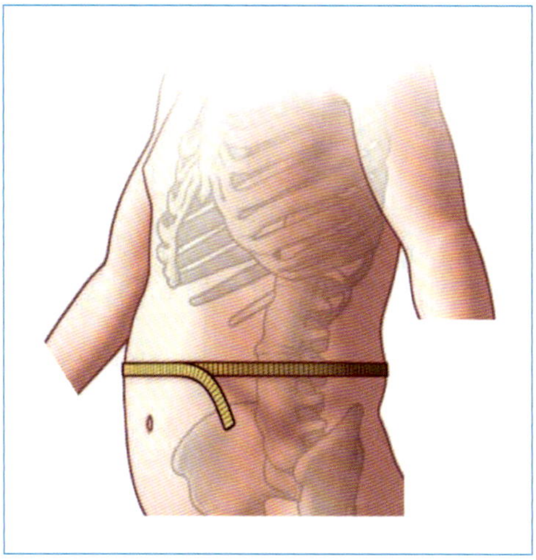

Fig. 3. Measurement of waist circumference. A measuring tape is placed around the trunk, at a point midway between the lower costal margin and the iliac crest, while the patient is standing with his/her feet approximately 25–30 cm apart. The measuring tape is fit snugly around the abdomen, but without compressing the underlying soft tissues. The waist circumference is recorded to the nearest 0.5 cm at the end of a normal expiration. After Douketis et al. [342], with permission.

oxygen saturation (Sao_2), was positively correlated with visceral fat, but not with BMI or total or subcutaneous fat [34]. The same group confirmed these findings in a subsequent study [36]. Similarly, a nuclear magnetic resonance imaging study suggested that AHI is significantly correlated with intra-abdominal fat, but not with subcutaneous fat in the neck region or parapharyngeal fat [35]. These findings suggest that the accumulation of visceral fat is a strong, independent risk indicator for OSA.

1.2.1 Visceral Obesity May Affect the Anatomy of the Upper Airway

Obesity increases adipose tissue deposits in tissues surrounding the pharyngeal airway. This contributes to the enlargement of soft tissues, including the tongue, soft palate, uvula [38, 39], lateral parapharyngeal fat pads [40–42] and the tissues bounded by the mandibular rami [40]. Obesity may also increase the quantity of muscle in the structures surrounding the upper airway; the volume of the surrounding pharyngeal airway structures may in turn be increased, resulting in a reduction in the pharyngeal airway space [38, 43]. This may contribute to: (1) enlargement of the neck circumference [40–43]; (2) reduction in the size of the upper airway (fig. 4); (3) change in the shape of the upper airway (fig. 4) [3, 39, 44–47], and (4) increase in the collapsibility of the upper airway (see below). The increase in neck circumference has been considered a better correlate of apnea severity than the BMI [41, 42].

1.2.2 Obesity and Upper Airway Collapsibility

OSA patients manifest partial or complete upper airway collapse during sleep in the retropalatal and retroglossal regions of the pharynx. Collapsibility may be assessed by measuring the critical closing pressure (P_{crit}), the concept of which arises from modeling the oropharynx as a simple collapsible tube (fig. 5) [48, 49]. The higher the P_{crit},

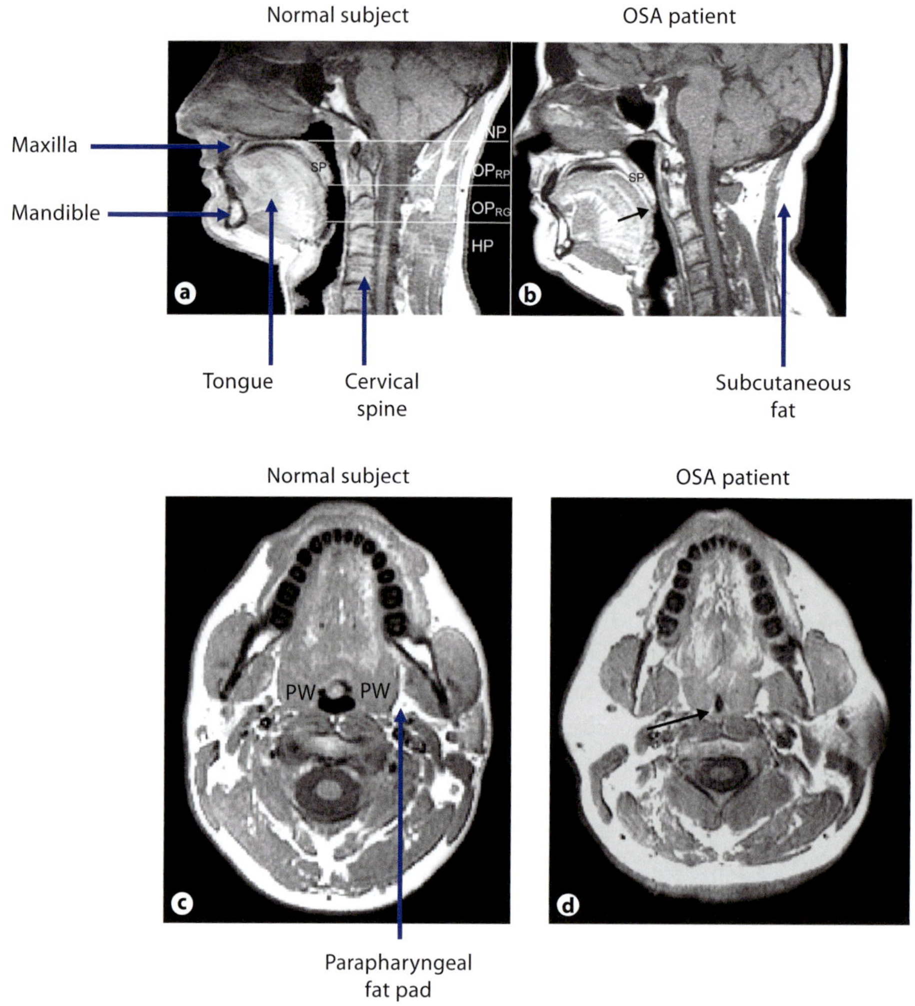

Fig. 4. Pharyngeal geometry in OSA patients and in normal subjects. **a**, **b** Midsagittal magnetic resonance images of the head of a normal subject (**a**) and an OSA patient (**b**). The airway is shown in black. **a** Note the 4 main anatomical regions of the upper airway: the nasopharynx (NP), the oropharynx adjacent to the retropalatal region (OP_{RP}), an oropharyngeal segment that is retroglossal (OP_{RG}) and the hypopharynx (HP). SP = Soft palate. **b** The airway narrowing is maximal at the low retropalatal and retroglossal regions (arrow). After Arens and Marcus [343], with permission. **c**, **d** Axial magnetic resonance images of the head at the retropalatal level of a normal subject (**c**) and a patient with OSA (**d**). The airway is shown in black. **c** The lateral pharyngeal wall (PW) is formed by soft tissues, including muscle and adipose tissue. **d** The pharyngeal narrowing is such that the anterior-posterior axis is longer than the lateral-lateral axis (arrow). After Arens and Marcus [343], with permission.

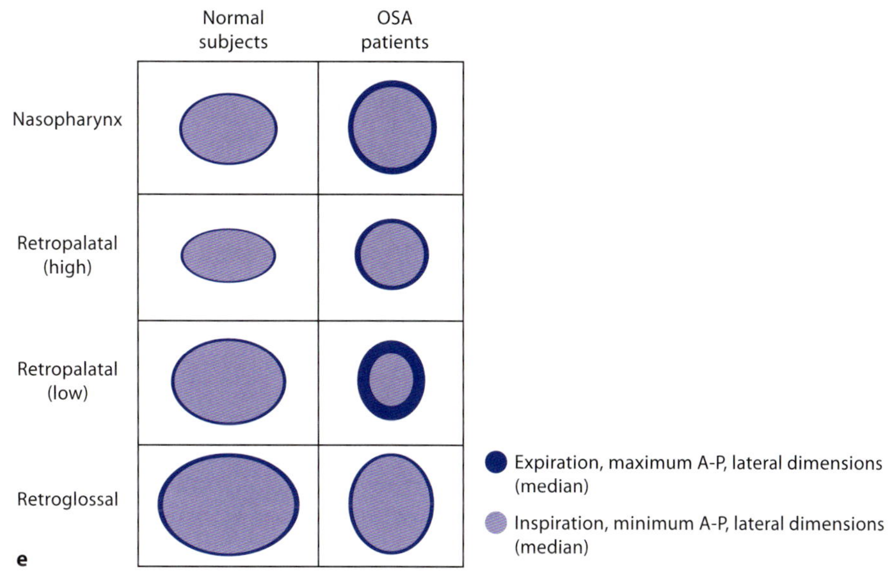

Fig. 4. e Schematic diagram of the respiratory changes in airway geometry using anterior-posterior (A-P) and lateral dimensions in normal subjects and OSA patients. Airway dimensions were measured with cine-computed tomography in 15 normal subjects and in 13 OSA patients in the supine position during wakeful nasal breathing. Axial slices were obtained at 4 anatomical levels (from the nasopharynx to the retroglossal region) during a respiratory cycle. The airway is drawn using the minimal anterior-posterior and lateral dimensions during inspiration, and the maximal anterior-posterior and lateral dimensions during expiration. The upper airway was significantly smaller in OSA patients than in normal subjects, especially at the lower retropalatal and retroglossal levels. The largest changes occurred in the OSA patients at the lower retropalatal level. The upper airway in OSA patients has an anterior-posterior configuration that differs from the normal airway at all 4 anatomical levels; the normal airway has a horizontal configuration, whereas the OSA airway is narrowed laterally. After Schwab et al. [44]. Reprinted with permission of the American Thoracic Society. © American Thoracic Society.

the more collapsible the airway (for a review, see Schwartz et al. [3, 6]). The increase in the collapsibility of the upper airway may be due to alterations in the mechanical properties of the upper airway and the neuromuscular control of upper airway patency. The collapsibility due to the mechanical properties of the airway and its surrounding tissue, called 'passive P_{crit}', has been measured in conditions where there is no neuromuscular control (e.g. in anesthetized patients [50–53]) or almost no neuromuscular control (e.g. during sleep) [54]. Alterations in upper airway neuromuscular control are assessed by measuring 'active P_{crit}', a composite parameter that represents the sum of 'passive P_{crit}' and the neuromuscular response to passive structural/anatomical loads. Therefore, dynamic neuromuscular responses are characterized by the difference between the active and passive P_{crit} levels [54]. For example, the relative contribution of mechanical loads and the dynamic neuromuscular responses to

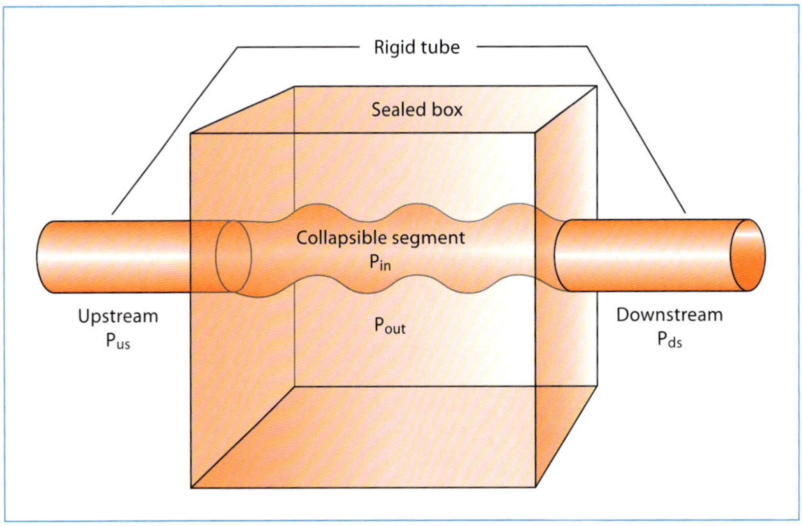

Fig. 5. Starling resistor model of OSA. The collapsible segment of the tube is bound by an upstream and downstream segment with corresponding upstream pressure (P_{us}), downstream pressure (P_{ds}), upstream resistance and downstream resistance. Airway occlusion occurs when the surrounding tissue pressure (P_{out}; from pharyngeal muscles, pharyngeal and submucosal fat, mucosal edema etc.) becomes greater than the intraluminal pressure (P_{in}). In this model of the upper airway, P_{us} is atmospheric at the airway opening, and P_{ds} is the tracheal pressure. The P_{crit} of the passive airway is defined as the pressure inside the airway (P_{in}) at which the airway collapses. The pressure gradient during airflow through the system is defined by $P_{us} - P_{crit}$ and remains independent of P_{ds}. Therefore, with increasing P_{crit}, as the differential between P_{us} and P_{crit} decreases, inspiratory airflow limitation will eventually develop, and when the P_{crit} is greater than P_{us}, complete airway occlusion occurs. After Dempsey et al. [5], with permission.

pharyngeal collapse during sleep were assessed in OSA patients (n = 16) and in normal subjects (n = 16) matched for age, sex and BMI (for a further description of the experimental procedure, see Patil et al. [54]). OSA patients had higher active and passive P_{crit} levels than normal subjects, suggesting that OSA patients have an increased upper airway mechanical load and a depressed dynamic response to upper airway obstruction compared with normal controls. It was proposed that increased upper airway mechanical load and blunted neuromuscular responses are both required for the development of OSA.

Weight loss has been associated with a decrease in upper airway collapsibility and OSA severity [3, 55]. A 17.4 ± 3.4% (mean ± SD) reduction in BMI in men with OSA was associated with a significant 5.5 cm H_2O decrease in P_{crit} and a significant 61% decrease in the respiratory disturbance index (RDI) during nonrapid eye movement (REM) sleep [55]. In contrast, in the weight-stable control group, no significant change in the disordered breathing rate and only a minimal reduction in P_{crit} were observed; the groups were matched for age, BMI, gender and non-REM disordered breathing rate.

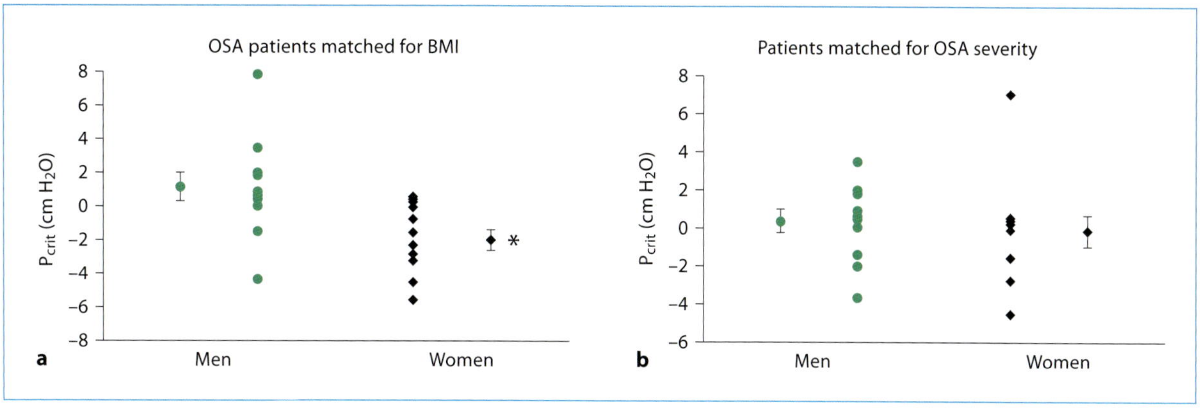

Fig. 6. Upper airway collapsibility in men and women with OSA matched for BMI (**a**) and severity of OSA (**b**). **a** This scatter plot shows the P_{crit} in 12 men and 12 women with OSA who were matched for BMI (within 2 points). Individual and group means (±SE) are presented. P_{crit} was significantly lower in women (–2.01 ± 0.62 cm H_2O) than men (1.16 ± 0.83 cm H_2O; p = 0.005). This shows that BMI-matched women with OSA have a less collapsible airway than BMI-matched men with OSA (the lower the P_{crit}, the less collapsible the upper airway). **b** This scatter plot shows P_{crit} in 11 men and 11 women matched for the severity of OSA. Individual and group means (±SE) are presented. There were no sex-specific significant differences in P_{crit}. After Jordan et al. [57], with permission.

The gender difference in the distribution of adipose tissue may contribute to the gender differences in OSA severity and upper airway collapsibility. For example, in a prospective case series observational sleep clinic study that assessed sex differences in the association between the AHI and measures of obesity in body regions defined using dual-energy absorptiometry and traditional anthropometric measures [56], the percentage of fat in the neck region and the BMI together explained 33% of the variance in the AHI in women, whereas, in men, the percentage of fat in the abdominal region and the neck-to-waist ratio together accounted for 37% of the variance in the AHI. It is suggested that regional obesity is associated with OSA severity, although differently in men and women. In women, a direct influence of neck fat on upper airway patency is implicated, while in men, abdominal obesity appears to be the predominant influence. Analysis of the severity of OSA with airway collapsibility in equally obese men and women indicated that the men had more severe OSA and a more collapsible airway than the women (fig. 6) [57]. Such a significant gender difference in upper airway collapsibility was not observed in men and women with equally severe OSA [57]. It is suggested that women may be protected from developing OSA by having a less collapsible upper airway for any given degree of obesity. A gender difference in the mechanical properties of the upper airway was also observed by measuring passive P_{crit} levels [58]. Passive P_{crit} was 1.9 cm H_2O lower in women than in men with OSA, after matching for BMI, age and disease severity. The magnitude of the change in P_{crit} per 10-point change in BMI was approximately 2-fold greater in men than in women. It is suggested that the mechanics of the upper airway are controlled differently in obese men and women with OSA.

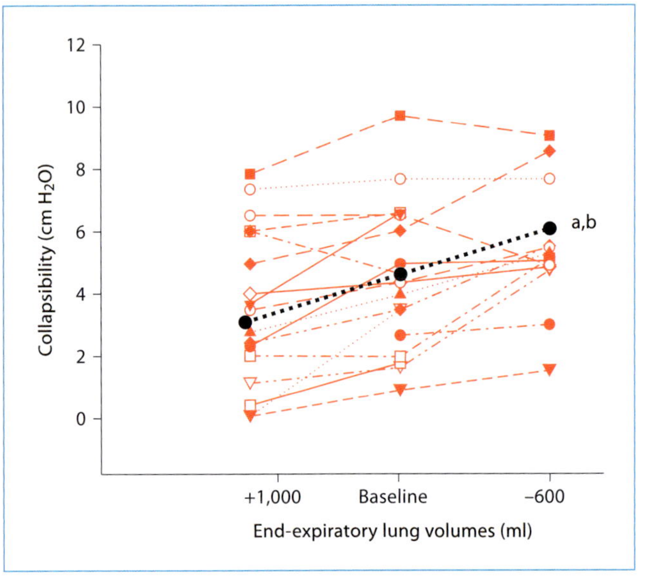

Fig. 7. Individual and group means for pharyngeal collapsibility measured at different end-expiratory lung volumes (EELV) (+1,000 ml: lung volume 1,000 ml above sleeping baseline EELV; –600 ml: lung volume 600 ml below sleeping baseline EELV). Mean values are presented as the largest circles with thick dashed lines. [a] $p < 0.05$ compared with baseline, [b] $p < 0.05$ compared with +1,000 ml EELV. After Stanchina et al. [69], with permission.

1.2.2.1 *Visceral Obesity Reduces Lung Volume and Tracheal Caudal Traction.* Visceral obesity contributes to the reduction of lung volume [59], and this is thought to be related to the loss of tracheal caudal and radial traction. The effects of reduced tracheal traction on the caliber and dynamics of the upper airway have been shown in animal models [60–63]. Inspiratory caudal displacement of the carina is thought to exert forces on the tracheal walls that, in turn, contribute to upper airway patency and stability [6, 60, 61, 64, 65]. Radial traction leads to a decompression of the tissues surrounding the upper airway [6, 64, 65], and its loss may also decrease the patency and collapsibility of the upper airway.

The experimental reduction in lung volume is associated with a decrease in airway caliber and an increase in airway resistance [66–68]. The reverse was observed when lung volume was increased. A reduction in lung volume also increases the collapsibility of the upper airway [69–71], OSA severity and continuous positive airway pressure (CPAP) requirements [72, 73]. For example, the effects of lung volume changes on pharyngeal pressure and collapsibility were assessed in normal individuals (n = 19) during stable non-REM sleep [69]. These experiments were carried out in a rigid head-out shell equipped with a variable positive/negative pressure attachment to manipulate the extrathoracic pressure and, thus, lung volume (the more negative the pressure, the more the volume increases). The change in end-expiratory lung volume and collapsibility of the pharynx in response to a brief pulse of negative pressure (–8 to –15 cm H_2O) was assessed under 3 conditions: baseline, increased end-expiratory lung volume (+1,000 ml) and decreased end-expiratory lung volume (–600 ml). Decreased lung volumes were observed to lead to an increase in upper airway resistance and collapsibility (fig. 7). The overall effect of lung volume on P_{crit} was recently quantified in healthy

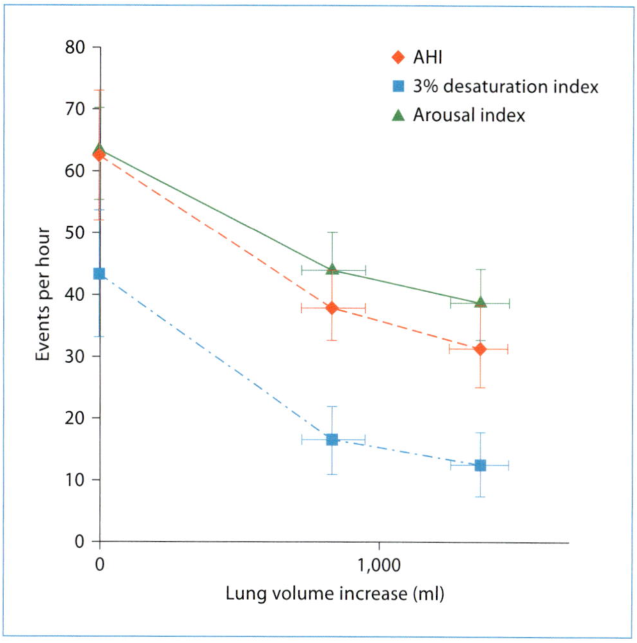

Fig. 8. Mean number (±SE) of respiratory events per hour (AHI), arousals per hour and number of 3% oxygen drops per hour at each lung volume. After Heinzer et al. [73], with permission.

subjects [74]: a 1-liter decrease in end-expiratory lung volume was accompanied by an increase of approximately 2.0 cm H_2O in P_{crit}, accounting for some of the effects of obesity on upper airway collapsibility. A similar device was used to assess the effects of changes in lung volume on sleep-disordered breathing (SDB) during non-REM sleep in OSA patients (n = 12) to determine the increase in lung volume due to CPAP (at a therapeutic level) [72, 73]. CPAP was then stopped and the subjects were studied under 3 conditions: (1) no treatment (baseline); (2) at 'CPAP lung volume', with the increased lung volume being reproduced by negative extrathoracic pressure alone, and (3) at 500 ml above the CPAP lung volume. Significant decreases were observed in the AHI, arousal index and 3% oxygen desaturation index when lung volume was increased (fig. 8) [73]. An increase in lung volume is also associated with a decrease in the CPAP required to prevent flow limitation [72]. Conversely, when the lung volume was reduced, the level of CPAP had to be increased.

Overall, these findings suggest that the reduction in lung volume and tracheal traction associated with visceral obesity may reduce the caliber of the upper airway and increase upper airway resistance and collapsibility. This, in turn, may increase the risk of development or aggravation of OSA and increase CPAP requirements [1, 3, 5, 6].

1.3 Adipose Tissue, an Endocrine Organ

After the discovery of adipokines, adipose tissue is now considered as an energy storage compartment and an endocrine and secretory organ [75, 76]. Adipocytes express and release inflammatory and bioactive substances termed adipokines, which include leptin, adiponectin and cytokines [76–80]. These substances may contribute to systemic and vascular inflammation, alterations in glucose metabolism and liver injury associated with OSA, and lead to the development and/or aggravation of metabolic and cardiovascular disorders associated with this condition. They have also been hypothesized to alter the control of breathing and increase susceptibility to OSA [81].

1.3.1 Leptin

Leptin is a 16-kDa protein secreted from white adipocytes. It is transported to the brain, where it regulates orexigenic and anorexigenic neuropeptides at the hypothalamic level, and to peripheral cellular targets, including adipocytes, skeletal muscle and pancreatic β-cells [82, 83].

1.3.1.1 Metabolic Effects of Leptin. Leptin contributes to the regulation of energy homeostasis [84–86], body adiposity, and acts as a satiety signal [87]. Serum leptin concentrations are significantly higher in obese patients than in normal subjects, and the levels correlate with the percentage of body fat [88]. As a consequence, it has been postulated that the apparent loss of the weight- and appetite-reducing effects of leptin in these subjects may result from leptin resistance [89, 90].

Leptin also contributes to the regulation of insulin secretion and sensitivity and glucose homeostasis. It is also involved in the regulation of the sympathetic nervous system, neuroendocrine functions, and immune and inflammatory responses [84, 86, 91].

1.3.1.2 Proatherogenic Effects of Leptin. Leptin may have direct proatherogenic effects on arterial wall cells [92–95]; however, it is unclear whether plasma leptin levels are independently linked with an increased risk of cardiovascular complications [96–99]. It is also unknown whether the possible proatherogenic effects of leptin contribute to the development of cardiovascular diseases associated with OSA.

1.3.1.3 Leptin and the Control of Breathing. Several studies have suggested that leptin may also be involved in the control of breathing [100–109]. In obese patients without OSA, circulating leptin levels are higher in hypercapnic subjects than in eucapnic subjects [106]. Similar findings have been reported in obese patients with OSA [107]. Noninvasive ventilation is associated with changes in serum leptin levels and the improvement in blood gas levels and CO_2 ventilatory response in obesity hypoventilation syndrome patients with or without OSA [108, 109]. Serum leptin levels were significantly lowered in patients with obesity hypoventilation syndrome treated with noninvasive ventilation administration (n = 9) for a median of 2.3 years, compared with those who did not use noninvasive ventilation (p = 0.001), without a change in the BMI. There was a trend for improved daytime hypercapnia and hypoxemia in the treated patients, while there were no changes in serum leptin, BMI or arterial blood gases in the nonusers [108]. Paradoxically, the opposite result was observed in a smaller number of hypoventilation syndrome patients without OSA (n = 6), i.e. an increase in leptin levels with ventilation [109]. Treatment for 6–20 months with nocturnal noninvasive mechanical ventilation was associated with an improvement

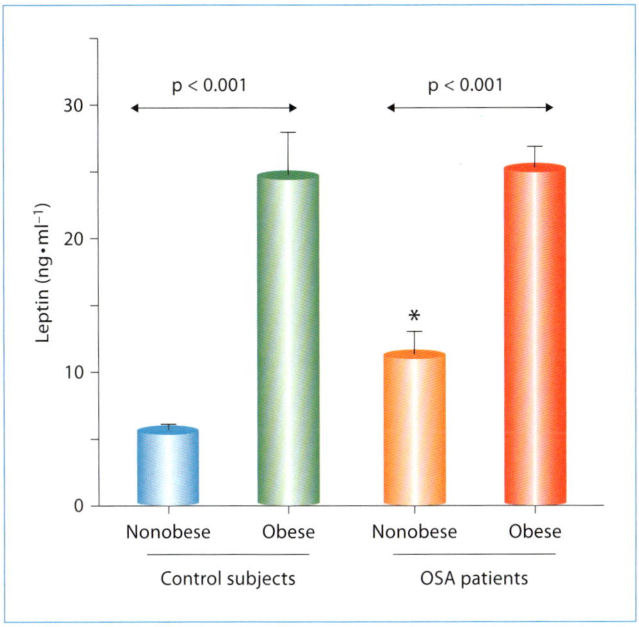

Fig. 9. Plasma leptin levels in 18 nonobese and 19 obese control subjects without OSA and in 24 nonobese and 23 obese patients with OSA: effects of obesity, OSA, and OSA plus obesity on plasma leptin levels. As for effects of obesity, obese control subjects had significantly higher leptin levels than nonobese control subjects ($p < 0.001$). As for effects of OSA, nonobese OSA patients had significantly higher leptin levels than nonobese control subjects (* $p < 0.01$). As for effects of OSA plus obesity, leptin levels were not significantly different between the control and OSA groups. Obesity was defined as having a BMI >30; nonobesity was defined as having a BMI <27. Data are shown as the mean ± SEM. After Barcelò et al. [114]. Reprinted with permission of the American Thoracic Society. © American Thoracic Society.

in blood gas exchange and CO_2 chemosensitivity and, paradoxically, with an increase in leptin levels [109]. Leptin levels correlate with a measure of CO_2 chemosensitivity. In obese subjects, log leptin levels were predictors for baseline $P_{0.1}$ (the mouth occlusion pressure at 0.1 s of inspiration, a measure of the ventilatory drive) and the hypercapnic response in males, but not in females [110]. Hyperleptinemia was associated with a reduction in the respiratory drive and hypercapnic response, irrespective of the amount of body fat [110]. However, in OSA, the increase in leptin levels has been suggested to be a consequence of hypoxemia [105, 110], indicating that it may be a consequence rather than a cause of hypoventilation [110]. It remains to be demonstrated whether leptin has an impact on the control of breathing and upper airway neuromuscular control, thereby increasing the susceptibility to OSA.

1.3.1.4 Leptin and OSA. The relationship between OSA and circulating leptin levels remains unresolved:

- Several studies have reported higher circulating leptin levels in OSA patients than in BMI-matched control subjects [96, 111–113], whereas other authors consider that the higher levels are mostly related to obesity (fig. 9) [114]. The severity of nocturnal hypoxemia has been associated with leptin levels, independently of obesity [115].

- Conversely, other studies have not found a significant association between circulating leptin levels and the AHI [116] after controlling for body fat and/or BMI [35, 117, 118].
- CPAP treatment reduces the circulating levels of leptin in OSA patients (BMI remained unchanged during the study period) [96, 113, 119–121]. A decrease in circulating leptin levels has been reported to occur only in nonobese OSA patients [114] or to be more pronounced in OSA patients with a BMI <30 than in obese OSA patients [122].

1.3.2 Adiponectin

Adiponectin is produced by adipocytes [123], and its biological functions include the improvement of lipid and glucose metabolism by increasing the oxidation of fatty acids and inhibiting glucose synthesis in the liver [124]. Serum adiponectin levels are high in healthy subjects [123] and low in patients with visceral obesity, insulin resistance, type 2 diabetes and cardiovascular diseases [125, 126]. Hypoadiponectinemia is associated with endothelial dysfunction and cardiovascular morbidity [127, 128].

As with leptin, the relationship between adiponectin levels and OSA remains to be clarified. Higher plasma adiponectin levels were observed in otherwise healthy obese male patients with OSA than in obesity-matched subjects without OSA [129]. In contrast, several studies have reported lower adiponectin levels in OSA patients than in control subjects. For example, in obese patients with and without OSA and normal-weight healthy subjects, OSA was associated with reduced levels of adiponectin, independently of insulin resistance and BMI [130]. However, it should be noted that the fasting homeostatic model assessment (HOMA) index is a poor measure of insulin resistance associated with sleep disturbances, i.e. no change in the fasting HOMA index does not mean there is no change in insulin sensitivity as assessed using the hyperinsulinemic-euglycemic clamp or intravenous glucose tolerance tests (see below) [131, 132]. Experimental studies in healthy young adults, in whom sleep duration or quality was manipulated and where insulin sensitivity (determined with the clamp or intravenous glucose tolerance tests) was the primary outcome measure, uniformly showed a decrease in insulin sensitivity, but no corresponding change in the fasting HOMA. Serum adiponectin levels were significantly lower in OSA patients than in simple snorers [133]. In a cohort of men without prevalent cardiovascular disease or diabetes mellitus, circulating adiponectin levels were reduced and correlated with the severity of OSA, independently of age and obesity [134]. Adiponectin levels were independently correlated with insulin resistance (assessed by the HOMA index) and sympathetic activation (measured by urine catecholamine levels) [134]. Reduced adiponectin levels have also been observed in patients with severe OSA and other comorbidities, compared with subjects without OSA [135–137]. Conversely, other reports have detected no significant independent relationship between plasma adiponectin levels and OSA [112, 138–140].

Studies assessing the effects of CPAP administration on adiponectin levels have also produced conflicting data. Several studies have shown reduced adiponectin levels in patients with severe OSA and other comorbidities, compared with subjects without OSA, while other studies have shown that the levels of adiponectin were significantly increased after a single night [136], 1 month [137], 2 months (the mean compliance rate with CPAP administration ± SE was 5.3 ± 1.7 h • night^{-1}) [141] or 3 months [142] of CPAP therapy. In an uncontrolled study, serum adiponectin levels were increased in OSA patients after 14 days of CPAP therapy (patients showed 'good compliance' to CPAP treatment, but the actual compliance rates were not reported) [143]. However, decreased serum adiponectin levels were observed after 2 days of CPAP treatment, followed by a return to baseline levels after 3 months of CPAP treatment (the mean duration of CPAP use per night ± SD was 5.15 ± 0.9 h) [144]. A randomized controlled study revealed no change in adiponectin levels after 3 months of CPAP treatment, compared with sham CPAP treatment, in men with severe OSA (the mean compliance with CPAP administration was <4 h • night^{-1} in both groups) [145]. Similarly, a study on the effect of therapeutic (n = 51) and subtherapeutic (n = 49) CPAP therapy in moderate-to-severe OSA patients on circulating inflammatory markers, including adiponectin (assessed at baseline and after 4 weeks of follow-up) [146], indicated that therapeutic CPAP did not significantly change the adiponectin levels compared with subtherapeutic CPAP therapy (the mean CPAP compliance ± SD was 3.9 ± 2.5 and 4.7 ± 2.1 h • night^{-1} in the subtherapeutic and therapeutic groups, respectively, $p > 0.05$). There is a need to emphasize the issue of compliance with CPAP when interpreting these data. Negative studies, such as that of West et al. [145], involved patients with very low compliance rates (e.g. less than 4 h of CPAP), and many studies have not monitored or reported the compliance rates. CPAP studies with optimum compliance may provide important evidence for a causative role of OSA in metabolic disturbances. Negative studies in which compliance was low or not reported may be considered as inconclusive rather than negative.

1.3.3 Cytokines

Adipose tissue expresses and releases cytokines such as tumor necrosis factor (TNF) α and interleukins (ILs). OSA is associated with increased levels of many of these mediators [see chapter 2, this vol., pp. 43–66; 147, 148], whose release may be triggered by chronic intermittent hypoxia and sleep loss and fragmentation [149, 150]. It remains to be demonstrated whether these mediators originate from the adipose tissue of OSA patients.

These cytokines are involved in the development of systemic and vascular inflammation, and may contribute to endothelial dysfunction, atherosclerosis and the development of vascular diseases associated with OSA [see chapters 4 and 6, this vol., pp. 139–169 and 197–265].

Table 3. Criteria for sleep-regulatory substances (SRS)

1	SRS should enhance a sleep phenotype, e.g. duration of non-REM sleep or EEG δ-wave power
2	Inhibition of SRS should reduce spontaneous sleep
3	SRS levels in the brain should correlate with sleep propensity
4	SRS should act on sleep-regulatory circuits
5	Levels of SRS during pathology should correlate with sleepiness

SRS criteria have been developed because sleep cannot be isolated as an independent variable from other variables, e.g. from body temperature or hormonal levels, which also change with sleep. EEG = Electroencephalogram. After Krueger et al. [151], with permission.

Several proinflammatory substances, including cytokines, have been classified as sleep-regulatory substances (table 3) [151]. For example, TNF-α, IL-1, IL-6 and IL-18 have been reported to promote non-REM sleep, while IL-4, IL-10, IL-13 and cytokine-associated substances (e.g. IL-1 receptor antagonist) inhibit spontaneous non-REM sleep. The effects of etanercept, a TNF-α antagonist, were assessed in a placebo-controlled, double-blind study on OSA severity and sleepiness in 8 obese male patients with OSA using nighttime polysomnography and multiple sleep latency tests [152]. There was a marked decrease in sleepiness with etanercept, which increased sleep latency during the multiple sleep latency test by 3.1 ± 1.0 min ($p < 0.05$) compared with placebo. The AHI was also significantly reduced by etanercept compared to placebo (52.8 ± 9.1 vs. 44.3 ± 10.3, respectively; adjusted difference, –8.4 ± 2.3; $p < 0.05$).

1.3.4 Other Adipokines

Resistin [153], visfatin, apelin, vaspin and hepcidin are adipokines that may be implicated in OSA, but their roles are unknown [147].

1.3.5 In Summary

The abnormal release of adipocytokines may be triggered by chronic intermittent hypoxia and sleep loss and fragmentation [149, 150]. However, it remains to be determined whether this occurs in OSA, contributes to the development or aggravation of metabolic and cardiovascular disorders associated with OSA, or increases susceptibility to OSA. There is evidence suggesting that both disorders contribute to an inflammatory state and that inflammatory cytokines can induce alterations in sleep and breathing patterns. It may be possible that the humoral effects of obesity aggravate OSA, as well as vice versa [3].

1.4 A Potentially Vicious Circle

Obesity is not only a risk factor for OSA, it may also be a consequence of OSA. OSA is associated with several changes that may promote overweight and obesity. Chronic intermittent hypoxia and sleep loss and fragmentation may contribute to alterations in adipokine secretion and glucose metabolism (see below), decreased energy expenditure and increased appetite [149, 154, 155].

Appetite is regulated by the appetite-stimulating and -inhibiting neuronal circuits in the arcuate nucleus of the hypothalamus [156, 157]. Several hormones that contribute to appetite regulation have been studied in OSA, including leptin (an appetite-inhibiting hormone, see above) and ghrelin (an appetite-stimulating hormone) [158]. As mentioned above, the hyperleptinemia observed in OSA patients is likely to be associated with central resistance to leptin (leptin is normally a satiety signal that should inhibit food intake); therefore, the ghrelin pathway may be more promising in terms of understanding the possible increased risk of obesity associated with OSA. Increased ghrelin levels have been reported in non-OSA subjects with partial sleep deprivation [157, 159], and plasma ghrelin levels are decreased in obese individuals and increased in lean individuals.

Unacylated ghrelin has a wide range of biological activities; however, binding to the growth hormone secretagogue receptor (needed to stimulate growth hormone release) and orexigenic effects are specific to acylated ghrelin [160, 161]. When the plasma levels of unacylated and acylated ghrelin were measured in OSA patients (n = 21) before and after 1 month of CPAP treatment, in untreated OSA patients (n = 14) and in an individual without OSA (n = 1) [162], baseline acylated and unacylated ghrelin levels were higher in OSA patients than in non-OSA subjects, and the levels of ghrelin were positively correlated with OSA severity. After 1 month of CPAP treatment, the acylated ghrelin levels were significantly decreased ($p = 0.02$), while a similar trend, albeit not significant, was observed for unacylated ghrelin levels ($p = 0.09$). Plasma ghrelin levels were significantly higher in OSA patients (n = 9) than in BMI-matched controls without OSA (n = 9; $p = 0.001$) [122]. After 2 days of CPAP treatment, plasma ghrelin levels decreased in the OSA patients, except 1 patient, to levels only slightly higher than those of the control subjects. However, other authors have not found significant differences in serum ghrelin levels between OSA patients and obese control subjects [163].

Other substances that contribute to appetite regulation, such as orexins and neuropeptide Y (NPY), have also been studied in OSA. Orexins (also called hypocretins) are appetite-stimulating neuropeptides produced in the lateral hypothalamus and the perifornical area. They contribute to the control of feeding, sleep, wakefulness, neuroendocrine homeostasis and autonomic regulation [164]. Orexins also play a role in disorders involving excessive daytime somnolence, e.g. in narcolepsy, plasma orexin levels are undetectable; however, the relationship between OSA and orexin levels is currently unresolved. Some reports have shown no significant difference in the levels of orexin in OSA patients compared with control subjects [165], whereas others have reported increased [166] or decreased orexin levels [167, 168]. Low plasma orexin A levels have been improved by CPAP treatment in patients with severe OSA [169]. Orexigenic neurons also activate the appetite-stimulating NPY neurons in the arcuate nucleus. Increased NPY levels were observed in OSA patients, independently of obesity, that were lowered after CPAP treatment (fig. 10) [114]. It is of note that the

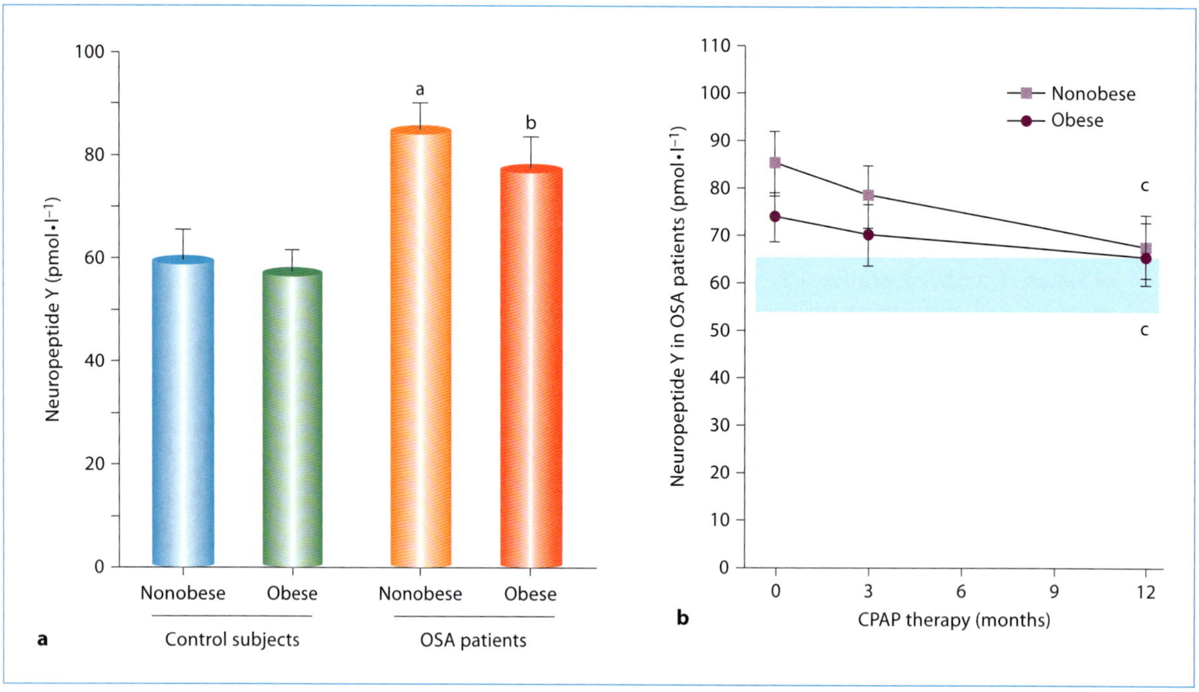

Fig. 10. Plasma neuropeptide Y levels in 19 obese and 18 nonobese control subjects without OSA and 23 obese and 24 nonobese patients with OSA: effect of CPAP treatment. **a** Plasma neuropeptide Y levels in the 4 groups studied. Levels were significantly increased in OSA patients ($p < 0.01$), independently of obesity. [a] $p < 0.01$ versus nonobese control subjects; [b] $p < 0.005$ versus obese control subjects. Data are shown as the mean ± SEM. **b** Effect of CPAP treatment on neuropeptide Y levels in OSA patients. CPAP treatment significantly reduced neuropeptide Y levels in all patients ($p < 0.01$). [c] $p < 0.05$ versus baseline (before treatment). Data are shown as the mean ± SEM. The shaded area represents the normal range of values in nonobese healthy subjects. After Barcelò et al. [114]. Reprinted with permission of the American Thoracic Society. © American Thoracic Society.

significance of the peripheral levels (as opposed to cerebrospinal fluid levels) of orexins and NPY relative to central activity is unclear.

In addition, although controversial [170], OSA is associated with a reduction in physical activity and performance [171–174] that may be the result of a lack of motivation, depression and excessive fatigue [171–173, 175].

Overall, these alterations may contribute to the development of overweight and obesity in OSA patients that, in turn, may aggravate OSA.

1.5 Conclusion

Obesity, especially visceral obesity, is the strongest risk factor for OSA. The increased deposits of adipose tissue around the pharyngeal airway, the reduction in lung volume and caudal traction on the upper airway associated with visceral obesity all contribute to reduce the size of the upper airway, to change its shape and increase its collapsibility.

Adipokines may contribute to the development of insulin resistance, inflammation, dysregulation of sleep and alterations in the control of breathing and body weight. Altogether, these alterations may result in OSA in obese patients. Treatment of obesity improves the severity of OSA, not only in patients with mild OSA, but also in those with moderate-to-severe OSA. However, as obesity accounts for only a small part of the variability in OSA severity, weight loss may not completely cure OSA.

Conversely, OSA may promote visceral adiposity. Chronic intermittent hypoxia, autonomic nervous system dysfunction, sleep loss and fragmentation, appetite dysregulation, reduced physical activity, endocrine dysfunction, chronic inflammation, and excessive daytime sleepiness and fatigue may all contribute to weight increase in OSA patients. A vicious cycle may therefore exist in obese patients with OSA, and it is often difficult to know which pathophysiological effects are attributable to OSA or to obesity.

2 Alterations in Glucose Metabolism and Obstructive Sleep Apnea

Recent research has provided strong evidence that OSA may increase the risk of developing alterations in glucose metabolism, including insulin resistance, glucose intolerance and type 2 diabetes mellitus. Conversely, alterations in glucose metabolism may also increase the risk of developing and/or aggravating OSA. The presence of confounders such as obesity increases the difficulty to establish a causal relationship between OSA and alterations in glucose metabolism and vice versa. However, the International Diabetes Federation recently published clinical practice recommendations suggesting that OSA patients should be routinely screened for markers of metabolic disturbance, including fasting glucose (table 4). Similarly, it recommended that the possibility of OSA should be considered in the assessment of all patients with type 2 diabetes. This section will describe evidence for the potential reciprocal links between OSA and alterations in glucose metabolism.

2.1 *Assessment of the Regulation of Glucose Metabolism*

2.1.1 Insulin Resistance

Glucose homeostasis results from a balance between the production of glucose in the liver and gut and the use of glucose by peripheral tissues. Glucose tolerance is the ability to return blood glucose levels to baseline after exogenous glucose has been metabolized [157]. Patients who need greater amounts of insulin than normal subjects to metabolize the same amount of glucose present with insulin resistance, i.e. reduced insulin sensitivity [157]. Insulin resistance plays a critical role in the occurrence and development of type 2 diabetes mellitus, as it is the precursor state of this disease.

The following tests are used to determine insulin resistance levels:

- The hyperinsulinemic-euglycemic clamp test is the gold standard method used to assess insulin sensitivity [176]. In this test, the plasma insulin concentration

Table 4. Clinical practices for health professionals working with type 2 diabetes and OSA to ensure that a patient presenting with one condition is considered for the other

Sleep services	OSA patients should be routinely screened for markers of metabolic disturbance and cardiovascular risk; minimum testing should include measurement of: waist circumference blood pressure fasting lipids fasting glucose
Diabetes services	The possibility of OSA should be considered in the assessment of all patients with type 2 diabetes and metabolic syndrome Patients should be assessed for symptoms of OSA: snoring, observed apnea during sleep and daytime somnolence There should be a low threshold for referral to establish the diagnosis because of the established benefits of therapy on hypertension and quality of life Management of OSA should focus initially on weight reduction for the overweight and obese; CPAP is the current best treatment for moderate-to-severe OSA and should be considered where appropriate

Clinical practices recommended by the International Diabetes Federation Task Force on Epidemiology and Prevention [184].

is acutely raised and maintained at a constant level by a prime-continuous infusion of insulin. The plasma glucose concentration is held constant at basal levels by a variable glucose infusion using the negative feedback principle. Under these steady-state conditions of euglycemia, the glucose infusion rate equals glucose uptake by all the tissues in the body and is, therefore, a measure of tissue sensitivity to exogenous insulin.

- The intravenous glucose tolerance test is a validated technique that uses a mathematical model [177]. Plasma insulin and glucose concentrations are assessed at 4-hour intervals during fasting and after intravenous glucose injection. In addition to measuring insulin resistance, this test also assesses glucose tolerance and β-cell responsiveness.
- The 15-min insulin tolerance test is a simple method to estimate insulin resistance by measuring the rate of fall of blood glucose following the intravenous administration of insulin [178–180].
- The HOMA index (the product of fasting serum insulin × fasting plasma glucose/22.5) is a validated estimate of insulin resistance [181]. An increased HOMA index indicates a high degree of insulin resistance.

2.1.2 Diabetes Mellitus

The classification of diabetes mellitus, according to the American Diabetes Association, includes 4 clinical classes [182]. Type 2 diabetes accounts for approximately 90–95% of

Table 5. Criteria for the diagnosis of prediabetes and diabetes, after the recommendations of the American Diabetes Association [182]

	Criteria for diagnosis
Prediabetes (impaired plasma glucose concentration)	Fasting plasma glucose concentration ranging from 100 to 125 $mg \cdot dl^{-1}$ (5.6–6.9 $mmol \cdot l^{-1}$) *or* oral glucose tolerance test resulting in a plasma glucose level ranging from 140 to 199 $mg \cdot dl^{-1}$ (7.8–11.0 $mmol \cdot l^{-1}$)
Diabetes	A casual plasma glucose concentration ≥200 $mg \cdot dl^{-1}$ (11.1 $mmol \cdot l^{-1}$) and symptoms of diabetes *or* fasting plasma glucose concentration ≥126 $mg \cdot dl^{-1}$ (7.0 $mmol \cdot l^{-1}$) *or* 2-hour plasma glucose concentration of 200 $mg \cdot dl^{-1}$ (11.1 $mmol \cdot l^{-1}$) during an oral glucose tolerance test

Prediabetes: hyperglycemia that is not sufficient to meet the diagnostic criteria for diabetes is categorized as either impaired fasting glucose or impaired glucose tolerance, depending on whether it is identified by fasting plasma glucose levels or an oral glucose tolerance test; in the absence of unequivocal hyperglycemia, these criteria should be confirmed by repeat testing on a different day; the oral glucose tolerance test is not recommended for routine clinical use but may be required in the evaluation of patients with impaired fasting glucose or when diabetes is still suspected despite normal fasting plasma glucose levels. 'Fasting' is defined as no caloric intake for at least 8 h. The oral glucose tolerance test should be performed as described by the WHO, using a glucose load containing the equivalent of 75 g anhydrous glucose dissolved in water. 'Casual' is defined as any time of day without regard to the time since the last meal. Reprinted with permission.

patients with diabetes mellitus. It usually occurs in middle-aged obese patients [182], and it encompasses patients with insulin resistance who usually have relative insulin deficiency.

The American Diabetes Association has recommended criteria for defining hyperglycemia (table 5) [183]. It has also recommended the measurement of hemoglobin (Hb) A_{1c} in a single blood sample to provide evidence of glucose control over the preceding 2–3 months [182].

2.2 *Evidence for Alterations in Glucose Metabolism in Obstructive Sleep Apnea*

2.2.1 Clinical and Epidemiological Studies

The association between OSA and type 2 diabetes is recognized [155, 184]. Cross-sectional studies suggest that up to 30% of patients with polysomnographically defined OSA have type 2 diabetes and that up to 86% of obese patients with type 2 diabetes (with a mean BMI of 36.5) have OSA [17, 185–188]. However, due to the presence of confounding variables, mainly overweight and obesity, it remains to be

Table 6. Frequency of impaired or diabetic glucose values as a function of the AHI in the Sleep Heart Health Study

	Prevalence of individuals with raised glucose levels, %	
	nonapneic subjects	patients with moderate-to-severe OSA
Impaired fasting glucose	8.7	17.5
Diabetic fasting glucose	4.0	8.8
Impaired 2-hour glucose level	29.1	36.0
Diabetic 2-hour glucose level	9.3	15.0

Nonapneic = AHI <5; moderate-to-severe OSA = AHI >15. After Punjabi et al. [201], with permission.

demonstrated whether there is a causal relationship between OSA and alterations in glucose metabolism [189, 190].

The majority of cross-sectional clinical studies [34, 112, 138, 186, 191–198] and cross-sectional and longitudinal population studies [185, 199–208] have shown an independent link between polysomnographically defined OSA and alterations in glucose metabolism. Hyperglycemia and insulin resistance may only occur in OSA patients presenting with excessive daytime somnolence [209, 210]. Only a few negative studies have been published [139, 211–213]. The following reports are of particular interest:

(1) The multicenter Sleep Heart Health Study, which took place in the USA, involved the participation of a large community sample of 2,656 subjects [201]. The frequencies of elevated fasting and 2-hour glucose levels measured during an oral glucose tolerance test were significantly higher in patients with moderate-to-severe OSA than in nonapneic subjects (table 6). Compared with nonapneic subjects, the AHI was independently associated with higher odds of elevated fasting and 2-hour glucose levels (table 7) and with the degree of insulin resistance (fig. 11). Sleep-related hypoxemia was also associated with insulin resistance and glucose intolerance, independently of age, gender, BMI and waist circumference. Disruption of nocturnal sleep continuity, as assessed by the frequency of arousals, was only associated with insulin resistance and not with glucose tolerance. Cross-sectional analysis of 2,588 participants without known diabetes confirmed that an AHI ≥10 was associated with alterations in glucose metabolism (occult diabetes, impaired fasting glucose, impaired glucose tolerance, and impaired fasting glucose plus impaired glucose tolerance) [205]. A 20–70% increase in the adjusted odds for impaired glucose metabolism was observed after adjusting for age, sex, race, BMI and waist circumference.

(2) The cross-sectional and longitudinal Wisconsin Sleep Cohort Study was performed on 1,387 participants [214]. This study reported that 14.7% of subjects with an AHI ≥15 had a diagnosis of diabetes, whereas only 2.8% of those with an AHI <5 had diabetes. Compared with non-OSA subjects, OSA patients (with an AHI ≥15)

Fig. 11. Risk of insulin resistance associated with OSA in participants of the Sleep Heart Health Study. Insulin resistance was assessed using the HOMA index (a raised HOMA index indicates a high degree of insulin resistance). Measurement of the index was not part of the baseline Sleep Heart Health Study examination, but it was performed at different time points. The figure shows the adjusted mean value of the HOMA index as a function of the AHI at the 3-month time point (n = 405). Compared with subjects with an AHI <5.0 and patients with mild OSA (AHI 5.0–14.9), those with moderate-to-severe OSA (AHI ≥15) were noted to have higher HOMA index values, indicating an insulin-resistant state. This was independent of age, gender, ethnicity, smoking status, BMI, waist circumference and sleep duration. After Punjabi et al. [201], with permission.

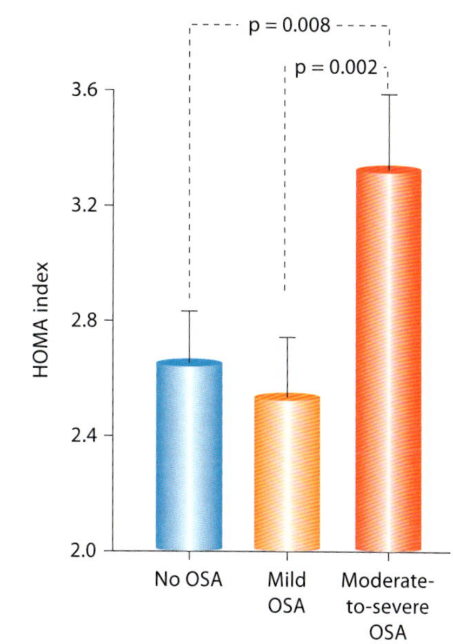

Table 7. Adjusted ORs for glucose intolerance based on fasting and 2-hour glucose levels, from the Sleep Heart Health Study, 1994–1999

Predictor	Fasting glucose level (n = 2,656)		Two-hour glucose level (n = 1,930)	
	OR	95% CI	OR	95% CI
AHI				
<5.0 events • h^{-1}	1.00		1.00	
5.0–14.9 events • h^{-1}	1.27	0.98–1.64	1.09	0.88–1.35
>15.0 events • h^{-1}	1.46	1.09–1.97	1.44	1.11–1.87
p for linear trend	0.0090		0.0096	

ORs and 95% CIs were based on multivariable ordinal logistic regression. Each row represents a distinct multivariate model that included adjustments for age, gender, race, BMI, waist circumference, smoking history, self-reported sleep duration and study site. Fasting glucose and 2-hour glucose levels were modeled as ordinal variables (normal, impaired and diabetic). The cutoff points were as follows: normal (fasting, <110 mg • dl^{-1}; 2 h, <140 mg • dl^{-1}); impaired (fasting, 110–125 mg • dl^{-1}; 2 h, 140–199 mg • dl^{-1}); diabetic (fasting, ≥126 mg • dl^{-1}; 2 h, ≥200 mg • dl^{-1}). After Punjabi et al. [201], with permission.

Table 8. ORs and 4-year follow-up incidence of prevalent physician-diagnosed diabetes for 2 levels of SDB (Wisconsin Sleep Cohort Study)

	OR	95% CI	p value
Diabetes prevalence			
AHI 5–15 vs. AHI <5	1.25	0.75–2.07	0.40
AHI ≥15 vs. AHI <5	2.30	1.28–4.11	0.005
Diabetes 4-year follow-up incidence			
AHI 5–15 vs. AHI <5	1.56	0.80–3.02	0.19
AHI ≥15 vs. AHI <5	1.62	0.67–3.65	0.24

ORs were adjusted for sex, age and body habitus. After Reichmuth et al. [214]. Reprinted with permission of the American Thoracic Society. © American Thoracic Society.

had a higher risk for diabetes mellitus after adjusting for age, sex and body habitus (table 8) [214]. However, no independent link was found between OSA and the incidence of diabetes mellitus at the 4-year follow-up when the data were adjusted for the same factors. Therefore, a causal role of OSA in the development of diabetes could not be established.

(3) Obese and nonobese patients with OSA were more resistant to insulin than non-OSA subjects, as indicated by higher levels of fasting serum insulin ($p = 0.001$) and the HOMA index ($p < 0.001$) in 270 participants (of whom 185 had an AHI ≥5) [199]. Stepwise multiple linear regression analysis demonstrated that OSA severity, assessed by AHI and minimum Sao_2, was an independent determinant of insulin resistance, but that obesity was the major determinant of insulin resistance.

(4) Using data from frequently sampled intravenous glucose tolerance tests, insulin sensitivity, the disposition index (an integrated measure of pancreatic β-cell function) and glucose effectiveness (a measure of the ability of glucose to mediate its own disposal) were assessed in nondiabetic patients with and without OSA (n = 118) [197]. The contribution of hyperglycemia to increased glucose disposal, i.e. the contribution of non-insulin-dependent glucose uptake, was assessed by measuring glucose effectiveness at zero insulin levels. SDB was associated with impairments in insulin sensitivity, glucose effectiveness and pancreatic β-cell function (fig. 12). These deficits are known to increase the predisposition for type 2 diabetes mellitus.

(5) A 4-year cohort study, the Australian Busselton Health Study (n = 399 at baseline), defined respiratory disturbances, measured using a portable home-monitoring device, as oxygen desaturation ≥3%, accompanied by either an increased heart rate ≥10 $beats{\cdot}min^{-1}$ and/or a burst of snoring [215]. Moderate-to-severe sleep apnea was a risk factor for the prevalence of diabetes and an independent risk factor for the 4-year incidence of diabetes. The longitudinal model used in this study remained significant after adjusting for confounding variables (table 9); however, it should be noted that the number of participants with moderate-to-severe OSA was very low in this study.

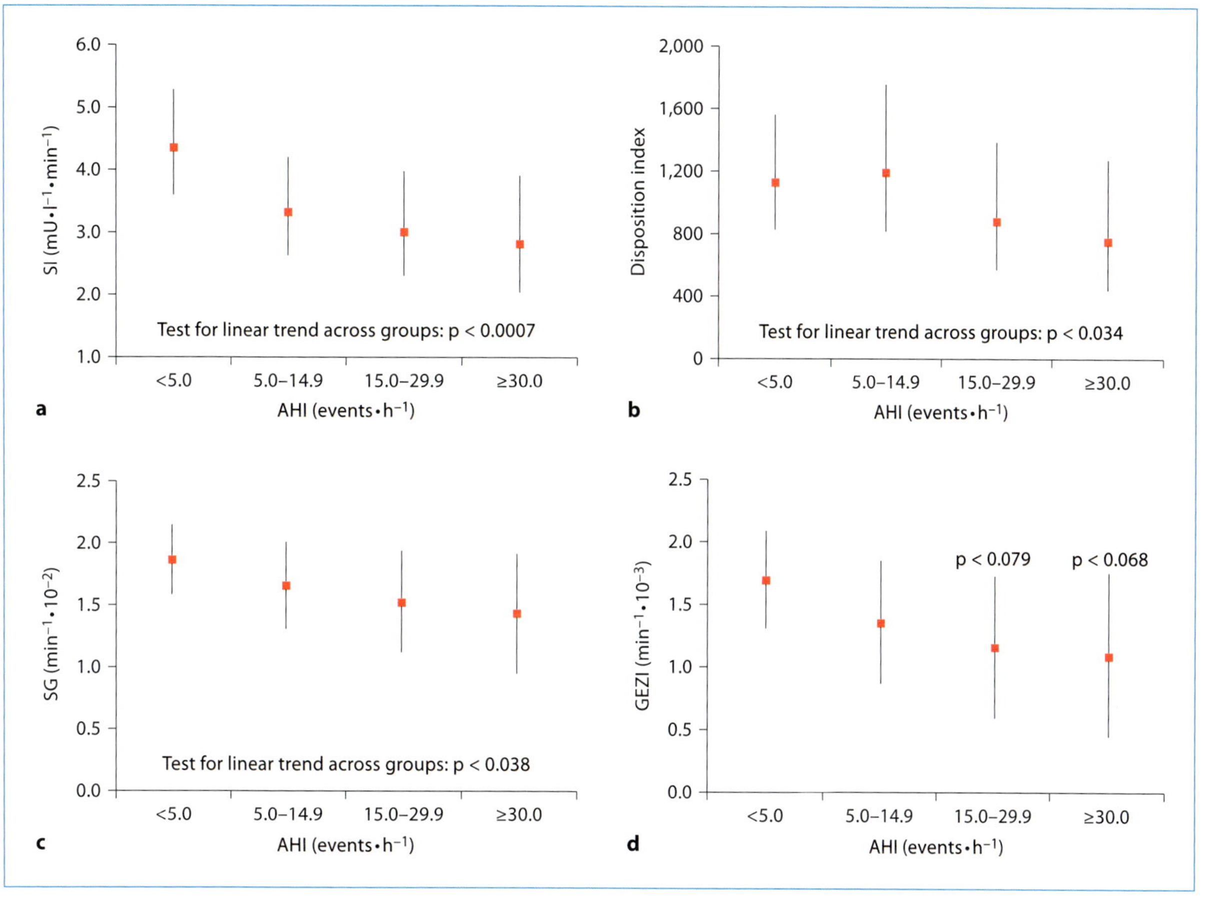

Fig. 12. Insulin sensitivity, deposition index and glucose effectiveness in nondiabetic subjects without or with mild, moderate or severe OSA. **a** Adjusted values of insulin sensitivity (average SI and 95% CI). **b** Disposition index (average and 95% CI). **c** Glucose effectiveness (median SG and 95% CI). **d** Glucose effectiveness at zero insulin (median GEZI and 95% CI). Values adjusted for age, sex, race and percent body fat. After Punjabi et al. [197]. Reprinted with permission of the American Thoracic Society. © American Thoracic Society.

(6) HbA_{1c} levels correlated with the AHI and oxygen desaturation levels in an observational study of nondiabetic patients with OSA [216].

Overall, these studies suggest an independent association between OSA and alterations in glucose metabolism; however, prospective studies of the incidence of diabetes have provided conflicting data [214, 215].

2.2.2 Therapeutic Studies

The effects of CPAP therapy on glucose metabolism alterations in OSA remain to be clarified [217]. The discrepancies between findings are probably due to methodological biases, e.g. lack of control groups or information on compliance with CPAP therapy, insufficient statistical power due to a small number of participants and short study

Table 9. Univariate and multivariate association of moderate-to-severe sleep apnea (RDI ≥15) with diabetes (Busselton Health Study)

	n	Cases of diabetes	Unadjusted OR	Partially adjusted OR	Fully adjusted OR
Association with diabetes at baseline					
No sleep apnea (RDI <5)	278	13 (4.7)	ref.	ref.	ref.
Mild sleep apnea (RDI 5 to <15)	77	4 (5.2)	1.12 [0.35–3.53]	0.83 [0.26–2.71]	0.84 [0.25–2.81]
Moderate-to-severe sleep apnea (RDI ≥15)	17	3 (17.7)	4.37 [1.12–17.12]	2.13 [0.48–9.50]	1.98 [0.41–9.55]
Association with incident diabetes					
No sleep apnea	226	5 (2.2)	ref.	ref.	ref.
Mild sleep apnea	59	2 (3.4)	1.47 [0.28–7.76]	1.31 [0.23–7.35]	1.51 [0.25–9.12]
Moderate-to-severe sleep apnea	10	2 (20)	11.20 [1.88–66.75]	8.62 [1.14–65.20]	13.45 [1.59–114.11]

Partially adjusted OR: adjusted for age, gender and waist circumference on the basis of the model presented from the Wisconsin Sleep Cohort [214]; fully adjusted OR: additionally adjusted for BMI, mean arterial pressure and high-density lipoprotein cholesterol. Figures in parentheses indicate percentages, those in square brackets show the 95% CI. After Marshall et al. [215], with permission.

duration [155, 189, 190, 218]. Good compliance with CPAP administration is likely to be necessary to demonstrate any significant effects of this treatment on glucose metabolism [219–222]. The negative findings of studies that assessed the effects of CPAP application have been hypothesized to be due to the impact of obesity, which may counterbalance the effect of the treatment [190, 223, 224]; however, this is controversial [225].

Several studies have shown an improvement of glucose metabolism with CPAP therapy, as presented below.

(1) An improvement in insulin sensitivity, fasting insulin levels and insulin secretion as assessed using the hyperinsulinemic-euglycemic clamp was observed in OSA patients with diabetes mellitus after up to 4 months of CPAP administration [223, 226]. Similar findings were observed in nonobese OSA patients without diabetes mellitus [227]. Insulin sensitivity was significantly increased after 2 days of CPAP treatment and remained stable after 3 months of treatment (fig. 13); however, the improvement in insulin sensitivity after 2 days was found to be much greater in nonobese patients than in obese patients (table 10). It is suggested that the improved insulin sensitivity after 2 days of treatment may reflect decreasing sympathetic activity, and that insulin sensitivity is mainly determined by obesity and, to a smaller extent, by OSA. When overweight male patients with moderate-to-severe OSA and no significant comorbidity were randomized to therapeutic or

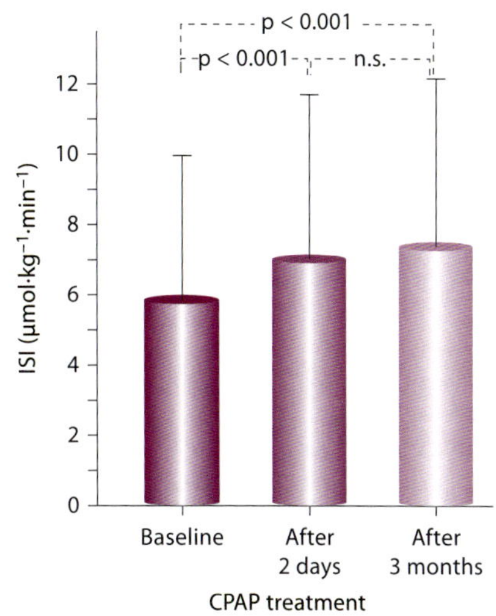

Fig. 13. Effect of CPAP treatment on insulin sensitivity in OSA patients. The insulin sensitivity index (ISI) was assessed with the hyperinsulinemic-euglycemic clamp method in OSA patients at baseline (n = 40), 2 days (n = 40) and 3 months after the onset of CPAP treatment (n = 31, as 9 of the 40 patients discontinued CPAP therapy). The ISI was significantly improved after 2 days of CPAP treatment. After 3 months, there was no further significant improvement of the ISI, but it was still significantly different from baseline. After Harsch et al. [227]. Reprinted with permission of the American Thoracic Society. © American Thoracic Society.

Table 10. Insulin sensitivity index ($\mu mol \cdot kg^{-1} \cdot min^{-1}$) before and during CPAP treatment in OSA patients with a BMI <30 or >30

	BMI <30 (n = 16; after 3 months, n = 13)	BMI >30 (n = 24; after 3 months, n = 18)
Baseline	8.53±4.48	3.89±2.80
After 2 days of CPAP therapy	10.47±5.09	4.33±2.87
Improvement compared with baseline	p = 0.001	p = 0.13
After 3 months of CPAP therapy	10.71±4.95	5.26±3.50
Improvement compared with baseline	p = 0.001	p = 0.03

After Harsch et al. [227]. Reprinted with permission of the American Thoracic Society. © American Thoracic Society.

sham CPAP treatment for 1 week followed by reassessment [225], an improvement in insulin sensitivity, estimated by the short insulin tolerance test, was observed after effective CPAP administration (n = 31), while there was no significant change in those receiving sham CPAP (n = 30; fig. 14). Those who received therapeutic CPAP were further evaluated at 12 weeks, and the improvement in insulin sensitivity was maintained at this time in those (n = 20) with a BMI ≥25, but not in the subjects (n = 9) with a BMI <25 or the entire group. This is in contrast with the findings of Harsch et al. [227]. An improvement in insulin sensitivity using the HOMA index was observed after 3 weeks of CPAP therapy in OSA patients with or

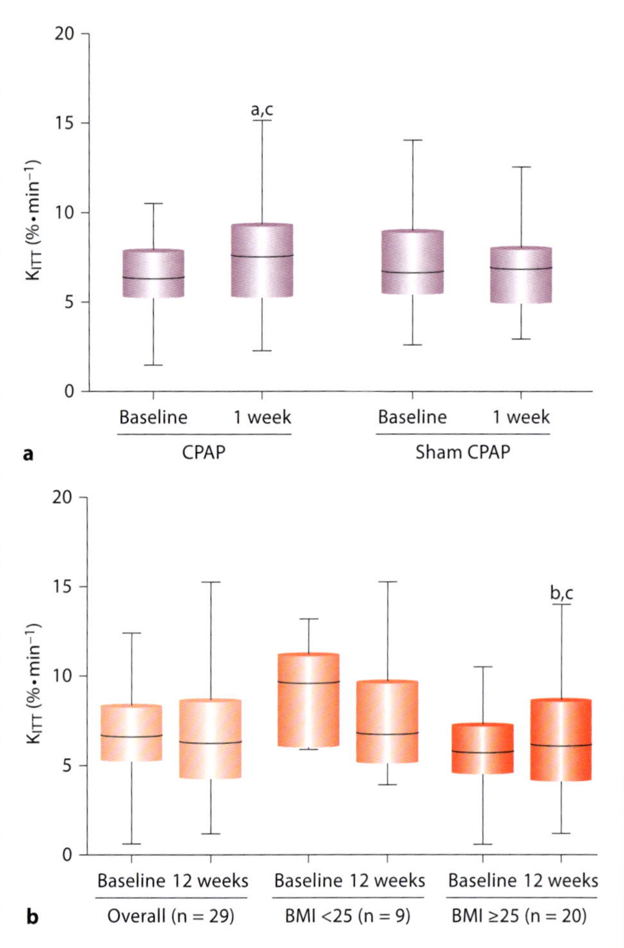

Fig. 14. Randomized controlled study of the effects of effective versus sham CPAP administration on insulin sensitivity. **a** Changes in the glucose disappearance rate for estimating insulin sensitivity (K_{ITT}) at baseline and after 1 week of effective CPAP and sham CPAP treatment. **b** Changes in K_{ITT} after 12 weeks of CPAP treatment overall (n = 29), with a BMI <25 (n = 9) and a BMI ≥25 (n = 20). [a] $p < 0.05$ for comparisons between groups; [b] $p < 0.05$ for comparisons between a BMI <25 and a BMI ≥25; [c] $p < 0.05$ for within-group comparisons. After Lam et al. [225], with permission. © European Respiratory Society.

without diabetes mellitus [228]. Similar findings have also been reported in patients with severe OSA and metabolic syndrome after 8 weeks of CPAP therapy for more than 4 h • night^{-1} (compared with baseline values) [220]. In addition, a reduction in fasting insulin levels and a decrease in insulin resistance have been reported after 3 weeks of CPAP treatment [228].

(2) An improvement in glucose levels was found after CPAP treatment. CPAP administration has been associated with: an improvement in 1-hour postprandial glucose levels in OSA patients with type 2 diabetes mellitus [219]; an improvement in glycemic control that was reflected by a decreased variability in glucose levels detected using continuous glucose monitoring techniques [229, 230], and decreased sleeping glucose levels [229].

(3) A decrease in HbA_{1c} levels has been linked with CPAP application [219, 231]. For example, a significant decrease in HbA_{1c} levels, but not of insulin resistance

(HOMA index), was observed in nondiabetic patients with OSA after 6 months of CPAP therapy [222]. This was only observed in those patients who received CPAP treatment for ≥4 h • day^{-1}.

Conversely, some studies have reported no significant effect on insulin sensitivity [145, 232–234], no change in fasting or nocturnal insulin levels [96, 232], an increase in nocturnal glucose [232] and no change in HbA_{1c} levels [145, 229] in OSA patients. Two randomized controlled studies of the effects of effective versus sham CPAP [145, 233] are of special interest. The first was a 6-week randomized controlled study in nondiabetic patients with OSA, where no significant changes were observed in glucose, lipids, insulin resistance or the proportion of patients with metabolic syndrome [233]. The second was a 3-month randomized controlled study in newly diagnosed OSA patients with type 2 diabetes that found no significant changes in HbA_{1c} levels, the HOMA index or insulin sensitivity assessed using the hyperinsulinemic-euglycemic clamp test in either the therapeutic or placebo groups [145]. It is of note that this study was marred by very low compliance rates (the mean hours per night of therapeutic or sham CPAP use were <4), and it was also underpowered. In both of these studies, CPAP administration was associated with an improvement of excessive daytime sleepiness. Effective CPAP was administered using autotitrating CPAP devices [145] or during CPAP titration performed in a sleep laboratory using the Autoset self-adjusting CPAP device (ResMed Autoscan) to obtain optimal CPAP pressure (defined as the pressure that abolished apnea and snoring) [233].

The effects of CPAP administration on insulin sensitivity may depend on the manner in which it is administered. When the effects of fixed and autoadjusting CPAP on cardiovascular risk factors, including insulin sensitivity measured using the HOMA index, were assessed [235], OSA indices were significantly reduced regardless of the CPAP administration method. Significant improvements in insulin sensitivity were observed in patients treated with fixed CPAP, but not in those treated with the autoadjusting device (fig. 15). The fixed CPAP titration was performed by a technician in a sleep laboratory until obstructive apnea, hypopnea, snoring and flow-limited breathing associated with arousals disappeared. It is suggested that, despite significant effects on OSA indices and symptoms, these methods do not improve metabolic alterations and cardiovascular risk factors in the same fashion.

2.2.3 In Summary

Whereas recent research provides strong evidence for an increased risk of alterations in glucose metabolism in OSA patients, the causal relationship between these conditions remains to be fully established [189, 190]. However, the International Diabetes Federation Task Force on Epidemiology and Prevention published the following clinical practice recommendations for health professionals working with type 2 diabetes and OSA patients: (1) to adopt clinical practices that ensure a patient presenting with one condition is considered for the other and (2) to develop locally appropriate clinical pathways for type 2 diabetes and sleep services (table 4) [184].

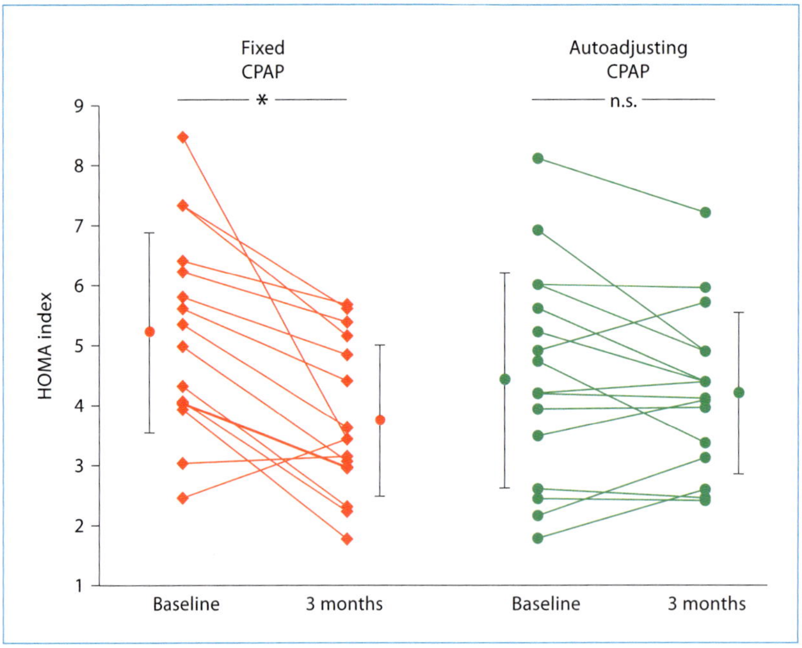

Fig. 15. Effects of fixed CPAP or autoadjusting CPAP on insulin sensitivity assessed by the HOMA index. Individual HOMA indices in obese patients with severe OSA (n = 31) at baseline and after either 3 months of fixed CPAP (n = 15) or autoadjusting CPAP (n = 16) administration. * $p < 0.05$. Average data are expressed as the mean ± SD. After Patruno et al. [235], with permission.

2.3 *Potential Mechanisms for the Development of Glucose Metabolism Alterations in Obstructive Sleep Apnea*

2.3.1 Inflammatory Dysfunction

The link between inflammation, the development of insulin resistance, and the pathogenesis of type 2 diabetes is well established [236, 237]. Before the critical role of adipose tissue in the development of alterations in glucose metabolism was discovered, type 2 diabetes was associated with increased levels of inflammatory markers, including fibrinogen, C-reactive protein, IL-6 and type 1 plasminogen activator inhibitor [236]. Adipocytes (and macrophages that infiltrate adipose tissue) are able to express and release inflammatory and bioactive substances that have a critical role in the pathogenesis of alterations in glucose metabolism [236]. These substances include TNF-α, IL-6 and leptin (fig. 16) [87, 236]. The local production of these substances promotes local chronic inflammation and potentially contributes to the systemic propagation of the inflammatory process (fig. 17) [236]. Increased levels of these bioactive substances, including TNF-α, macrophage chemotactic protein 1 and IL-8, and oxidative stress have been reported in OSA patients [see chapter 2, this vol.,

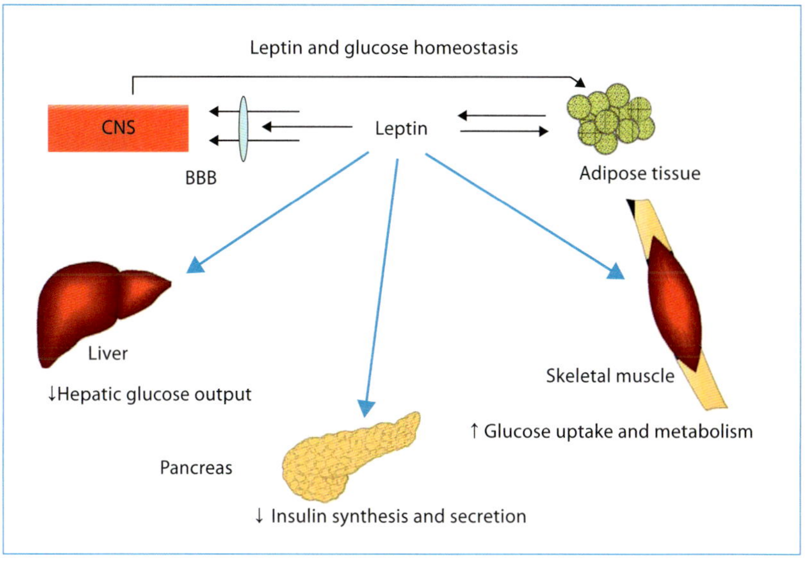

Fig. 16. Effects of leptin on glucose homeostasis. Leptin crosses the blood-brain barrier (BBB) by a saturable transport system, and reaches the arcuate nucleus of the hypothalamus where it controls food intake, energy expenditure and neuroendocrine function. Circulating leptin also has direct peripheral effects: (1) decreases hepatic glucose output, (2) increases glucose uptake and metabolism in skeletal muscle and (3) decreases insulin synthesis and secretion by pancreatic β-cells. CNS = Central nervous system. After Yildiz and Haznedaroglu [87], with permission.

pp. 45–66]. However, it remains to be elucidated whether they originate from adipose tissue and how they may alter glucose metabolism.

Activation of the nuclear factor (NF) κB pathway by inflammatory markers may be of critical importance in the development of alterations in glucose metabolism in OSA because the NF-κB target gene products are potentially involved in the pathogenesis of insulin resistance (the additional involvement of NF-κB in OSA pathogenesis is discussed in chapter 2 [this vol., pp. 43–66]) [236, 238]. Several transcription factors and kinases are involved in the inflammatory processes associated with insulin resistance and diabetes mellitus [236, 237]. Obesity and a high-fat diet activate certain transcription factors, including the NF-κB inflammatory pathway, in adipocytes, hepatocytes and associated macrophages (fig. 18). Stimuli that activate these pathways during metabolic dysregulation include the ligands for TNF-α, IL-1, Toll, advanced glycation end-products (AGEs) and intracellular stresses including reactive oxygen species (ROS). AGEs are a heterogeneous group of compounds derived from sugars, such as glucose, that can be engaged by specific cell surface receptors, i.e. receptors for AGEs, and can subsequently activate the NF-κB pathway [239, 240]. They have been implicated in the progression of age-related diseases such as diabetes mellitus and atherosclerosis [241, 242]. The serum levels of AGEs were increased in nondiabetic subjects with OSA and were associated with the severity of OSA [243]. The levels of AGEs may

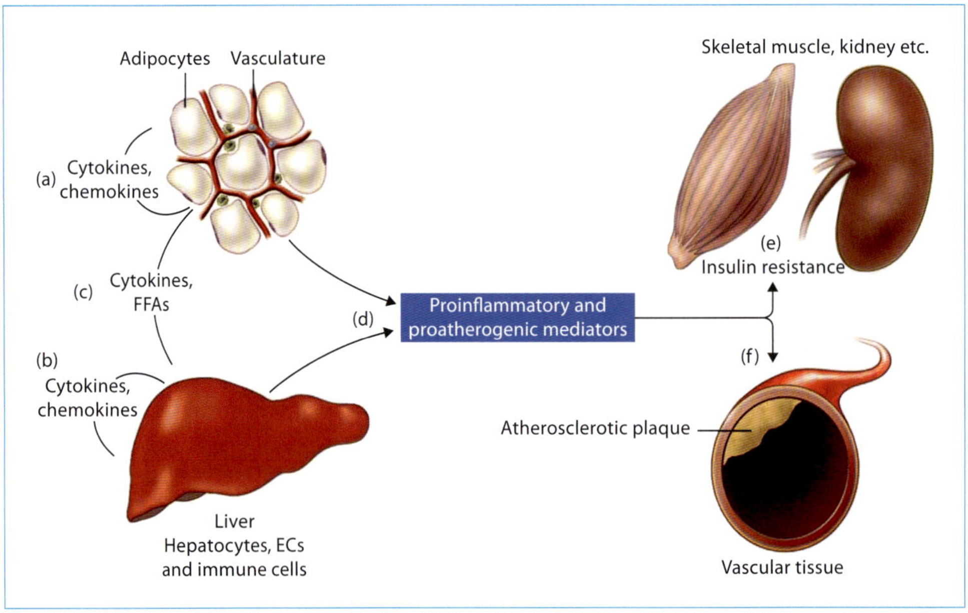

Fig. 17. Local, portal and systemic effects of inflammation in insulin resistance and atherogenesis. Increasing adiposity activates inflammatory responses in adipose tissue (a) and liver (b), with associated increases in the production of cytokines and chemokines. Immune cells, including monocytes and macrophages, are recruited and/or activated, resulting in local insulin resistance. Portal delivery of abdominal fat-derived cytokines and lipids (c) contributes to hepatic inflammation and insulin resistance. Proinflammatory and proatherogenic mediators are produced in the adipose tissue, liver and associated immune cells (d). This creates a predisposition to a systemic inflammatory reaction that promotes insulin resistance in skeletal muscle, the kidney and other tissues (e), and atherogenesis in the vasculature (f). ECs = Liver sinusoid endothelial cells; FFAs = free fatty acids. After Shoelson et al. [236], with permission.

increase for several reasons including hyperglycemia, excessive ROS production and diet (food products cooked at high temperatures and those with high caloric content contain high levels of AGEs) [244]. However, the mechanisms that may increase the levels in AGEs in OSA and how they contribute to the development of alterations in glucose metabolism associated with OSA remain to be determined.

Chronic intermittent hypoxia and sleep fragmentation may be the link between OSA and the development of alterations in glucose metabolism as described below.

2.3.2 Chronic Intermittent Hypoxia

The severity of hypoxemia related to OSA has been associated with indices of insulin resistance in epidemiological studies, suggesting that chronic intermittent hypoxia may adversely affect glucose metabolism [199–201]. Experimental studies in humans [245, 246] and in murine models [247, 248] have provided further evidence for this hypothesis. The contribution of autonomic function to hypoxia-induced insulin resistance was suggested in a study of healthy subjects in which

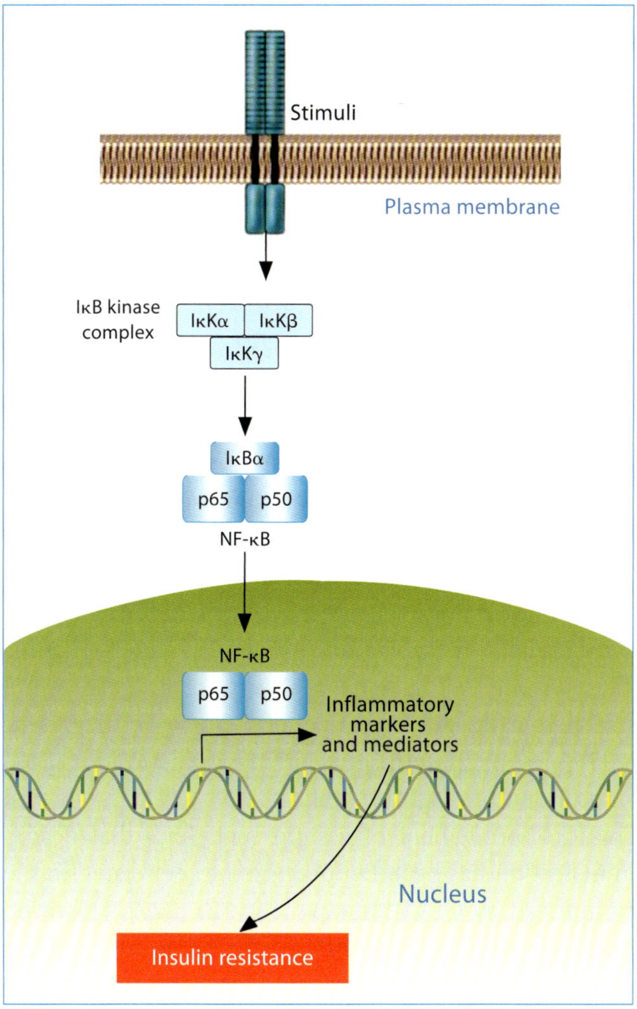

Fig. 18. Simplified scheme of potential cellular mechanisms for the activation of inflammatory signaling that may contribute to the development of insulin resistance. NF-κB is a generic name for a family of dimeric transcription factors composed of several proteins including p50 and p65. p50 and p65 share a domain for DNA binding and the binding of the NF-κB inhibitor (IκB) [344–347]. In unstimulated cells, NF-κB remains inactive in the cytoplasm due to its interaction with IκB. In response to multiple stimuli, NF-κB is activated. This activation is achieved by the phosphorylation of IκB by the IκB kinase complex (IκK complex, which contains several subunits including 2 related catalytic subunits, IκKα and IκKβ, and a regulatory subunit, IκKγ [346]). The phosphorylation of IκB frees NF-κB from its inhibitor. The freed NF-κB can then translocate to the nucleus, where it activates transcription of a variety of target genes involved in the inflammatory process, which may, in turn, cause insulin resistance. After Shoelson et al. [236], with permission.

the effects of sustained hypoxia for 30 min on insulin resistance (assessed using the hyperinsulinemic-euglycemic clamp method) and neurohormonal stress response (evaluated by measuring plasma epinephrine levels and heart rate) were assessed [245]. Compared with control subjects who received oxygen at 96% saturation, subjects receiving gas at 75% oxygen saturation showed significant insulin resistance, increased plasma epinephrine levels and an increased heart rate [245]. The effects of 5 h of intermittent hypoxia or normoxia (24.3 events • h^{-1}) on glucose metabolism were assessed in awake healthy volunteers (n = 13); this study was performed in a randomized order on 2 separate days using minimal model analysis of frequently sampled intravenous glucose tolerance tests [246]. Compared with the normoxic condition, intermittent hypoxia was associated with a significant decrease in insulin sensitivity and glucose effectiveness (the ability of glucose to facilitate its disposal independently of an insulin response). Pancreatic insulin secretion and serum cortisol levels were comparable between the 2 conditions. Analysis of heart rate variability showed that the intermittent hypoxia was associated with a shift in the sympathovagal balance toward an increase in the activity of the sympathetic nervous system. It is suggested that intermittent hypoxemia may be a central mechanism for metabolic dysfunction in OSA patients, and that the sympathetic nervous system is a putative mediator of this process.

It remains to be determined whether the adverse effect of hypoxia on the alterations in glucose metabolism in OSA is linked to the effect of sympathetic activation; however, it is known that chronic autonomic dysfunction may adversely alter glucose homeostasis [249–251]. The rapid improvement of insulin sensitivity that occurs after only 2 days of CPAP administration has been hypothesized to be related to the decreased sympathetic activity induced by CPAP therapy (fig. 13) [227]. However, in a murine model, insulin sensitivity was decreased after exposure to intermittent hypoxia, and it was not restored by blocking the autonomic nervous system [247]. The insulin resistance associated with chronic intermittent hypoxia was suggested to occur independently of the activation of the sympathetic nervous system.

Hypoxic adipose tissue has been hypothesized to play a critical role in the development of the diseases associated with obesity, particularly type 2 diabetes and metabolic syndrome [76, 150]. Chronic intermittent hypoxia increases the formation of ROS and proinflammatory cytokines that, in turn, may contribute to the development of alterations in glucose metabolism. ROS suppress insulin secretion and worsen insulin sensitivity [252, 253], while proinflammatory cytokines, such as IL-6 and TNF-α, are involved in the pathogenesis of insulin resistance and type 2 diabetes [236]. The molecular mechanisms by which adipocytes sense and respond to hypoxia involve several transcription factors, including NF-κB [75, 76]. NF-κB activation in adipocytes mediates the expression of inflammatory molecules such as TNF-α, a cytokine with a critical role in the development of alterations in glucose metabolism [75]. It remains to be demonstrated whether NF-κB activation contributes to the development of such alterations in OSA patients.

2.3.3 Sleep Loss and Fragmentation

The sleep of OSA patients is characterized by increased fragmentation and reduced slow-wave and REM sleep. Poor and short sleep are considered risk factors for adverse cardiovascular and metabolic events, including the development of hypertension, alterations in glucose metabolism and obesity [149, 254]. Chronic inflammation could be an intermediate mechanism linking the sleep loss and fragmentation associated with OSA and the later development of cardiovascular disorders. However, this remains to be demonstrated, and it is important to distinguish sleep deprivation per se from sleep fragmentation secondary to sleep apnea because the former can occur without the coexistence of sleep apnea.

Clinical and epidemiological studies, as well as controlled laboratory studies in healthy subjects, indicate that sleep fragmentation and reduced total sleep time in the absence of known SDB are independently associated with alterations in glucose metabolism and increase the risk of developing diabetes [149]. Other researchers have partially confirmed or have not confirmed these findings. For example, a population-based, cross-sectional multicenter study indicated that short (≤6 h) and long (≥8 h) sleep duration are related to an increased risk of type 2 diabetes in middle-aged women (n = 1,434), but not in men (n = 1,336) [255]. A median 4.2-year follow-up study in Japan revealed, after adjusting for confounders, an association between a higher risk of developing diabetes mellitus with difficulty in self-reported sleep initiation, but not with sleep maintenance or duration [256].

A meta-analysis of prospective studies associating the assessment of sleep disturbances at baseline and the incidence of type 2 diabetes with a follow-up >3 years was performed to assess the relationship between habitual sleep disturbances and the incidence of type 2 diabetes [257]. Ten studies were included in the analysis: 13 independent cohort samples; 107,756 male and female participants; follow-up range 4.2–32 years, and 3,586 incident cases of type 2 diabetes. For a short sleep duration (≤5–6 h • night^{-1}), the relative risk was 1.28 (95% CI 1.03–1.60; p = 0.024, heterogeneity p = 0.015); for a long sleep duration (>8–9 h • night^{-1}), the relative risk was 1.48 (95% CI 1.13–1.96; p = 0.005); for difficulty in initiating sleep, it was 1.57 (95% CI 1.25–1.97; p < 0.0001), and for difficulty in maintaining sleep, the relative risk was 1.84 (95% CI 1.39–2.43; p < 0.0001). It is suggested that the quantity and quality of sleep consistently and significantly predict the risk of developing type 2 diabetes. The largest prospective study of sleep duration and diabetes risk published to date examined whether day napping or short night sleeping is associated with a higher risk of diabetes in a prospective study of hours of day napping and night sleeping assessed in 1996–1997 in relation to diabetes diagnosed between 2000 and 2006 (n = 10,143) among 174,542 participants in the National Institutes of Health-AARP (formerly known as the American Association of Retired Persons) Diet and Health Study [258]. Longer day napping was associated with a higher risk of diabetes. After adjustment for potential confounders, ORs were 1.23 (95% CI 1.18–1.29) for those reporting <1 h and 1.55 (95% CI 1.45–1.66) for those reporting ≥1 h of napping compared with individuals who did not nap [p (trend) <0.0001]. For night sleeping, with 7–8 h as the reference, the OR was 1.46 (95% CI 1.31–1.63) for <5 h, 1.11 (1.06–1.16) for 5–6 h and 1.11 (0.99–1.24) for ≥9 h. In both analyses, additional adjustment for BMI only modestly attenuated the associations. Further analysis showed a statistically significant interaction between hours of napping and sleeping on diabetes [p (interaction) < 0.0001]. Among participants with no napping, only short night sleeping was associated with a higher occurrence of diabetes, whereas among those with ≥1 h of napping, long and short sleeping times were associated with a higher risk. It is suggested that day napping and short night sleeping are associated with a higher risk of diabetes; therefore, the association between sleep duration and diabetes may be modified by napping habits.

Overall, these studies may be relevant to OSA because many OSA patients present with complaints of insomnia (particularly females) and OSA is often associated with either short sleep or long sleep (where patients attempt to compensate for poor sleep quality with longer sleep duration).

2.3.3.1 Potential Mechanisms Linking Sleep Loss and Fragmentation with Alterations in Glucose Metabolism. OSA is associated with a reduced total sleep time and increased sleep fragmentation that may cause adverse effects on glucose metabolism. These effects may be due to slow-wave sleep deprivation, an increase in sympathetic activity and changes in appetite regulation [132, 157, 218].

Deep sleep is characterized by slow waves on encephalograms. In young healthy adults (n = 9), the all-night selective suppression of slow-wave sleep, without any change in total sleep time, results in marked decreases in insulin sensitivity [132]. The reduction in insulin sensitivity was associated with raised daytime sympathetic activity, as assessed by heart rate variability. It was also strongly correlated with a reduction in slow-wave sleep, but not with measures of sleep fragmentation. Under normal circumstances, when insulin sensitivity decreases, the amount of insulin released by β-cells should increase reciprocally so that the disposition index (a marker of the risk for diabetes, calculated as insulin sensitivity × insulin release) remains constant and glucose tolerance is maintained [259]; however, after the suppression of slow-wave sleep, a decrease in insulin sensitivity is compensated by an increase in insulin release, as insulin release remained virtually unchanged (fig. 19a, b). This resulted in an approximately 20% fall in the disposition index (fig. 19c), leading to reduced glucose tolerance (fig. 19d) and to a potentially increased risk of diabetes [132]. Glucose tolerance was within the range reported in older adults with impaired glucose tolerance [260]. These findings provide evidence for a restorative role of slow-wave sleep on metabolic function [132].

2.4 A Potentially Vicious Circle

Some observational studies have assessed whether diabetes mellitus is a risk factor for OSA using type 4 monitoring, polygraphy or polysomnography [17, 187, 188, 261–263]:

(1) Questionnaires and overnight pulse oximetry were used to identify men with diabetes mellitus at a low and high risk for OSA (the results were verified by detailed

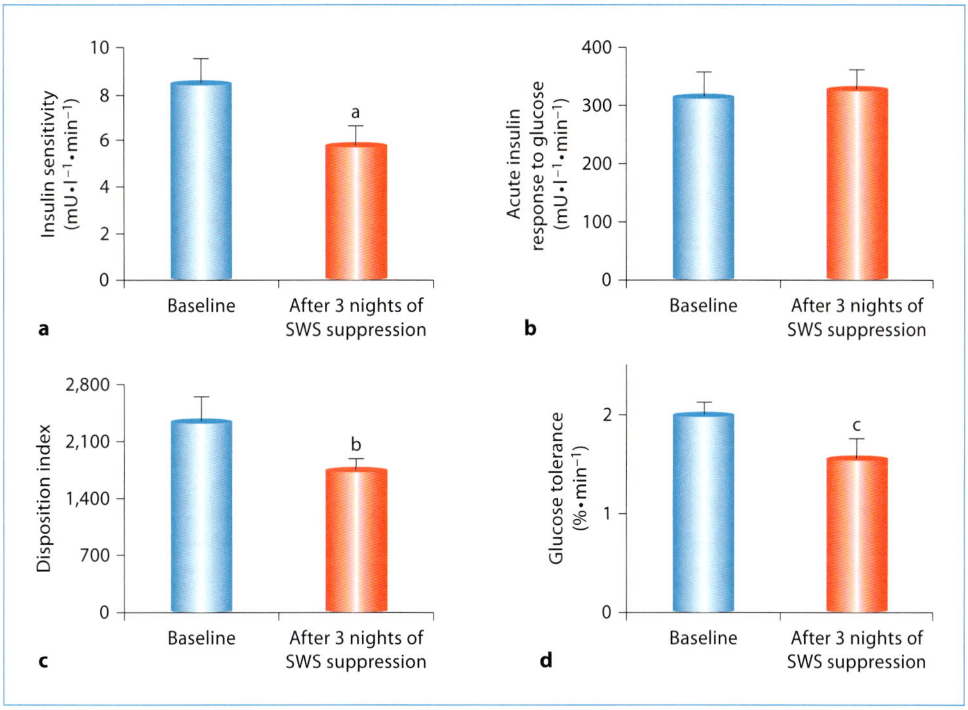

Fig. 19. Insulin sensitivity, insulin release and glucose tolerance at baseline and after 3 nights of slow-wave sleep (SWS) suppression in healthy subjects. **a** Insulin sensitivity: after 3 nights of experimental suppression of SWS, insulin sensitivity was decreased by approximately 25%. [a] p = 0.009. **b, c** Insulin response to the decrease in insulin sensitivity: the decrease in insulin sensitivity was not compensated for by an increase in insulin release, as insulin release remained virtually unchanged (p = 0.73; **b**), resulting in an approximately 20% fall in the disposition index, a marker of diabetes risk (**c**). [b] p = 0.02. **d** Glucose tolerance was reduced by approximately 23%. [c] p = 0.03. Data are the mean ± SEM (n = 9); significant differences were determined by the paired t test. After Tasali et al. [132], with permission. © 2008 National Academy of Sciences, USA.

sleep studies) [262]. The prevalence of OSA, assessed using oximetry, was significantly higher in the participants than in a control population from a previous study (17 vs. 6%, respectively; $p < 0.001$); therefore, diabetes was an independent predictor of OSA.

(2) Using a single-channel recording device that measures disordered breathing events from a nasal cannula airflow signal, the overall prevalence of OSA (defined by an AHI ≥15 events • h^{-1}) was 36% (49% in males and 21% in females) in patients from a diabetes clinic (n = 279) [187]. Age ≥62 years, male sex, BMI ≥30, snoring and reports of breathing interruption during sleep were associated with sleep apnea.

(3) In 303 consecutive patients hospitalized for poorly controlled type 2 diabetes [188] assessed using polygraphy, 34% had mild sleep apnea (RDI 5–15), 19% had moderate sleep apnea (RDI 16–29), and 10% had severe sleep apnea (RDI ≥30). The

sleep apnea was obstructive in 99% of the apneic patients. Patients with severe or moderate sleep apnea had significantly higher BMI and waist and neck circumference values than nonapneic patients. It is of note that the percentage of patients with excessive daytime sleepiness (Epworth Sleepiness Scale >10), fatigue or nocturia did not significantly differ among patients with severe, moderate or mild sleep apnea syndrome versus nonapneic patients.

(4) Cross-sectional data from the Sleep Heart Health Study indicated a 57.7% prevalence for SDB (assessed using in-home polysomnography) in diabetic patients, whereas it was 42.6% in nondiabetic patients. There was a significant difference in the distribution of diabetes across RDI categories, with proportionally more diabetic individuals in the higher categories (e.g. 23.8% of diabetic subjects were in the RDI ≥15 group, compared with 15.6% of nondiabetic subjects; $p < 0.001$). After adjusting for the usual confounding variables, including the BMI, no significant differences were observed in the levels of obstructive respiratory events between diabetic and nondiabetic participants [261]. Diabetes was associated with periodic breathing (OR for diabetic subjects vs. nondiabetic subjects 1.80; 95% CI 1.02–3.15). It is suggested that diabetes is associated with periodic breathing, a respiratory abnormality associated with alterations in the central control of ventilation. It has been hypothesized that autonomic neuropathy may be responsible for the dysfunction of central respiratory control [264–266]; however, it is possible that the patients may have been misdiagnosed, as the diagnosis of diabetes did not rely on objective data, but was obtained from self-reporting or on the use of oral hypoglycemic medications or insulin [266].

(5) In a study of 306 obese patients with type 2 diabetes, over 86% had OSA with an AHI ≥5 diagnosed using unattended polysomnography [17]. The mean AHI was 20.5 ± 16.8. A total of 30.5% of the participants had moderate OSA ($15 \leq AHI < 30$) and 22.6% had severe OSA (AHI ≥30). Waist circumference was significantly related to the presence of OSA (OR 1.1; 95% CI 1.0–1.1; $p = 0.03$). Severe OSA was most likely in individuals with a higher BMI (OR 1.1; 95% CI 1.0–1.2; $p = 0.03$).

(6) In patients with diabetes mellitus and untreated OSA (assessed using polysomnography studies), the adjusted mean HbA_{1c} level was increased by 1.49% ($p = 0.0028$) in patients with mild OSA, 1.93% ($p = 0.0033$) in patients with moderate OSA, and 3.69% ($p < 0.0001$) in patients with severe OSA ($p < 0.0001$ for the linear trend) compared to patients without OSA, and after controlling for confounding variables (fig. 20) [263]. It is suggested that in patients with type 2 diabetes, increasing severity of OSA is associated with poorer glucose control, independently of confounders, with effect sizes comparable to those of widely used hypoglycemic drugs.

Overall, these findings suggest that OSA is highly prevalent in diabetic patients, is related to abdominal obesity, and may not be predicted using clinical data. Although it is possible that diabetes mellitus may cause or aggravate OSA, the evidence to support this hypothesis is limited.

Fig. 20. Adjusted mean HbA_{1c} values for patients with no, mild, moderate and severe OSA. Data were adjusted for age, gender, race, BMI, number of antidiabetic medications taken, level of exercise, years of diabetes and total sleep time on polysomnography. Bars represent standard errors. After Aronsohn et al. [263]. Reprinted with permission of the American Thoracic Society. © American Thoracic Society.

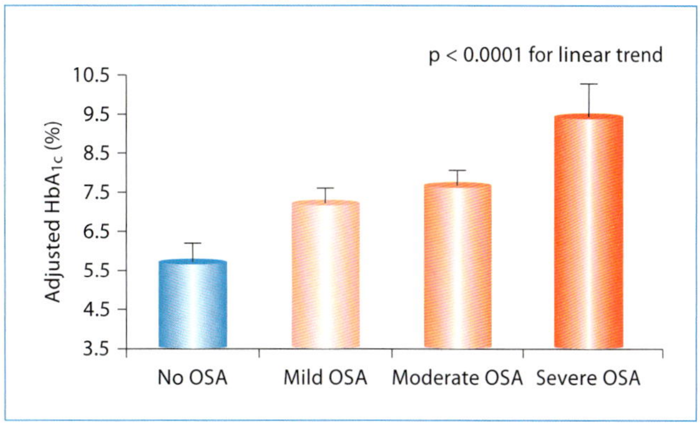

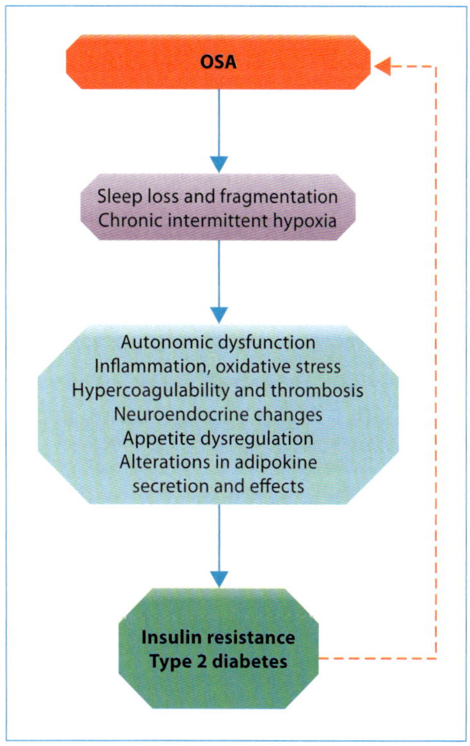

Fig. 21. Schematic description of potential mechanisms linking OSA, chronic intermittent hypoxia, sleep loss and fragmentation, and alterations in glucose metabolism.

2.5 Conclusion

Recent research provides strong evidence that there is an increased risk of alterations in glucose metabolism in OSA patients, including insulin resistance, glucose intolerance and diabetes mellitus (fig. 21). Such alterations may contribute to the development of cardiovascular diseases associated with OSA. Although the cause-and-effect relationships between OSA and diabetes remain to be fully established,

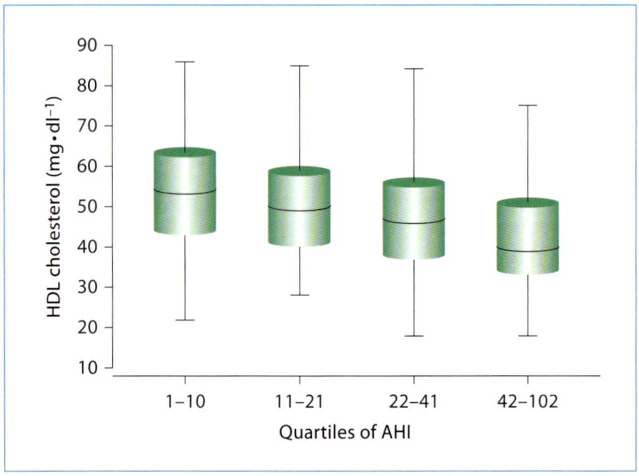

Fig. 22. Distribution of HDL cholesterol (n = 366, $p < 0.001$) in different quartiles of the AHI in OSA patients. After Börgel et al. [273], with permission. © European Respiratory Society.

recommendations have been published to adopt clinical practices to ensure that a patient presenting with one condition is considered for the other (table 4).

3 Dyslipidemia and Obstructive Sleep Apnea

Chronic intermittent hypoxia is associated with dyslipidemia in rodent models [267–270]; however, it is unclear whether OSA, and especially chronic intermittent hypoxia associated with OSA, is a risk factor for dyslipidemia in humans. Extensive reviews devoted to this topic have recently been published [271, 272].

3.1 Population and Clinical Studies of the Link between Obstructive Sleep Apnea and Dyslipidemia

Data from the Sleep Heart Health Study indicated that total cholesterol levels were positively associated with the RDI in men, after adjusting for age and BMI [16]. In women, high-density lipoprotein (HDL) cholesterol levels were inversely associated and triglyceride levels were positively associated with the RDI. It is suggested that obesity alone does not explain the association between dyslipidemia and OSA. A significant association between the AHI and serum HDL cholesterol levels was observed in OSA patients (n = 366), independent of age, sex, BMI, diabetes and lipid-lowering medication (fig. 22) [273]. There were no independent associations with total cholesterol, triglyceride and low-density lipoprotein (LDL) cholesterol serum levels. The majority of the other clinical studies addressing the link between OSA and dyslipidemia have included a much lower number of participants. Compared with non-OSA subjects, these studies have shown lipid level abnormalities in OSA patients (including lower serum HDL cholesterol levels), independently of confounders [112, 192, 274], and higher serum triglyceride levels [96, 275]. In addition, a higher total cholesterol-to-HDL ratio [96, 192] and higher serum total cholesterol levels were observed in OSA patients [112]. Obese patients with OSA exhibiting nocturnal oxyhemoglobin desaturation had higher plasma triglyceride and LDL cholesterol levels than subjects without hypoxemia [270]. Compared with nondesaturating OSA patients, these patients presented with higher levels of a hepatic enzyme for lipoprotein secretion, coenzyme A desaturase 1; the levels of this enzyme correlated with the degree of nocturnal hypoxemia ($r = 0.68$; $p = 0.001$). Conversely, other authors have not observed abnormal lipid levels in OSA patients [195, 274].

OSA may also alter the function of HDL. OSA patients ($n = 128$) had increased levels of oxidized LDL and total 8-isoprostane plasma levels, and a decreased ability of HDL to inhibit LDL oxidation ex vivo, compared with control subjects [276]. The AHI was the main determinant of HDL dysfunction. These observations suggest that HDL may be dysfunctional in OSA patients, partly contributing to their increased cardiovascular risk.

3.2 *Effects of Continuous Positive Airway Pressure Administration on Dyslipidemia*

Effective bilevel or CPAP therapy significantly increased the mean HDL cholesterol serum levels by approximately 5.8% within 6 months of treatment [273]. An independent relationship was found between the change in the AHI and the change in HDL cholesterol or triglyceride levels. Significant decreases in the levels of total cholesterol ($p = 0.021$), the ratio of total cholesterol to HDL cholesterol ($p = 0.018$) and the ratio of apolipoprotein A–I to B ($p = 0.021$) were observed in patients who complied with their CPAP treatment for 4 h or more per night [277]. No significant changes were observed in patients with poor compliance with CPAP therapy (<4 $h \bullet night^{-1}$) or who refused the treatment (fig. 23). Similar findings were reported by other authors [220]. Randomized studies have been used to assess the effects of CPAP administration on serum lipid levels, e.g. the effects of effective versus subtherapeutic CPAP administration for 1 month were assessed in 220 OSA patients [278]. A trend toward a significant fall in total cholesterol was observed in patients treated with therapeutic CPAP ($p = 0.06$) compared with those who received subtherapeutic CPAP. In the therapeutic group, there was a clinically significant mean fall of 0.28 $mmol \bullet l^{-1}$ in total cholesterol levels (95% CI 0.11–0.45; $p = 0.001$). However, in a randomized controlled study of effective CPAP versus sham CPAP administration for 6 weeks ($n = 34$), there was no CPAP-induced change in lipid levels [233]. It is of note that subjects who received CPAP first spent significantly more time on CPAP than the subtherapeutic alternative [3.9 (0–6.2) vs. 1.9 $h \bullet night^{-1}$ (0–5.5); $p < 0.01$]. Conversely, subjects who received CPAP second used each treatment for a similar length of time [4 (0–7.4) for active CPAP vs. 3.3 $h \bullet night^{-1}$ (0–7.5) for subtherapeutic CPAP; $p < 0.22$]. In addition, no significant treatment effect on serum lipid levels was observed in 2 randomized studies that assessed the effects of CPAP treatment versus no treatment in a small number of OSA participants for

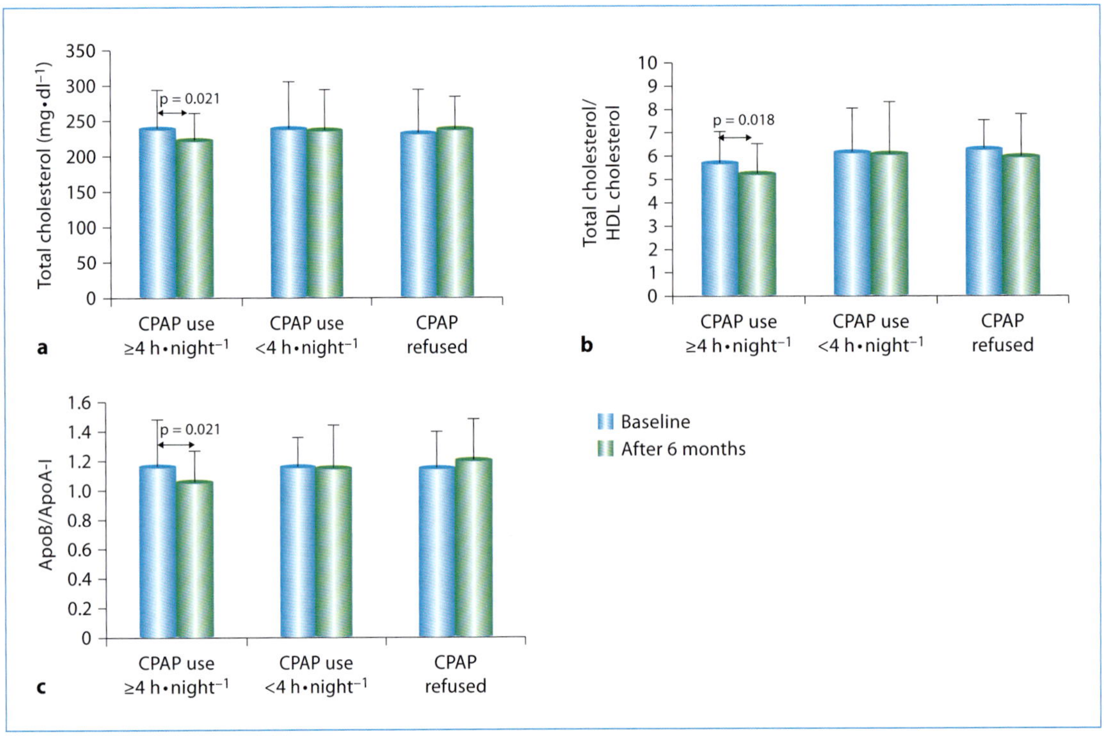

Fig. 23. Changes in total cholesterol levels (**a**), total cholesterol/HDL cholesterol ratio (**b**), and the apolipoprotein (Apo) B/ApoA–I ratio (**c**) in OSA patients who have either adhered to ≥4 h•night^{-1} CPAP therapy (n = 20), adhered to <4 h•night^{-1} CPAP therapy (n = 19) or refused CPAP therapy (n = 14) over 6 months. After Steiropoulos et al. [277], with permission.

4 weeks (n = 13, mean compliance with CPAP therapy was 5.53 h•night^{-1}) [234] and 4 months in 24 patients compliant with CPAP treatment (CPAP was used for 6 ± 0.6 h•night^{-1}, range 5–6.6) [279].

3.3 Conclusion

Overall, methodological biases have made the interpretation of studies assessing the relationship between OSA and dyslipidemia difficult [272]. These biases include the presence of confounders such as obesity, short study duration, inadequate power and lack of controls. Some studies suggest that OSA may be associated with a decrease in serum HDL cholesterol levels and an increase in serum triglyceride levels [16, 192, 280], but not with abnormal serum levels of total and LDL cholesterol [272]. Only 1 randomized study [278] has reported a significant decrease in serum total cholesterol levels after CPAP, whereas the others [233, 234, 279] have shown no significant changes in serum lipid levels after CPAP administration. Therefore, it remains to be determined whether OSA is a risk factor for dyslipidemia and whether CPAP administration (in compliant patients) alleviates dyslipidemia.

4 Metabolic Syndrome and Obstructive Sleep Apnea

The association of OSA and metabolic syndrome has been termed 'syndrome Z' [281]. It has been suggested that OSA is a manifestation of metabolic syndrome [282–284]; indeed, both conditions share common intermediate pathogenic pathways including alterations in the regulation of the autonomic nervous system, increased inflammatory activity, alterations in adipokine levels and endothelial dysfunction [189, 190, 285]. These mechanisms may be involved in the interplay between these 2 conditions. Extensive reviews devoted to this topic have recently been published [147, 148, 189, 190, 271, 286, 287].

4.1 Definition and Prevalence of Metabolic Syndrome

Metabolic syndrome is composed of risk factors for cardiovascular disorders and type 2 diabetes mellitus. It refers to the association of the 5 following components: obesity (especially central adiposity), raised blood pressure, elevated glucose and triglyceride levels, and low HDL cholesterol levels [288]. It is considered to predict diabetes and cardiovascular diseases better than any of its individual components [288, 289]. Although it is beyond the scope of this chapter to review evidence for the usefulness of considering metabolic syndrome as a specific entity [288, 289], it is of note that this has been questioned by some authors [290–292].

Several definitions of metabolic syndrome have been proposed. In 1998, the WHO definition required a glucose tolerance test or a measure of insulin resistance using clamp studies as an essential part of its diagnosis [293]. According to the National Cholesterol Education Program (NCEP) Adult Treatment Panel III (ATP III) [294], the diagnosis of metabolic syndrome required the presence of 3 of the following 5 factors: abdominal obesity, elevated triglycerides, reduced HDL cholesterol, elevated blood pressure and elevated fasting glucose (the demonstration of insulin resistance was not required). In 2005, the International Diabetes Federation proposed a definition that was similar to that of the ATP III, but used cutoff values for waist circumference that differed according to ethnicity [289, 295]. In 2009, several professional organizations published a joint paper in an attempt to unify the diagnostic criteria [288], in which the association of 5 components was assessed, where 3 abnormal findings out of 5 were sufficient for the diagnosis of metabolic syndrome. A single threshold value was defined for each of the 4 following components: raised blood pressure, raised triglycerides, lowered HDL cholesterol and raised fasting glucose (table 11). The fifth component, visceral obesity, is assessed by measuring waist circumference (fig. 3) and classed using national or regional cutoff points (table 12) [288].

Metabolic syndrome is common. Its prevalence varies between populations and is increasing in developed and developing countries, as observed for obesity [285, 296–298]. For example, using the NCEP ATP III definition, the age-adjusted prevalence of metabolic syndrome in the USA was (mean ± SE) 34.6 ± 0.9% (men,

Table 11. Criteria for the clinical diagnosis of metabolic syndrome according to the International Diabetes Federation Task Force on Epidemiology and Prevention

Measure	Categorical cutoff points
Raised triglycerides	≥150 mg • dl^{-1} (1.7 mmol • l^{-1})
Lowered HDL cholesterol	<40 mg • dl^{-1} (1.0 mmol • l^{-1}) in males; <50 mg • dl^{-1} (1.3 mmol • l^{-1}) in females
Raised fasting glucose	≥100 mg • dl^{-1}
Raised blood pressure	systolic ≥130 and/or diastolic ≥85 mm Hg
Increased waist circumference	population- and country-specific definitions

Three abnormal findings out of 5 would qualify a person for metabolic syndrome. Triglycerides: drug treatment for raised triglycerides is an alternate indicator; HDL cholesterol: drug treatment for lowered HDL cholesterol is an alternate indicator. The most commonly used drugs for raised triglycerides and lowered HDL cholesterol are fibrates and nicotinic acid. A patient taking 1 of these drugs can be presumed to have high triglycerides and low HDL cholesterol. Similarly, the taking of high-dose ω-3 fatty acids presumes high triglycerides. Glucose: drug treatment for raised glucose is an alternate indicator. Following the proposed criteria, most patients with type 2 diabetes mellitus will have metabolic syndrome. Blood pressure: antihypertensive drug treatment in a patient with a history of hypertension is an alternate indicator; waist circumference: it is recommended that the International Diabetes Federation cutoff points be used for non-Europeans and either theirs or the cutoff points of the American Heart Association/National Heart, Lung and Blood Institute be used for people of European origin until more data become available. The International Diabetes Federation Task Force was comprised of experts from the National Heart, Lung and Blood Institute, the American Heart Association, the World Heart Federation, the International Atherosclerosis Society and the International Association for the Study of Obesity. After Alberti et al. [288], with permission.

34.4 ± 1.5%; women, 34.5 ± 1.4%) [298]. In Europe, using a modification of the WHO definition, the age-standardized prevalence of metabolic syndrome was slightly higher in men (15.7%) than in women (14.2%) [299]. These epidemiological data show how this major cardiometabolic risk factor is a burden for patients and society.

4.2 *Obstructive Sleep Apnea and the Risk for Metabolic Syndrome*

4.2.1 Prevalence of Metabolic Syndrome in Obstructive Sleep Apnea Patients

The association between SDB and the prevalence of metabolic syndrome (defined using the NCEP definition) was examined in a subset of participants from the Wisconsin Sleep Cohort Study [283]. Compared with those with an AHI <5, the age- and sex-adjusted ORs of metabolic syndrome associated with mild and moderate-to-severe SDB were 4.0 (95% CI 2.6–6.3) and 5.3 (95% CI 3.2–8.8), respectively. These associations were weaker after adjusting for BMI, but they remained statistically significant. It is suggested that SDB may be considered as an integral component of metabolic

Table 12. Current recommended waist circumference thresholds for abdominal obesity, by organization

Population	Organization	Men, cm	Women, cm
Europid	IDF [295]	≥94	≥80
Caucasian	WHO [350]	≥94 (increased risk) ≥102 (still higher risk)	≥80 (increased risk) ≥88 cm (still higher risk)
USA	AHA/NHLBI (ATP III)[1] [351]	≥102	≥88
Canada	Health Canada [352, 353]	≥102	≥88
Europe	European Cardiovascular Societies [354]	≥102	≥88
Asia (including Japan)	IDF [295]	≥90	≥80
Asia	WHO [355]	≥90	≥80
Japan	Japanese Obesity Society [356]	≥85	≥90
China	Cooperative Task Force [357]	≥85	≥80
Middle East, Mediterranean	IDF [295]	≥94	≥80
Sub-Saharan Africa	IDF [295]	≥94	≥80
Ethnic Central and South America	IDF [295]	≥90	≥80

IDF = International Diabetes Federation; AHA/NHLBI = American Heart Association/National Heart, Lung and Blood Institute. After Alberti et al. [288], with permission. © 2009 American Heart Association Inc.

[1] Recent AHA/NHLBI guidelines for metabolic syndrome recognize an increased risk for cardiovascular disease and diabetes at waist circumference thresholds of ≥94 cm in men and ≥80 cm in women, and identify these as optional cutoff points for individuals or populations with increased insulin resistance.

syndrome. Two studies [192, 202], in which the NCEP ATP III metabolic syndrome definition was used, reported that an AHI >5 [202] and an AHI >15 [192] were significantly associated with a 5- [202] and 9-fold [192] increased risk for metabolic syndrome, respectively. OSA was associated with a 6-fold increased risk for metabolic syndrome when the International Diabetes Federation metabolic syndrome definition was used [300]. OSA was independently associated with metabolic syndrome in men, but not in women when the metabolic syndrome diagnostic criteria for the Japanese population were used [301]. Men with OSA (AHI ≥5) had a higher risk of metabolic syndrome compared with control subjects (OR 3.47; 95% CI 1.84–6.53). In a retrospective examination of the records of 250 consecutive patients referred for the evaluation of OSA, the frequency of metabolic syndrome was significantly greater in patients with OSA than in those without OSA (60 vs. 40%, respectively; $p = 0.004$) [302]. Conversely, obesity, and not OSA, is associated with metabolic abnormalities [139] or the presence of metabolic syndrome [303].

Overall, these studies suggest that OSA is a risk factor for metabolic syndrome.

4.2.2 Effects of Obstructive Sleep Apnea on the Early Signs of Atherosclerosis in Metabolic Syndrome Patients

When the relative impact of OSA on the development of atherosclerosis was assessed in consecutive metabolic syndrome patients (n = 81), those with OSA (AHI ≥15) had higher levels of carotid intima-media thickness, carotid-femoral pulse wave velocity and carotid artery diameter than metabolic syndrome patients without OSA (AHI <15; fig. 24) [304]. AHI was independently associated with all of the studied vascular parameters, suggesting that OSA has an additive effect on the development of atherosclerosis in metabolic syndrome patients. Moreover, vascular parameters did not significantly differ when metabolic syndrome patients with OSA were sleepy or not. These observations may suggest that metabolic syndrome patients should be routinely assessed for OSA, whether they have excessive daytime sleepiness or not [305]. Conversely, excessive daytime sleepiness was an independent predictor of carotid atherosclerosis in patients referred for sleep studies [306].

4.2.3 Effects of Continuous Positive Airway Pressure Administration on Metabolic Syndrome

In an observational study of patients with severe OSA and metabolic syndrome, 8 weeks of CPAP application (>4 h • night^{-1}) significantly reduced systolic and diastolic blood pressure, insulin resistance, systemic inflammation, oxidative stress and the global cardiovascular risk [220]. No significant changes were detected in patients who used CPAP for <4 h • night^{-1}. When cardiovascular and metabolic outcomes were assessed after 6 weeks of therapeutic and sham CPAP in 34 obese patients with OSA in a randomized, placebo-controlled, blinded crossover study, no significant changes to the levels of glucose, lipids and insulin resistance or the proportion of patients with metabolic syndrome were associated with CPAP administration [233]. To our knowledge, only 1 study has shown that treatment of OSA was associated with a significant reduction in the proportion of metabolic syndrome, where autoadjusting positive airway pressure administration was associated with an approximately 16% reduction in the frequency of metabolic syndrome, mainly in patients with less severe OSA and with a better therapeutic compliance [307].

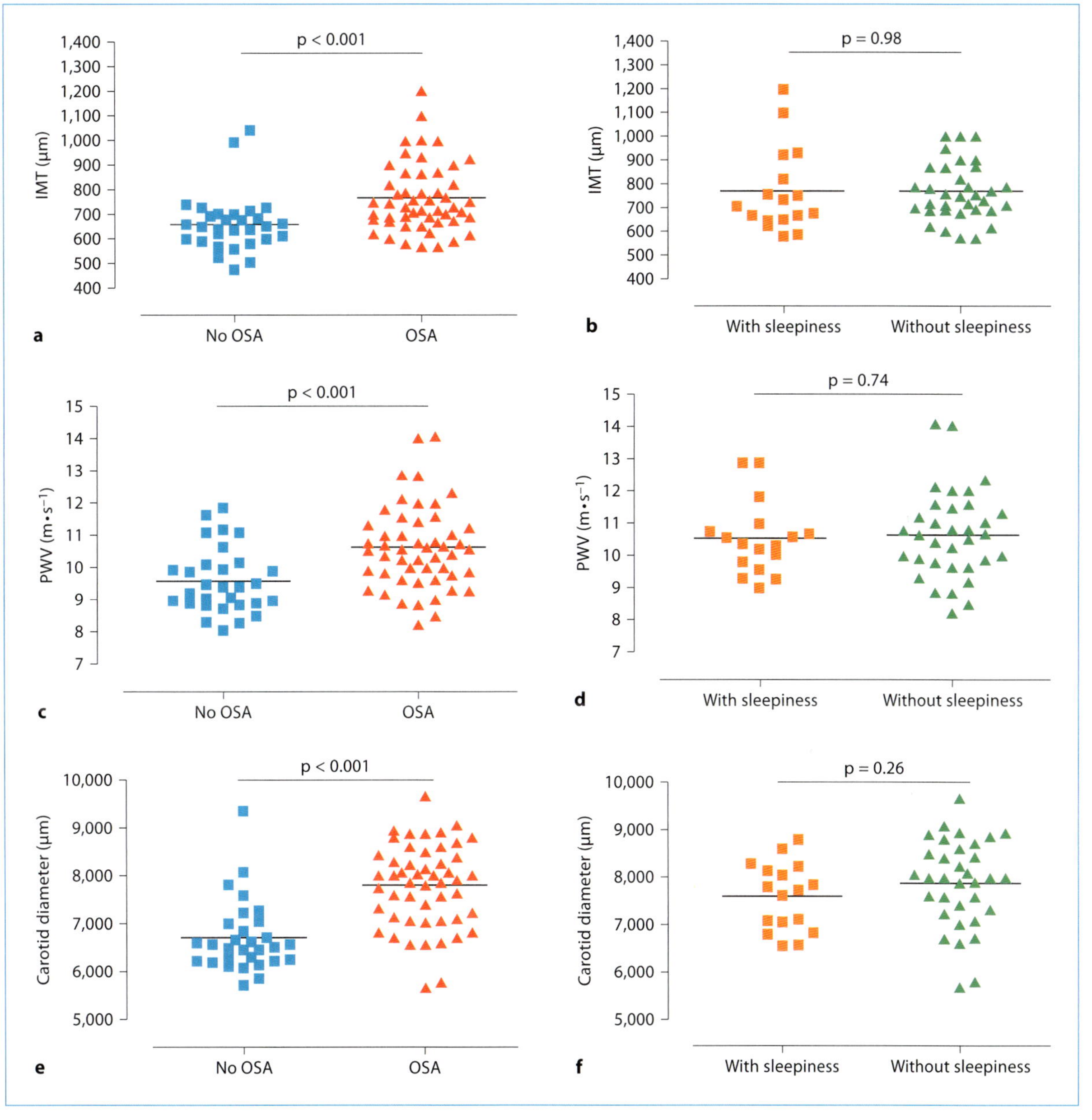

Fig. 24. Incremental role of OSA for markers of atherosclerosis in patients with metabolic syndrome. **a** Individual values of intima-media thickness (IMT) in metabolic syndrome patients without and with OSA. **c** Individual values of carotid-femoral pulse wave velocity (PWV) in metabolic syndrome patients without and with OSA. **e** Individual values of carotid artery diameter in metabolic syndrome patients without and with OSA. **b** Individual values of intima-media thickness in metabolic syndrome patients with OSA according to the presence or absence of subjective daytime sleepiness. **d** Individual values of carotid-femoral pulse wave velocity in metabolic syndrome patients with OSA according to the presence or absence of subjective daytime sleepiness. **f** Individual values of carotid artery diameter in metabolic syndrome patients with OSA according to the presence or absence of subjective daytime sleepiness. After Drager et al. [304], with permission.

Overall, the effects of CPAP administration on metabolic syndrome remain to be demonstrated.

4.3 Metabolic Syndrome and the Risk for Obstructive Sleep Apnea

The association between metabolic syndrome and OSA may be different for ethnic groups who have different definitions of metabolic syndrome [308]. A significant relationship between the severity of OSA and the prevalence of metabolic syndrome ($p < 0.001$) was detected in 275 Japanese men working for an urban company [303]; however, this association did not remain significant after adjusting for age and BMI. Severe OSA was 7.8 times more likely to be present in subjects with metabolic syndrome (16.2% of all 68 metabolic syndrome subjects) than in those without metabolic syndrome (2.4% of 207 non-metabolic-syndrome subjects; $p < 0.001$). The Berlin questionnaire [309], obesity and resistant hypertension were not reliable indicators of OSA in hypertensive patients due to either poor sensitivity or poor specificity; however, metabolic syndrome was associated with a high sensitivity and specificity for OSA (0.86 and 0.85, respectively) and was independently associated with OSA (OR 19.04; 95% CI 5.25–69.03) [310]. It is suggested that the presence of metabolic syndrome is an important marker for OSA among patients with hypertension.

4.4 Conclusion

OSA and metabolic syndrome frequently coexist. OSA may be a risk factor for the development or aggravation of metabolic syndrome. There is also compelling evidence demonstrating that metabolic syndrome is a strong predictor for OSA. These observations suggest that patients with metabolic syndrome should be routinely evaluated for OSA, whether they present with excessive daytime sleepiness or not [310].

5 Liver Injury and Obstructive Sleep Apnea

Nonalcoholic fatty liver disease (NAFLD) is a manifestation of metabolic syndrome (obesity, diabetes mellitus, hypertension and dyslipidemia are risk factors for NAFLD) [311–314]. NAFLD, metabolic syndrome and OSA frequently coexist [5, 272, 315, 316]. Several studies have provided evidence suggesting that OSA may contribute to the development and/or aggravation of NAFLD [196, 270, 271, 316–320].

5.1 Characteristics of Nonalcoholic Fatty Liver Disease

NAFLD is characterized by the accumulation of triglycerides in hepatocytes in the absence of excessive alcohol consumption or other known liver diseases. NAFLD includes a spectrum of diseases ranging from isolated fatty liver, nonalcoholic steatohepatitis (NASH) and fibrosis, and end-stage liver cirrhosis [313, 321–324]. A liver biopsy is the only reliable method to diagnose and stage NAFLD [325, 326]. The histopathological changes associated with NAFLD include simple fatty liver (hepatic steatosis), hepatocyte ballooning, lobular inflammation and lobular necrosis associated with hepatic steatosis, with or without fibrosis (NASH) and liver fibrosis.

5.2 *The 'Two-Hit' Theory*

A 'two-hit' theory has been proposed to explain the development of NAFLD [321]. The progression from a normal liver to hepatic steatosis is thought to be related to insulin resistance and triglyceride accumulation in hepatocytes (the 'first hit') [314], and the progression from steatosis to NASH is thought to be mediated by oxidative and cytokine-induced liver injury (the 'second hit') [321]. NASH develops in approximately 10–30% of NAFLD patients [321, 322, 327, 328; for a review of this subject, see 314].

5.3 *Obstructive Sleep Apnea and Liver Injury*

5.3.1 Hepatic Enzyme Levels in Obstructive Sleep Apnea

NAFLD may be associated with abnormal hepatic enzyme levels; however, normal hepatic enzyme levels do not rule out the diagnosis of NAFLD [196]. Several studies have reported increased plasma levels of hepatic enzymes in OSA [317, 318, 329–331]. For example, severe OSA (AHI >50) was an independent predictor of elevated liver enzymes (OR 5.9; 95% CI 1.2–29) [317]. In a cohort of morbidly obese patients requiring bariatric surgery (n = 62; BMI 47.8), OSA severity was a risk factor for elevated liver enzymes, but not for NASH [330]. In a retrospective case series of obese patients with OSA (n = 109), a significant correlation was observed between serum aminotransferase levels and the lowest Spo_2 level (r = –0.307 to –0.316) and the time below 90% saturation (r = 0.307–0.376), whereas there was no correlation with the AHI and BMI [331]. In patients with moderately severe OSA, nocturnal hypoxia explained a greater amount of variance in serum aminotransferase levels than did markers of metabolic syndrome. In contrast, other authors have not observed elevated liver enzyme levels in OSA patients [196, 332].

The effects of CPAP administration on liver enzyme levels are controversial. In an uncontrolled study, mean (±SD) aspartate aminotransferase levels were higher in the morning than in the previous afternoon (before sleep: 34 ± 20 $IU \bullet l^{-1}$; after sleep: 39 ± 28 $IU \bullet l^{-1}$; p = 0.006) [329]. After the first night of CPAP administration, the overnight increases in aspartate and alanine aminotransferase levels were significantly less marked (p = 0.0003 and p = 0.006, respectively). The effects of 4 weeks of CPAP administration on alanine and aspartate aminotransferase levels were observed in patients with moderate-to-severe OSA (n = 94) who were randomized for therapeutic or subtherapeutic CPAP treatment [320]. Alanine aminotransferase levels decreased in patients treated with therapeutic CPAP, but they also decreased in those treated with subtherapeutic CPAP (difference between mean changes: –3.4; 95% CI –7.8–1.0 $IU \bullet l^{-1}$; p = 0.13 between groups). Aspartate aminotransferase levels did not change significantly with therapeutic CPAP or with subtherapeutic CPAP, suggesting that 4 weeks of active CPAP had no beneficial effect on aminotransferase levels when compared with subtherapeutic CPAP in OSA patients.

Overall, it remains to be determined whether OSA is independently associated with abnormal plasma hepatic enzyme levels.

5.3.2 Histopathological Evidence Linking Obstructive Sleep Apnea and Nonalcoholic Fatty Liver Disease

Several authors have assessed the histopathological changes in the livers of obese patients with OSA and raised liver enzymes [317] or requiring bariatric surgery [196, 318, 333]. When 85 patients were assessed who had a liver biopsy performed at the time of obesity surgery (51% had OSA), a trend toward a higher prevalence of OSA was detected in those with evidence of progressive liver disease, as indicated by inflammation plus fibrosis (11/15; 73%), compared with those with inflammation alone (22/48; 46%; $p = 0.06$) [318]. The percentage of hepatic steatosis and the lobular necrosis score were positively correlated with the AHI, independently of age and BMI [317]. Hepatic immunostaining, used as an indirect marker of hypoxia, was not different between patients with or without severe OSA. The authors suggested that OSA may be a risk factor for liver injury, but did not provide evidence for a pathogenic role of chronic intermittent hypoxia in its development. Conversely, in individuals undergoing bariatric surgery, patients with NASH had significantly lower desaturation levels (77 vs. 85%; $p = 0.006$), lower mean nocturnal oxygen saturation levels (91 vs. 93%; $p = 0.05$), higher AHI (35 vs. 22; $p = 0.03$), higher RDI (46 vs. 21; $p = 0.02$) and a higher alanine aminotransferase/aspartate aminotransferase ratio (1.4 vs. 1.3, $p = 0.05$) than non-NASH control patients, respectively [333]. The lowest desaturation level was independently associated with histological NASH, while the lowest desaturation and mean nocturnal oxygen saturation levels were significantly lower in subjects with fibrosis. It is suggested that the frequent nocturnal hypoxic episodes in NAFLD patients may be a risk factor for developing NASH. Liver biopsies were obtained from 20 severely obese patients presenting for bariatric surgery ($n = 90$, without concomitant diabetes mellitus or a preexistent diagnosis of sleep apnea or liver disease), and OSA (RDI >5) was diagnosed in 81.1% of these patients [196]. It was suggested that significant nocturnal desaturation may predispose to hepatic inflammation, hepatocyte ballooning and liver fibrosis (fig. 25). In addition, oxygen desaturation levels greater than 4.6% were associated with a 1.5-fold increase in insulin resistance, assessed according to the HOMA index. There was no relationship between the RDI and insulin resistance or liver histopathology. It is suggested that the hypoxic stress of sleep apnea may be implicated in the development of insulin resistance and steatohepatitis in severe obesity.

Overall, these findings suggest that OSA may be a risk factor for NAFLD. Further investigations are required to determine whether OSA is an independent risk factor for NAFLD, and these investigations should also assess the effects of CPAP treatment on liver injury.

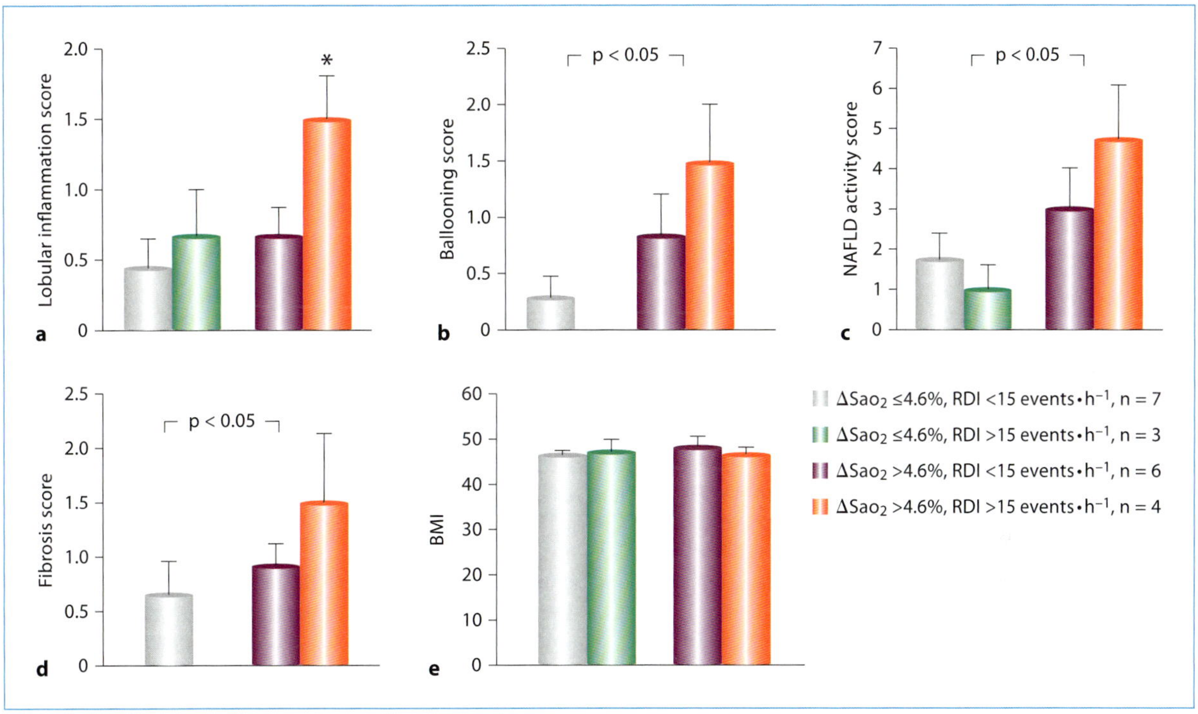

Fig. 25. Relationships between hepatic histopathology and the severity of OSA, as measured by the RDI (<15 or >15 events•h^{-1}) and the average fall in oxyhemoglobin saturation during apneic events (ΔSao_2 <4.6 and ≥4.6%). **a** Hepatic lobular inflammation score. **b** Hepatocyte ballooning score. **c** NAFLD activity score defined as the sum of steatosis, lobular inflammation and ballooning score [348]. **d** Hepatic fibrosis score. **e** BMI. * $p < 0.05$ between the group of patients with RDI <15 events•h^{-1} and ΔSao_2 <4.6% and the group of patients with RDI >15 events•h^{-1} and ΔSao_2 ≥4.6%. After Polotsky et al. [196]. Reprinted with permission of the American Thoracic Society. © American Thoracic Society.

5.3.3 Is Liver Injury in Obstructive Sleep Apnea Consistent with the 'Two-Hit' Theory?

Intermediate mechanisms that may lead to the development or aggravation of NAFLD appear to be present in OSA patients, especially in those who are obese. In addition, evidence suggests that OSA may be associated with an increased risk for insulin resistance (see above). Furthermore, the dyslipidemia observed in OSA may be similar to that observed in NAFLD, e.g. decreased HDL cholesterol and increased triglyceride levels [314, 334, 335]. Finally, OSA is associated with increased inflammatory and oxidative activities [see chapter 2, this vol., pp. 43–66]. The interplay between the mechanisms for these conditions has been studied in animal models. For example, a mouse model was developed to assess the relationship between chronic intermittent hypoxia, diet and NAFLD [269, 319, 336]. Chronic intermittent hypoxia was demonstrated to lead to mild liver injury, but not to NASH, in the absence of obesity [319], and that lobular inflammation, fibrosis and lipid peroxidation in the liver occurred only in mice pretreated with a high-fat, high-cholesterol diet. It is hypothesized that the 'first hit' may be related

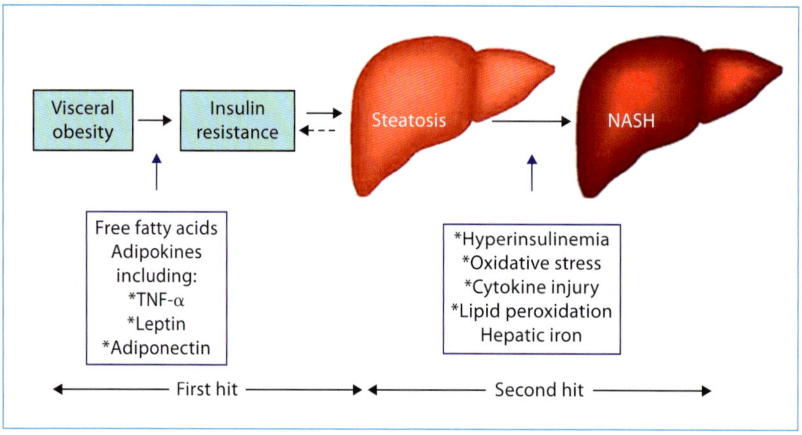

Fig. 26. Mechanisms by which OSA may influence the development of NAFLD. This figure represents a scheme for the pathogenesis of steatosis and steatohepatitis. The 'two-hit' theory has been proposed to explain the evolution of NAFLD [321]. The 'first hit' is the result of insulin resistance and triglyceride accumulation in hepatocytes. Insulin resistance may be due to visceral obesity and adipokine secretion; it has also been considered to be the consequence of NAFLD (dashed arrow) [314]. The 'second hit' may be the result of oxidative stress, which may produce liver inflammation and fibrosis. Asterisks indicate variables that are presumed to be altered by OSA and thus contribute to the development and/or aggravation of NAFLD. Reprinted from Shifflet and Wu [313] with permission from Elsevier.

to severe obesity, which may contribute to the progression of a normal liver to hepatic steatosis, and the 'second hit' may be due to the chronic intermittent hypoxia of OSA, which may contribute to the progression of hepatic steatosis to NASH [196]. However, it remains to be demonstrated whether this occurs in OSA patients [for a review, see 271].

5.4 Conclusion

Research on the link between OSA and NAFLD is at a very early stage, and it remains to be demonstrated whether OSA is a risk factor for NAFLD. Obesity may be responsible for the progression from a normal liver to hepatic steatosis, whereas the chronic intermittent hypoxia associated with OSA may contribute to the tendency toward NASH in some patients (fig. 26).

NAFLD has been hypothesized to be an independent risk factor for cardiovascular disorders and type 2 diabetes mellitus [for a review, see 337–340]. If this is so, NAFLD may then be another confounding variable in OSA, making it even more difficult to assess the link between OSA and cardiovascular and metabolic diseases.

6 Conclusion and Future Perspectives

Compelling evidence links OSA and metabolic disorders. To date, only one causal link has been definitely established, obesity, which is the strongest risk factor for

OSA. Metabolic syndrome is also very likely to be an independent risk factor for OSA. Conversely, OSA itself may be a risk factor for insulin resistance/diabetes mellitus and metabolic syndrome that, in turn, may increase the risk for OSA. It remains to be determined whether OSA is associated with dyslipidemia or NAFLD.

The interplay between OSA and metabolic disorders raises numerous pathophysiological, diagnostic and prognostic issues. Common intermediate mechanisms are activated by OSA and metabolic disorders. An important milestone would be to identify which intermediate pathways specifically contribute to the adverse effects of these conditions. Assessing overnight changes in relevant biomarkers across the sleep period has been proposed as an optimal strategy to address this issue [147].

Further research and guidelines are still needed to: (1) more specifically define diagnostic strategies according to clinical, biological and genetic profiles; (2) identify which patients are likely to develop specific adverse metabolic effects related to OSA, and (3) quantify the possible synergistic adverse effects of metabolic disorders on cardiovascular disorders associated with OSA [147].

Clinical practice recommendations have been published for the diagnosis of OSA in patients with diabetes mellitus and metabolic syndrome, and for the diagnosis of cardiovascular and metabolic risk in OSA patients (table 4). Awareness of OSA-related issues in patients with metabolic disorders may be improved in: (1) physicians, by enhancing medical education; (2) patients, by enhancing their education and support, and (3) in the public, by improving available information (using the lay press, internet resources etc.) [341]. Although our knowledge as to the nature and causes of OSA has progressed over the last 2 decades, a considerable amount of work remains to be done.

7 References

1 Pillar G, Shehadeh N: Abdominal fat and sleep apnea: the chicken or the egg? Diabetes Care 2008;31(suppl 2):S303–S309.

2 Vgontzas AN: Does obesity play a major role in the pathogenesis of sleep apnoea and its associated manifestations via inflammation, visceral adiposity, and insulin resistance? Arch Physiol Biochem 2008; 114:211–223.

3 Schwartz AR, Patil SP, Laffan AM, Polotsky V, Schneider H, Smith PL: Obesity and obstructive sleep apnea: pathogenic mechanisms and therapeutic approaches. Proc Am Thorac Soc 2008;5:185–192.

4 Shah N, Roux F: The relationship of obesity and obstructive sleep apnea. Clin Chest Med 2009;30: 455–465, vii.

5 Dempsey JA, Veasey SC, Morgan BJ, O'Donnell CP: Pathophysiology of sleep apnea. Physiol Rev 2010; 90:47–112.

6 Schwartz AR, Patil SP, Squier S, Schneider H, Kirkness JP, Smith PL: Obesity and upper airway control during sleep. J Appl Physiol 2010;108: 430–435.

7 World Health Organization: Global database on body mass index. 2010. http://apps.who.int/bmi/index.jsp.

8 McClean KM, Kee F, Young IS, Elborn JS: Obesity and the lung. 1. Epidemiology. Thorax 2008;63:649–654.

9 Ogden CL, Fryar CD, Carroll MD, Flegal KM: Mean body weight, height, and body mass index, United States 1960–2002. Adv Data 2004;347:1–17.

10 Charles MA, Eschwege E, Basdevant A: Monitoring the obesity epidemic in France: the Obepi surveys 1997–2006. Obesity (Silver Spring) 2008;16:2182–2186.

11 Ogden CL, Carroll MD, Curtin LR, McDowell MA, Tabak CJ, Flegal KM: Prevalence of overweight and obesity in the United States, 1999–2004. JAMA 2006;295:1549–1555.

12 Flegal KM, Carroll MD, Ogden CL, Curtin LR: Prevalence and trends in obesity among US adults, 1999–2008. JAMA 2010;303:235–241.

13 Young T, Palta M, Dempsey J, Skatrud J, Weber S, Badr S: The occurrence of sleep-disordered breathing among middle-aged adults. N Engl J Med 1993; 328:1230–1235.

14 Nieto FJ, Young TB, Lind BK, Shahar E, Samet JM, Redline S, D'Agostino RB, Newman AB, Lebowitz MD, Pickering TG: Association of sleep-disordered breathing, sleep apnea, and hypertension in a large community-based study. Sleep Heart Health Study. JAMA 2000;283:1829–1836.

15 Peppard PE, Young T, Palta M, Dempsey J, Skatrud J: Longitudinal study of moderate weight change and sleep-disordered breathing. JAMA 2000;284: 3015–3021.

16 Newman AB, Nieto FJ, Guidry U, Lind BK, Redline S, Pickering TG, Quan SF: Relation of sleep-disordered breathing to cardiovascular disease risk factors: the Sleep Heart Health Study. Am J Epidemiol 2001;154:50–59.

17 Foster GD, Sanders MH, Millman R, Zammit G, Borradaile KE, Newman AB, Wadden TA, Kelley D, Wing RR, Sunyer FX, Darcey V, Kuna ST: Obstructive sleep apnea among obese patients with type 2 diabetes. Diabetes Care 2009;32:1017–1019.

18 Young T, Peppard PE, Taheri S: Excess weight and sleep-disordered breathing. J Appl Physiol 2005;99: 1592–1599.

19 Newman AB, Foster G, Givelber R, Nieto FJ, Redline S, Young T: Progression and regression of sleep-disordered breathing with changes in weight: the Sleep Heart Health Study. Arch Intern Med 2005; 165:2408–2413.

20 Young T, Peppard PE, Gottlieb DJ: Epidemiology of obstructive sleep apnea: a population health perspective. Am J Respir Crit Care Med 2002;165:1217–1239.

21 Grunstein RR, Stenlof K, Hedner JA, Peltonen M, Karason K, Sjostrom L: Two year reduction in sleep apnea symptoms and associated diabetes incidence after weight loss in severe obesity. Sleep 2007;30:703–710.

22 Lam B, Sam K, Mok WY, Cheung MT, Fong DY, Lam JC, Lam DC, Yam LY, Ip MS: Randomised study of three non-surgical treatments in mild to moderate obstructive sleep apnoea. Thorax 2007;62: 354–359.

23 Foster GD, Borradaile KE, Sanders MH, Millman R, Zammit G, Newman AB, Wadden TA, Kelley D, Wing RR, Pi-Sunyer FX, Reboussin D, Kuna ST: A randomized study on the effect of weight loss on obstructive sleep apnea among obese patients with type 2 diabetes: the Sleep AHEAD study. Arch Intern Med 2009;169:1619–1626.

24 Johansson K, Neovius M, Lagerros YT, Harlid R, Rossner S, Granath F, Hemmingsson E: Effect of a very low energy diet on moderate and severe obstructive sleep apnoea in obese men: a randomised controlled trial. BMJ 2009;339:b4609.

25 Tuomilehto HP, Seppa JM, Partinen MM, Peltonen M, Gylling H, Tuomilehto JO, Vanninen EJ, Kokkarinen J, Sahlman JK, Martikainen T, Soini EJ, Randell J, Tukiainen H, Uusitupa M: Lifestyle intervention with weight reduction: first-line treatment in mild obstructive sleep apnea. Am J Respir Crit Care Med 2009;179:320–327.

26 Tuomilehto H, Gylling H, Peltonen M, Martikainen T, Sahlman J, Kokkarinen J, Randell J, Tukiainen H, Vanninen E, Partinen M, Tuomilehto J, Uusitupa M, Seppa J: Sustained improvement in mild obstructive sleep apnea after a diet- and physical activity-based lifestyle intervention: postinterventional follow-up. Am J Clin Nutr 2010;92:688–696.

27 Buchwald H, Avidor Y, Braunwald E, Jensen MD, Pories W, Fahrbach K, Schoelles K: Bariatric surgery: a systematic review and meta-analysis. JAMA 2004;292:1724–1737.

28 Greenburg DL, Lettieri CJ, Eliasson AH: Effects of surgical weight loss on measures of obstructive sleep apnea: a meta-analysis. Am J Med 2009;122: 535–542.

29 Mokhlesi B, Gozal D: Update in sleep medicine 2009. Am J Respir Crit Care Med 2010;181:545–549.

30 Jordan AS, McEvoy RD: Gender differences in sleep apnea: epidemiology, clinical presentation and pathogenic mechanisms. Sleep Med Rev 2003;7:377–389.

31 Bixler EO, Vgontzas AN, Lin HM, Ten Have T, Rein J, Vela-Bueno A, Kales A: Prevalence of sleep-disordered breathing in women: effects of gender. Am J Respir Crit Care Med 2001;163:608–613.

32 Millman RP, Carlisle CC, McGarvey ST, Eveloff SE, Levinson PD: Body fat distribution and sleep apnea severity in women. Chest 1995;107:362–366.

33 Shinohara E, Kihara S, Yamashita S, Yamane M, Nishida M, Arai T, Kotani K, Nakamura T, Takemura K, Matsuzawa Y: Visceral fat accumulation as an important risk factor for obstructive sleep apnoea syndrome in obese subjects. J Intern Med 1997;241: 11–18.

34 Vgontzas AN, Papanicolaou DA, Bixler EO, Hopper K, Lotsikas A, Lin HM, Kales A, Chrousos GP: Sleep apnea and daytime sleepiness and fatigue: relation to visceral obesity, insulin resistance, and hypercytokinemia. J Clin Endocrinol Metab 2000;85:1151–1158.

35 Schafer H, Pauleit D, Sudhop T, Gouni-Berthold I, Ewig S, Berthold HK: Body fat distribution, serum leptin, and cardiovascular risk factors in men with obstructive sleep apnea. Chest 2002;122:829–839.

36 Vgontzas AN, Zoumakis E, Bixler EO, Lin HM, Collins B, Basta M, Pejovic S, Chrousos GP: Selective effects of CPAP on sleep apnoea-associated manifestations. Eur J Clin Invest 2008;38:585–595.

37 Soriano-Co M, Vanhecke TE, Franklin BA, Sangal RB, Hakmeh B, McCullough PA: Increased central adiposity in morbidly obese patients with obstructive sleep apnea. Intern Med J 2011;41:560–566.

38 Stauffer JL, Buick MK, Bixler EO, Sharkey FE, Abt AB, Manders EK, Kales A, Cadieux RJ, Barry JD, Zwillich CW: Morphology of the uvula in obstructive sleep apnea. Am Rev Respir Dis 1989;140:724–728.

39 Schwab RJ: Upper airway imaging. Clin Chest Med 1998;19:33–54.

40 Shelton KE, Gay SB, Hollowell DE, Woodson H, Suratt PM: Mandible enclosure of upper airway and weight in obstructive sleep apnea. Am Rev Respir Dis 1993;148:195–200.

41 Schwab RJ, Gupta KB, Gefter WB, Metzger LJ, Hoffman EA, Pack AI: Upper airway and soft tissue anatomy in normal subjects and patients with sleep-disordered breathing: significance of the lateral pharyngeal walls. Am J Respir Crit Care Med 1995; 152:1673–1689.

42 Mortimore IL, Marshall I, Wraith PK, Sellar RJ, Douglas NJ: Neck and total body fat deposition in nonobese and obese patients with sleep apnea compared with that in control subjects. Am J Respir Crit Care Med 1998;157:280–283.

43 Schwab RJ, Kuna ST, Remmers JE: Anatomy and physiology of upper airway obstruction; in Kryger MH, Roth T, Dement WC (eds): Principles and Practice of Sleep Medicine, ed 4 online. Philadelphia, Saunders, 2005, pp 983–1000.

44 Schwab RJ, Gefter WB, Hoffman EA, Gupta KB, Pack AI: Dynamic upper airway imaging during awake respiration in normal subjects and patients with sleep disordered breathing. Am Rev Respir Dis 1993;148:1385–1400.

45 Whittle AT, Marshall I, Mortimore IL, Wraith PK, Sellar RJ, Douglas NJ: Neck soft tissue and fat distribution: comparison between normal men and women by magnetic resonance imaging. Thorax 1999;54:323–328.

46 Schwab RJ, Pasirstein M, Pierson R, Mackley A, Hachadoorian R, Arens R, Maislin G, Pack AI: Identification of upper airway anatomic risk factors for obstructive sleep apnea with volumetric magnetic resonance imaging. Am J Respir Crit Care Med 2003;168:522–530.

47 Schwab RJ: Genetic determinants of upper airway structures that predispose to obstructive sleep apnea. Respir Physiol Neurobiol 2005;147:289–298.

48 Gold AR, Schwartz AR: The pharyngeal critical pressure: the whys and hows of using nasal continuous positive airway pressure diagnostically. Chest 1996;110:1077–1088.

49 Boudewyns A, Punjabi N, Van de Heyning PH, De Backer WA, O'Donnell CP, Schneider H, Smith PL, Schwartz AR: Abbreviated method for assessing upper airway function in obstructive sleep apnea. Chest 2000;118:1031–1041.

50 Isono S, Remmers JE, Tanaka A, Sho Y, Sato J, Nishino T: Anatomy of pharynx in patients with obstructive sleep apnea and in normal subjects. J Appl Physiol 1997;82:1319–1326.

51 Eastwood PR, Szollosi I, Platt PR, Hillman DR: Comparison of upper airway collapse during general anaesthesia and sleep. Lancet 2002;359:1207–1209.

52 Eastwood PR, Szollosi I, Platt PR, Hillman DR: Collapsibility of the upper airway during anesthesia with isoflurane. Anesthesiology 2002;97:786–793.

53 Oliven A, Aspandiarov E, Gankin I, Gaitini L, Tov N: Collapsibility of the relaxed pharynx and risk of sleep apnoea. Eur Respir J 2008;32:1309–1315.

54 Patil SP, Schneider H, Marx JJ, Gladmon E, Schwartz AR, Smith PL: Neuromechanical control of upper airway patency during sleep. J Appl Physiol 2007; 102:547–556.

55 Schwartz AR, Gold AR, Schubert N, Stryzak A, Wise RA, Permutt S, Smith PL: Effect of weight loss on upper airway collapsibility in obstructive sleep apnea. Am Rev Respir Dis 1991;144:494–498.

56 Simpson L, Mukherjee S, Cooper MN, Ward KL, Lee JD, Fedson AC, Potter J, Hillman DR, Eastwood P, Palmer LJ, Kirkness J: Sex differences in the association of regional fat distribution with the severity of obstructive sleep apnea. Sleep 2010;33:467–474.

57 Jordan AS, Wellman A, Edwards JK, Schory K, Dover L, MacDonald M, Patel SR, Fogel RB, Malhotra A, White DP. Respiratory control stability and upper airway collapsibility in men and women with obstructive sleep apnea. J Appl Physiol 2005;99: 2020–2027.

58 Kirkness JP, Schwartz AR, Schneider H, Punjabi NM, Maly JJ, Laffan AM, McGinley BM, Magnuson T, Schweitzer M, Smith PL, Patil SP: Contribution of male sex, age, and obesity to mechanical instability of the upper airway during sleep. J Appl Physiol 2008;104:1618–1624.
59 Sharp JT, Henry JP, Sweany SK, Meadows WR, Pietras RJ: Effects of mass loading the respiratory system in man. J Appl Physiol 1964;19:959–966.
60 Van de Graaff WB: Thoracic influence on upper airway patency. J Appl Physiol 1988;65:2124–2131.
61 Van de Graaff WB: Thoracic traction on the trachea: mechanisms and magnitude. J Appl Physiol 1991;70:1328–1336.
62 Thut DC, Schwartz AR, Roach D, Wise RA, Permutt S, Smith PL: Tracheal and neck position influence upper airway airflow dynamics by altering airway length. J Appl Physiol 1993;75:2084–2090.
63 Kairaitis K, Byth K, Parikh R, Stavrinou R, Wheatley JR, Amis TC: Tracheal traction effects on upper airway patency in rabbits: the role of tissue pressure. Sleep 2007;30:179–186.
64 Rowley JA, Permutt S, Willey S, Smith PL, Schwartz AR: Effect of tracheal and tongue displacement on upper airway airflow dynamics. J Appl Physiol 1996;80:2171–2178.
65 Schwartz AR, Rowley JA, Thut DC, Permutt S, Smith PL: Structural basis for alterations in upper airway collapsibility. Sleep 1996;19:S184–S188.
66 Begle RL, Badr S, Skatrud JB, Dempsey JA: Effect of lung inflation on pulmonary resistance during NREM sleep. Am Rev Respir Dis 1990;141:854–860.
67 Series F, Cormier Y, Desmeules M: Influence of passive changes of lung volume on upper airways. J Appl Physiol 1990;68:2159–2164.
68 Series F, Marc I: Influence of lung volume dependence of upper airway resistance during continuous negative airway pressure. J Appl Physiol 1994;77:840–844.
69 Stanchina ML, Malhotra A, Fogel RB, Trinder J, Edwards JK, Schory K, White DP: The influence of lung volume on pharyngeal mechanics, collapsibility, and genioglossus muscle activation during sleep. Sleep 2003;26:851–856.
70 Tagaito Y, Isono S, Remmers JE, Tanaka A, Nishino T: Lung volume and collapsibility of the passive pharynx in patients with sleep-disordered breathing. J Appl Physiol 2007;103:1379–1385.
71 Owens RL, Malhotra A, Eckert DJ, White DP, Jordan AS: The influence of end-expiratory lung volume on measurements of pharyngeal collapsibility. J Appl Physiol 2010;108:445–451.
72 Heinzer RC, Stanchina ML, Malhotra A, Fogel RB, Patel SR, Jordan AS, Schory K, White DP: Lung volume and continuous positive airway pressure requirements in obstructive sleep apnea. Am J Respir Crit Care Med 2005;172:114–117.
73 Heinzer RC, Stanchina ML, Malhotra A, Jordan AS, Patel SR, Lo YL, Wellman A, Schory K, Dover L, White DP: Effect of increased lung volume on sleep disordered breathing in patients with sleep apnoea. Thorax 2006;61:435–439.
74 Squier SB, Patil SP, Schneider H, Kirkness JP, Smith PL, Schwartz AR: Effect of end-expiratory lung volume on upper airway collapsibility in sleeping men and women. J Appl Physiol 2010;109:977–985.
75 Ye J, Gao Z, Yin J, He Q: Hypoxia is a potential risk factor for chronic inflammation and adiponectin reduction in adipose tissue of ob/ob and dietary obese mice. Am J Physiol Endocrinol Metab 2007;293:E1118–E1128.
76 Trayhurn P, Wang B, Wood IS: Hypoxia in adipose tissue: a basis for the dysregulation of tissue function in obesity? Br J Nutr 2008;100:227–235.
77 Fried SK, Bunkin DA, Greenberg AS: Omental and subcutaneous adipose tissues of obese subjects release interleukin-6: depot difference and regulation by glucocorticoid. J Clin Endocrinol Metab 1998;83:847–850.
78 Hotamisligil GS: Mechanisms of TNF-alpha-induced insulin resistance. Exp Clin Endocrinol Diabetes 1999;107:119–125.
79 Weisberg SP, McCann D, Desai M, Rosenbaum M, Leibel RL, Ferrante AW Jr: Obesity is associated with macrophage accumulation in adipose tissue. J Clin Invest 2003;112:1796–1808.
80 Hopkins TA, Ouchi N, Shibata R, Walsh K: Adiponectin actions in the cardiovascular system. Cardiovasc Res 2007;74:11–18.
81 Schwartz AR, Patil SP, Schneider H, Smith PL: Modelling pathogenic mechanisms of upper airway dysfunction in the molecular age. Eur Respir J 2008;32:255–258.
82 Jequier E: Leptin signaling, adiposity, and energy balance. Ann NY Acad Sci 2002;967:379–388.
83 Paracchini V, Pedotti P, Taioli E: Genetics of leptin and obesity: a HuGE review. Am J Epidemiol 2005;162:101–114.
84 Steiner AA, Romanovsky AA: Leptin: at the crossroads of energy balance and systemic inflammation. Prog Lipid Res 2007;46:89–107.
85 Anubhuti, Arora S: Leptin and its metabolic interactions: an update. Diabetes Obes Metab 2008;10:973–993.

86 Lago R, Gomez R, Lago F, Gomez-Reino J, Gualillo O: Leptin beyond body weight regulation – current concepts concerning its role in immune function and inflammation. Cell Immunol 2008;252:139–145.
87 Yildiz BO, Haznedaroglu IC: Rethinking leptin and insulin action: therapeutic opportunities for diabetes. Int J Biochem Cell Biol 2006;38:820–830.
88 Considine RV, Sinha MK, Heiman ML, Kriauciunas A, Stephens TW, Nyce MR, Ohannesian JP, Marco CC, McKee LJ, Bauer TL, et al: Serum immunoreactive-leptin concentrations in normal-weight and obese humans. N Engl J Med 1996;334: 292–295.
89 Bravo PE, Morse S, Borne DM, Aguilar EA, Reisin E: Leptin and hypertension in obesity. Vasc Health Risk Manag 2006;2:163–169.
90 Shimizu H, Oh IS, Okada S, Mori M: Leptin resistance and obesity. Endocr J 2007;54:17–26.
91 Lam QL, Lu L: Role of leptin in immunity. Cell Mol Immunol 2007;4:1–13.
92 Bouloumie A, Marumo T, Lafontan M, Busse R: Leptin induces oxidative stress in human endothelial cells. Faseb J 1999;13:1231–1238.
93 Shin HJ, Oh J, Kang SM, Lee JH, Shin MJ, Hwang KC, Jang Y, Chung JH: Leptin induces hypertrophy via p38 mitogen-activated protein kinase in rat vascular smooth muscle cells. Biochem Biophys Res Commun 2005;329:18–24.
94 Wolk R, Deb A, Caplice NM, Somers VK: Leptin receptor and functional effects of leptin in human endothelial progenitor cells. Atherosclerosis 2005; 183:131–139.
95 Fantuzzi G, Mazzone T: Adipose tissue and atherosclerosis: exploring the connection. Arterioscler Thromb Vasc Biol 2007;27:996–1003.
96 Ip MS, Lam KS, Ho C, Tsang KW, Lam W: Serum leptin and vascular risk factors in obstructive sleep apnea. Chest 2000;118:580–586.
97 Berg AH, Scherer PE: Adipose tissue, inflammation, and cardiovascular disease. Circ Res 2005;96:939–949.
98 Wannamethee SG, Tchernova J, Whincup P, Lowe GD, Kelly A, Rumley A, Wallace AM, Sattar N: Plasma leptin: associations with metabolic, inflammatory and haemostatic risk factors for cardiovascular disease. Atherosclerosis 2007;191:418–426.
99 Reis JP, Macera CA, Wingard DL, Araneta MR, Lindsay SP, Marshall SJ: The relation of leptin and insulin with obesity-related cardiovascular risk factors in US adults. Atherosclerosis 2008;200:150–160.
100 O'Donnell CP, Schaub CD, Haines AS, Berkowitz DE, Tankersley CG, Schwartz AR, Smith PL: Leptin prevents respiratory depression in obesity. Am J Respir Crit Care Med 1999;159:1477–1484.
101 Tankersley CG, O'Donnell C, Daood MJ, Watchko JF, Mitzner W, Schwartz A, Smith P: Leptin attenuates respiratory complications associated with the obese phenotype. J Appl Physiol 1998;85:2261–2269.
102 O'Donnell CP, Tankersley CG, Polotsky VP, Schwartz AR, Smith PL: Leptin, obesity, and respiratory function. Respir Physiol 2000;119:163–170.
103 Polotsky VY, Wilson JA, Smaldone MC, Haines AS, Hurn PD, Tankersley CG, Smith PL, Schwartz AR, O'Donnell CP: Female gender exacerbates respiratory depression in leptin-deficient obesity. Am J Respir Crit Care Med 2001;164:1470–1475.
104 Ambrosini G, Nath AK, Sierra-Honigmann MR, Flores-Riveros J: Transcriptional activation of the human leptin gene in response to hypoxia: involvement of hypoxia-inducible factor 1. J Biol Chem 2002;277:34601–34609.
105 Grosfeld A, Andre J, Hauguel-De Mouzon S, Berra E, Pouyssegur J, Guerre-Millo M: Hypoxia-inducible factor 1 transactivates the human leptin gene promoter. J Biol Chem 2002;277:42953–42957.
106 Phipps PR, Starritt E, Caterson I, Grunstein RR: Association of serum leptin with hypoventilation in human obesity. Thorax 2002;57:75–76.
107 Shimura R, Tatsumi K, Nakamura A, Kasahara Y, Tanabe N, Takiguchi Y, Kuriyama T: Fat accumulation, leptin, and hypercapnia in obstructive sleep apnea-hypopnea syndrome. Chest 2005;127:543–549.
108 Yee BJ, Cheung J, Phipps P, Banerjee D, Piper AJ, Grunstein RR: Treatment of obesity hypoventilation syndrome and serum leptin. Respiration 2006;73: 209–212.
109 Redolfi S, Corda L, La Piana G, Spandrio S, Prometti P, Tantucci C: Long-term non-invasive ventilation increases chemosensitivity and leptin in obesity-hypoventilation syndrome. Respir Med 2007;101:1191–1195.
110 Campo A, Fruhbeck G, Zulueta JJ, Iriarte J, Seijo LM, Alcaide AB, Galdiz JB, Salvador J: Hyperleptinaemia, respiratory drive and hypercapnic response in obese patients. Eur Respir J 2007; 30:223–231.
111 Phillips BG, Kato M, Narkiewicz K, Choe I, Somers VK: Increases in leptin levels, sympathetic drive, and weight gain in obstructive sleep apnea. Am J Physiol Heart Circ Physiol 2000;279:H234–H237.
112 McArdle N, Hillman D, Beilin L, Watts G: Metabolic risk factors for vascular disease in obstructive sleep apnea: a matched controlled study. Am J Respir Crit Care Med 2007;175:190–195.
113 Drummond M, Winck JC, Guimaraes JT, Santos AC, Almeida J, Marques JA: Autoadjusting-CPAP effect on serum leptin concentrations in obstructive sleep apnoea patients. BMC Pulm Med 2008;8:21.

114 Barcelò A, Barbe F, Llompart E, de la Pena M, Duran-Cantolla J, Ladaria A, Bosch M, Guerra L, Agusti AG: Neuropeptide Y and leptin in patients with obstructive sleep apnea syndrome: role of obesity. Am J Respir Crit Care Med 2005;171:183–187.
115 Kapsimalis F, Varouchakis G, Manousaki A, Daskas S, Nikita D, Kryger M, Gourgoulianis K: Association of sleep apnea severity and obesity with insulin resistance, C-reactive protein, and leptin levels in male patients with obstructive sleep apnea. Lung 2008;186:209–217.
116 Yamamoto Y, Fujiuchi S, Hiramatsu M, Nishigaki Y, Takeda A, Fujita Y, Yamazaki Y: Resistin is closely related to systemic inflammation in obstructive sleep apnea. Respiration 2008;76:377–385.
117 Patel SR, Palmer LJ, Larkin EK, Jenny NS, White DP, Redline S: Relationship between obstructive sleep apnea and diurnal leptin rhythms. Sleep 2004;27:235–239.
118 Tatsumi K, Kasahara Y, Kurosu K, Tanabe N, Takiguchi Y, Kuriyama T: Sleep oxygen desaturation and circulating leptin in obstructive sleep apnea-hypopnea syndrome. Chest 2005;127:716–721.
119 Chin K, Shimizu K, Nakamura T, Narai N, Masuzaki H, Ogawa Y, Mishima M, Nakamura T, Nakao K, Ohi M: Changes in intra-abdominal visceral fat and serum leptin levels in patients with obstructive sleep apnea syndrome following nasal continuous positive airway pressure therapy. Circulation 1999;100: 706–712.
120 Sanner BM, Kollhosser P, Buechner N, Zidek W, Tepel M: Influence of treatment on leptin levels in patients with obstructive sleep apnoea. Eur Respir J 2004;23:601–604.
121 Cuhadaroglu C, Utkusavas A, Ozturk L, Salman S, Ece T: Effects of nasal CPAP treatment on insulin resistance, lipid profile, and plasma leptin in sleep apnea. Lung 2009;187:75–81.
122 Harsch IA, Konturek PC, Koebnick C, Kuehnlein PP, Fuchs FS, Pour Schahin S, Wiest GH, Hahn EG, Lohmann T, Ficker JH: Leptin and ghrelin levels in patients with obstructive sleep apnoea: effect of CPAP treatment. Eur Respir J 2003;22:251–257.
123 Arita Y, Kihara S, Ouchi N, Takahashi M, Maeda K, Miyagawa J, Hotta K, Shimomura I, Nakamura T, Miyaoka K, Kuriyama H, Nishida M, Yamashita S, Okubo K, Matsubara K, Muraguchi M, Ohmoto Y, Funahashi T, Matsuzawa Y: Paradoxical decrease of an adipose-specific protein, adiponectin, in obesity. Biochem Biophys Res Commun 1999;257:79–83.
124 Chiarugi P, Fiaschi T: Adiponectin in health and diseases: from metabolic syndrome to tissue regeneration. Expert Opin Ther Targets 2010;14:193–206.
125 Kawano J, Arora R. The role of adiponectin in obesity, diabetes, and cardiovascular disease. J Cardiometab Syndr 2009;4:44–49.
126 Goldstein BJ, Scalia RG, Ma XL: Protective vascular and myocardial effects of adiponectin. Nat Clin Pract Cardiovasc Med 2009;6:27–35.
127 Pischon T: Use of obesity biomarkers in cardiovascular epidemiology. Dis Markers 2009;26:247–263.
128 Pischon T, Girman CJ, Hotamisligil GS, Rifai N, Hu FB, Rimm EB: Plasma adiponectin levels and risk of myocardial infarction in men. JAMA 2004;291:1730–1737.
129 Wolk R, Svatikova A, Nelson CA, Gami AS, Govender K, Winnicki M, Somers VK: Plasma levels of adiponectin, a novel adipocyte-derived hormone, in sleep apnea. Obes Res 2005;13:186–190.
130 Masserini B, Morpurgo PS, Donadio F, Baldessari C, Bossi R, Beck-Peccoz P, Orsi E: Reduced levels of adiponectin in sleep apnea syndrome. J Endocrinol Invest 2006;29:700–705.
131 Buxton OM, Pavlova M, Reid EW, Wang W, Simonson DC, Adler GK: Sleep restriction for 1 week reduces insulin sensitivity in healthy men. Diabetes 2010;59:2126–2133.
132 Tasali E, Leproult R, Ehrmann DA, Van Cauter E: Slow-wave sleep and the risk of type 2 diabetes in humans. Proc Natl Acad Sci USA 2008;105:1044–1049.
133 Zhang XL, Yin KS, Wang H, Su S: Serum adiponectin levels in adult male patients with obstructive sleep apnea hypopnea syndrome. Respiration 2006;73:73–77.
134 Lam JC, Xu A, Tam S, Khong PI, Yao TJ, Lam DC, Lai AY, Lam B, Lam KS, Mary SM: Hypoadiponectinemia is related to sympathetic activation and severity of obstructive sleep apnea. Sleep 2008;31:1721–1727.
135 Kanbay A, Kokturk O, Ciftci TU, Tavil Y, Bukan N: Comparison of serum adiponectin and tumor necrosis factor-alpha levels between patients with and without obstructive sleep apnea syndrome. Respiration 2008;76:324–330.
136 Nakagawa Y, Kishida K, Kihara S, Sonoda M, Hirata A, Yasui A, Nishizawa H, Nakamura T, Yoshida R, Shimomura I, Funahashi T: Nocturnal reduction in circulating adiponectin concentrations related to hypoxic stress in severe obstructive sleep apnea-hypopnea syndrome. Am J Physiol Endocrinol Metab 2008;294:E778–E784.
137 Takahashi K, Chin K, Nakamura H, Morita S, Sumi K, Oga T, Matsumoto H, Niimi A, Fukuhara S, Yodoi J, Mishima M: Plasma thioredoxin, a novel oxidative stress marker, in patients with obstructive sleep apnea before and after nasal continuous positive airway pressure. Antioxid Redox Signal 2008;10:715–726.

138 Makino S, Handa H, Suzukawa K, Fujiwara M, Nakamura M, Muraoka S, Takasago I, Tanaka Y, Hashimoto K, Sugimoto T: Obstructive sleep apnoea syndrome, plasma adiponectin levels, and insulin resistance. Clin Endocrinol (Oxf) 2006;64:12–19.
139 Sharma SK, Kumpawat S, Goel A, Banga A, Ramakrishnan L, Chaturvedi P: Obesity, and not obstructive sleep apnea, is responsible for metabolic abnormalities in a cohort with sleep-disordered breathing. Sleep Med 2007;8:12–17.
140 Tokuda F, Sando Y, Matsui H, Koike H, Yokoyama T: Serum levels of adipocytokines, adiponectin and leptin, in patients with obstructive sleep apnea syndrome. Intern Med 2008;47:1843–1849.
141 De Lima AM, Franco CM, de Castro CM, Bezerra Ade A, Ataide L Jr, Halpern A: Effects of nasal continuous positive airway pressure treatment on oxidative stress and adiponectin levels in obese patients with obstructive sleep apnea. Respiration 2010;79: 370–376.
142 Carneiro G, Togeiro SM, Ribeiro-Filho FF, Truksinas E, Ribeiro AB, Zanella MT, Tufik S: Continuous positive airway pressure therapy improves hypoadiponectinemia in severe obese men with obstructive sleep apnea without changes in insulin resistance. Metab Syndr Relat Disord 2009;7:537–542.
143 Zhang XL, Yin KS, Li C, Jia EZ, Li YQ, Gao ZF: Effect of continuous positive airway pressure treatment on serum adiponectin level and mean arterial pressure in male patients with obstructive sleep apnea syndrome. Chin Med J (Engl) 2007;120:1477–1481.
144 Harsch IA, Wallaschofski H, Koebnick C, Pour Schahin S, Hahn EG, Ficker JH, Lohmann T. Adiponectin in patients with obstructive sleep apnea syndrome: course and physiological relevance. Respiration 2004;71:580–586.
145 West SD, Nicoll DJ, Wallace TM, Matthews DR, Stradling JR: Effect of CPAP on insulin resistance and HbA_{1c} in men with obstructive sleep apnoea and type 2 diabetes. Thorax 2007;62:969–974.
146 Kohler M, Ayers L, Pepperell JC, Packwood KL, Ferry B, Crosthwaite N, Craig S, Siccoli MM, Davies RJ, Stradling JR: Effects of continuous positive airway pressure on systemic inflammation in patients with moderate to severe obstructive sleep apnoea: a randomised controlled trial. Thorax 2009;64:67–73.
147 Arnardottir ES, Mackiewicz M, Gislason T, Teff KL, Pack AI: Molecular signatures of obstructive sleep apnea in adults: a review and perspective. Sleep 2009;32:447–470.
148 Lavie L, Lavie P. Molecular mechanisms of cardiovascular disease in OSAHS: the oxidative stress link. Eur Respir J 2009;33:1467–84.
149 Spiegel K, Tasali E, Leproult R, Van Cauter E: Effects of poor and short sleep on glucose metabolism and obesity risk. Nat Rev Endocrinol 2009;5:253–261.
150 Ye J. Emerging role of adipose tissue hypoxia in obesity and insulin resistance. Int J Obes (Lond) 2009;33:54–66.
151 Krueger JM, Rector DM, Churchill L. Sleep and Cytokines. Sleep Med Clin 2007;2:161–169.
152 Vgontzas AN, Zoumakis E, Lin HM, Bixler EO, Trakada G, Chrousos GP: Marked decrease in sleepiness in patients with sleep apnea by etanercept, a tumor necrosis factor-alpha antagonist. J Clin Endocrinol Metab 2004;89:4409–4413.
153 Wysocka E, Cofta S, Dziegielewska S, Gozdzik J, Torlinski L, Batura-Gabryel H: Adipocytokines in sleep apnea syndrome. Eur J Med Res 2009;14(suppl 4):255–258.
154 Knutson KL, Spiegel K, Penev P, Van Cauter E: The metabolic consequences of sleep deprivation. Sleep Med Rev 2007;11:163–178.
155 Tasali E, Leproult R, Spiegel K: Reduced sleep duration or quality: relationships with insulin resistance and type 2 diabetes. Prog Cardiovasc Dis 2009;51: 381–391.
156 Gale SM, Castracane VD, Mantzoros CS: Energy homeostasis, obesity and eating disorders: recent advances in endocrinology. J Nutr 2004;134:295–298.
157 Knutson KL: Impact of sleep and sleep loss on glucose homeostasis and appetite regulation. Sleep Med Clin 2007;2:187–197.
158 Yildiz BO, Suchard MA, Wong ML, McCann SM, Licinio J: Alterations in the dynamics of circulating ghrelin, adiponectin, and leptin in human obesity. Proc Natl Acad Sci USA 2004;101:10434–10439.
159 Spiegel K, Tasali E, Penev P, Van Cauter E: Brief communication: sleep curtailment in healthy young men is associated with decreased leptin levels, elevated ghrelin levels, and increased hunger and appetite. Ann Intern Med 2004;141:846–850.
160 Ukkola O: Ghrelin and metabolic disorders. Curr Protein Pept Sci 2009;10:2–7.
161 Granata R, Baragli A, Settanni F, Scarlatti F, Ghigo E: Unraveling the role of the ghrelin gene peptides in the endocrine pancreas. J Mol Endocrinol 2010; 45:107–118.
162 Takahashi K, Chin K, Akamizu T, Morita S, Sumi K, Oga T, Matsumoto H, Niimi A, Tsuboi T, Fukuhara S, Kangawa K, Mishima M: Acylated ghrelin level in patients with OSA before and after nasal CPAP treatment. Respirology 2008;13:810–816.
163 Ulukavak Ciftci T, Kokturk O, Bukan N, Bilgihan A: Leptin and ghrelin levels in patients with obstructive sleep apnea syndrome. Respiration 2005;72:395–401.

164 Sakurai T: Roles of orexins and orexin receptors in central regulation of feeding behavior and energy homeostasis. CNS Neurol Disord Drug Targets 2006;5:313–325.
165 Snow A, Gozal E, Malhotra A, Tiosano D, Perlman R, Vega C, Shahar E, Gozal D, Hochberg Z, Pillar G: Severe hypersomnolence after pituitary/hypothalamic surgery in adolescents: clinical characteristics and potential mechanisms. Pediatrics 2002;110:e74.
166 Igarashi N, Tatsumi K, Nakamura A, Sakao S, Takiguchi Y, Nishikawa T, Kuriyama T: Plasma orexin-A levels in obstructive sleep apnea-hypopnea syndrome. Chest 2003;124:1381–1385.
167 Nishijima T, Sakurai S, Arihara Z, Takahashi K: Plasma orexin-A-like immunoreactivity in patients with sleep apnea hypopnea syndrome. Peptides 2003;24:407–411.
168 Busquets X, Barbe F, Barcelo A, de la Pena M, Sigritz N, Mayoralas LR, Ladaria A, Agusti A: Decreased plasma levels of orexin-A in sleep apnea. Respiration 2004;71:575–579.
169 Sakurai S, Nishijima T, Takahashi S, Yamauchi K, Arihara Z, Takahashi K: Low plasma orexin-A levels were improved by continuous positive airway pressure treatment in patients with severe obstructive sleep apnea-hypopnea syndrome. Chest 2005;127: 731–737.
170 Rizzi CF, Cintra F, Risso T, Pulz C, Tufik S, de Paola A, Poyares D: Exercise capacity and obstructive sleep apnea in lean subjects. Chest 2010;137:109–114.
171 Aguillard RN, Riedel BW, Lichstein KL, Grieve FG, Johnson CT, Noe SL: Daytime functioning in obstructive sleep apnea patients: exercise tolerance, subjective fatigue, and sleepiness. Appl Psychophysiol Biofeedback 1998;23:207–217.
172 Grote L, Hedner J, Peter JH: The heart rate response to exercise is blunted in patients with sleep-related breathing disorder. Cardiology 2004;102:93–99.
173 Basta M, Lin HM, Pejovic S, Sarrigiannidis A, Bixler E, Vgontzas AN: Lack of regular exercise, depression, and degree of apnea are predictors of excessive daytime sleepiness in patients with sleep apnea: sex differences. J Clin Sleep Med 2008;4:19–25.
174 Vasquez MM, Goodwin JL, Drescher AA, Smith TW, Quan SF: Associations of dietary intake and physical activity with sleep disordered breathing in the Apnea Positive Pressure Long-Term Efficacy Study (APPLES). J Clin Sleep Med 2008;4:411–418.
175 Peppard PE, Szklo-Coxe M, Hla KM, Young T: Longitudinal association of sleep-related breathing disorder and depression. Arch Intern Med 2006;166: 1709–1715.
176 De Fronzo RA, Tobin JD, Andres R: Glucose clamp technique: a method for quantifying insulin secretion and resistance. Am J Physiol 1979;237: E214–E223.
177 Bergman RN, Finegood DT, Ader M: Assessment of insulin sensitivity in vivo. Endocr Rev 1985;6:45–86.
178 Bonora E, Moghetti P, Zancanaro C, Cigolini M, Querena M, Cacciatori V, Corgnati A, Muggeo M: Estimates of in vivo insulin action in man: comparison of insulin tolerance tests with euglycemic and hyperglycemic glucose clamp studies. J Clin Endocrinol Metab 1989;68:374–378.
179 Akinmokun A, Selby PL, Ramaiya K, Alberti KG: The short insulin tolerance test for determination of insulin sensitivity: a comparison with the euglycaemic clamp. Diabet Med 1992;9:432–437.
180 Hirst S, Phillips DI, Vines SK, Clark PM, Hales CN. Reproducibility of the short insulin tolerance test. Diabet Med 1993;10:839–842.
181 Matthews DR, Hosker JP, Rudenski AS, Naylor BA, Treacher DF, Turner RC: Homeostasis model assessment: insulin resistance and beta-cell function from fasting plasma glucose and insulin concentrations in man. Diabetologia 1985;28:412–419.
182 Standards of medical care in diabetes – 2007. Diabetes Care 2007;30(suppl 1):S4–S41.
183 Diagnosis and classification of diabetes mellitus. Diabetes Care 2006;29(suppl 1):S43–S48.
184 Shaw JE, Punjabi NM, Wilding JP, Alberti KG, Zimmet PZ: Sleep-disordered breathing and type 2 diabetes: a report from the International Diabetes Federation Task Force on Epidemiology and Prevention. Diabetes Res Clin Pract 2008;81:2–12.
185 Elmasry A, Lindberg E, Berne C, Janson C, Gislason T, Awad Tageldin M, Boman G: Sleep-disordered breathing and glucose metabolism in hypertensive men: a population-based study. J Intern Med 2001; 249:153–161.
186 Meslier N, Gagnadoux F, Giraud P, Person C, Ouksel H, Urban T, Racineux JL: Impaired glucose-insulin metabolism in males with obstructive sleep apnoea syndrome. Eur Respir J 2003;22:156–160.
187 Einhorn D, Stewart DA, Erman MK, Gordon N, Philis-Tsimikas A, Casal E: Prevalence of sleep apnea in a population of adults with type 2 diabetes mellitus. Endocr Pract 2007;13:355–362.
188 Laaban JP, Daenen S, Leger D, Pascal S, Bayon V, Slama G, Elgrably F: Prevalence and predictive factors of sleep apnoea syndrome in type 2 diabetic patients. Diabetes Metab 2009;35:372–377.
189 Tasali E, Ip MS: Obstructive sleep apnea and metabolic syndrome: alterations in glucose metabolism and inflammation. Proc Am Thorac Soc 2008;5: 207–217.

190 Levy P, Bonsignore MR, Eckel J: Sleep, sleep-disordered breathing and metabolic consequences. Eur Respir J 2009;34:243–260.
191 Tassone F, Lanfranco F, Gianotti L, Pivetti S, Navone F, Rossetto R, Grottoli S, Gai V, Ghigo E, Maccario M: Obstructive sleep apnoea syndrome impairs insulin sensitivity independently of anthropometric variables. Clin Endocrinol (Oxf) 2003;59:374–379.
192 Coughlin SR, Mawdsley L, Mugarza JA, Calverley PM, Wilding JP: Obstructive sleep apnoea is independently associated with an increased prevalence of metabolic syndrome. Eur Heart J 2004;25:735–741.
193 Peled N, Kassirer M, Shitrit D, Kogan Y, Shlomi D, Berliner AS, Kramer MR: The association of OSA with insulin resistance, inflammation and metabolic syndrome. Respir Med 2007;101:1696–1701.
194 Peltier AC, Consens FB, Sheikh K, Wang L, Song Y, Russell JW: Autonomic dysfunction in obstructive sleep apnea is associated with impaired glucose regulation. Sleep Med 2007;8:149–155.
195 Kono M, Tatsumi K, Saibara T, Nakamura A, Tanabe N, Takiguchi Y, Kuriyama T: Obstructive sleep apnea syndrome is associated with some components of metabolic syndrome. Chest 2007;131:1387–1392.
196 Polotsky VY, Patil SP, Savransky V, Laffan A, Fonti S, Frame LA, Steele KE, Schweizter MA, Clark JM, Torbenson MS, Schwartz AR: Obstructive sleep apnea, insulin resistance, and steatohepatitis in severe obesity. Am J Respir Crit Care Med 2009;179:228–234.
197 Punjabi NM, Beamer BA: Alterations in Glucose Disposal in Sleep-disordered Breathing. Am J Respir Crit Care Med 2009;179:235–240.
198 Keckeis M, Lattova Z, Maurovich-Horvat E, Beitinger PA, Birkmann S, Lauer CJ, Wetter TC, Wilde-Frenz J, Pollmacher T: Impaired glucose tolerance in sleep disorders. PLoS One 2010;5:e9444.
199 Ip MS, Lam B, Ng MM, Lam WK, Tsang KW, Lam KS: Obstructive sleep apnea is independently associated with insulin resistance. Am J Respir Crit Care Med 2002;165:670–676.
200 Punjabi NM, Sorkin JD, Katzel LI, Goldberg AP, Schwartz AR, Smith PL: Sleep-disordered breathing and insulin resistance in middle-aged and overweight men. Am J Respir Crit Care Med 2002;165:677–682.
201 Punjabi NM, Shahar E, Redline S, Gottlieb DJ, Givelber R, Resnick HE: Sleep-disordered breathing, glucose intolerance, and insulin resistance: the Sleep Heart Health Study. Am J Epidemiol 2004;160:521–530.
202 Lam JC, Lam B, Lam CL, Fong D, Wang JK, Tse HF, Lam KS, Ip MS: Obstructive sleep apnea and the metabolic syndrome in community-based Chinese adults in Hong Kong. Respir Med 2006;100:980–987.
203 Okada M, Takamizawa A, Tsushima K, Urushihata K, Fujimoto K, Kubo K: Relationship between sleep-disordered breathing and lifestyle-related illnesses in subjects who have undergone health-screening. Intern Med 2006;45:891–896.
204 Sulit L, Storfer-Isser A, Kirchner HL, Redline S: Differences in polysomnography predictors for hypertension and impaired glucose tolerance. Sleep 2006;29:777–783.
205 Seicean S, Kirchner HL, Gottlieb DJ, Punjabi NM, Resnick H, Sanders M, Budhiraja R, Singer M, Redline S: Sleep-disordered breathing and impaired glucose metabolism in normal-weight and overweight/obese individuals: the Sleep Heart Health Study. Diabetes Care 2008;31:1001–1006.
206 Stamatakis K, Sanders MH, Caffo B, Resnick HE, Gottlieb DJ, Mehra R, Punjabi NM: Fasting glycemia in sleep disordered breathing: lowering the threshold on oxyhemoglobin desaturation. Sleep 2008;31:1018–1024.
207 Theorell-Haglow J, Berne C, Janson C, Lindberg E: Obstructive sleep apnoea is associated with decreased insulin sensitivity in females. Eur Respir J 2008;31:1054–1060.
208 Botros N, Concato J, Mohsenin V, Selim B, Doctor K, Yaggi HK: Obstructive sleep apnea as a risk factor for type 2 diabetes. Am J Med 2009;122:1122–1127.
209 Barcelo A, Barbe F, de la Pena M, Martinez P, Soriano JB, Pierola J, Agusti AG: Insulin resistance and daytime sleepiness in patients with sleep apnoea. Thorax 2008;63:946–950.
210 Ronksley PE, Hemmelgarn BR, Heitman SJ, Hanly PJ, Faris PD, Quan H, Tsai WH: Obstructive sleep apnoea is associated with diabetes in sleepy subjects. Thorax 2009;64:834–839.
211 Davies RJ, Turner R, Crosby J, Stradling JR: Plasma insulin and lipid levels in untreated obstructive sleep apnoea and snoring: their comparison with matched controls and response to treatment. J Sleep Res 1994;3:180–185.
212 Barcelo A, Barbe F, Llompart E, Mayoralas LR, Ladaria A, Bosch M, Agusti AG: Effects of obesity on C-reactive protein level and metabolic disturbances in male patients with obstructive sleep apnea. Am J Med 2004;117:118–121.
213 Mahmood K, Akhter N, Eldeirawi K, Onal E, Christman JW, Carley DW, Herdegen JJ: Prevalence of type 2 diabetes in patients with obstructive sleep apnea in a multi-ethnic sample. J Clin Sleep Med 2009;5:215–221.

214 Reichmuth KJ, Austin D, Skatrud JB, Young T: Association of sleep apnea and type II diabetes: a population-based study. Am J Respir Crit Care Med 2005;172:1590–1595.

215 Marshall NS, Wong KK, Phillips CL, Liu PY, Knuiman MW, Grunstein RR: Is sleep apnea an independent risk factor for prevalent and incident diabetes in the Busselton Health Study? J Clin Sleep Med 2009;5:15–20.

216 Papanas N, Steiropoulos P, Nena E, Tzouvelekis A, Maltezos E, Trakada G, Bouros D: HbA_{1c} is associated with severity of obstructive sleep apnea hypopnea syndrome in nondiabetic men. Vasc Health Risk Manag 2009;5:751–756.

217 Steiropoulos P, Papanas N, Nena E, Maltezos E, Bouros D: Continuous positive airway pressure treatment in patients with sleep apnoea: does it really improve glucose metabolism? Curr Diabetes Rev 2010;6:156–166.

218 Punjabi NM, Polotsky VY: Disorders of glucose metabolism in sleep apnea. J Appl Physiol 2005;99: 1998–2007.

219 Babu AR, Herdegen J, Fogelfeld L, Shott S, Mazzone T: Type 2 diabetes, glycemic control, and continuous positive airway pressure in obstructive sleep apnea. Arch Intern Med 2005;165:447–452.

220 Dorkova Z, Petrasova D, Molcanyiova A, Popovnakova M, Tkacova R: Effects of continuous positive airway pressure on cardiovascular risk profile in patients with severe obstructive sleep apnea and metabolic syndrome. Chest 2008;134:686–692.

221 Schahin SP, Nechanitzky T, Dittel C, Fuchs FS, Hahn EG, Konturek PC, Ficker JH, Harsch IA: Long-term improvement of insulin sensitivity during CPAP therapy in the obstructive sleep apnoea syndrome. Med Sci Monit 2008;14:CR117–CR121.

222 Steiropoulos P, Papanas N, Nena E, Tsara V, Fitili C, Tzouvelekis A, Christaki P, Maltezos E, Bouros D: Markers of glycemic control and insulin resistance in non-diabetic patients with obstructive sleep apnea hypopnea syndrome: does adherence to CPAP treatment improve glycemic control? Sleep Med 2009;10:887–891.

223 Harsch IA, Schahin SP, Bruckner K, Radespiel-Troger M, Fuchs FS, Hahn EG, Konturek PC, Lohmann T, Ficker JH: The effect of continuous positive airway pressure treatment on insulin sensitivity in patients with obstructive sleep apnoea syndrome and type 2 diabetes. Respiration 2004;71: 252–259.

224 Harsch IA, Hahn EG, Pour Schahin S: Effect of CPAP on insulin resistance in patients with obstructive sleep apnoea and type 2 diabetes. Thorax 2008;63:384–385, author reply 385.

225 Lam JC, Lam B, Yao TJ, Lai AY, Ooi CG, Tam S, Lam KS, Ip MS: A randomised controlled trial of nasal continuous positive airway pressure on insulin sensitivity in obstructive sleep apnoea. Eur Respir J 2010;35:138–145.

226 Brooks B, Cistulli PA, Borkman M, Ross G, McGhee S, Grunstein RR, Sullivan CE, Yue DK: Obstructive sleep apnea in obese noninsulin-dependent diabetic patients: effect of continuous positive airway pressure treatment on insulin responsiveness. J Clin Endocrinol Metab 1994;79:1681–1685.

227 Harsch IA, Schahin SP, Radespiel-Troger M, Weintz O, Jahreiss H, Fuchs FS, Wiest GH, Hahn EG, Lohmann T, Konturek PC, Ficker JH: Continuous positive airway pressure treatment rapidly improves insulin sensitivity in patients with obstructive sleep apnea syndrome. Am J Respir Crit Care Med 2004;169:156–162.

228 Lindberg E, Berne C, Elmasry A, Hedner J, Janson C: CPAP treatment of a population-based sample – what are the benefits and the treatment compliance? Sleep Med 2006;7:553–560.

229 Dawson A, Abel SL, Loving RT, Dailey G, Shadan FF, Cronin JW, Kripke DF, Kline LE: CPAP therapy of obstructive sleep apnea in type 2 diabetics improves glycemic control during sleep. J Clin Sleep Med 2008;4:538–542.

230 Pallayova M, Donic V, Tomori Z: Beneficial effects of severe sleep apnea therapy on nocturnal glucose control in persons with type 2 diabetes mellitus. Diabetes Res Clin Pract 2008;81:e8–e11.

231 Hassaballa HA, Tulaimat A, Herdegen JJ, Mokhlesi B: The effect of continuous positive airway pressure on glucose control in diabetic patients with severe obstructive sleep apnea. Sleep Breath 2005;9:176–180.

232 Czupryniak L, Loba J, Pawlowski M, Nowak D, Bialasiewicz P: Treatment with continuous positive airway pressure may affect blood glucose levels in nondiabetic patients with obstructive sleep apnea syndrome. Sleep 2005;28:601–603.

233 Coughlin SR, Mawdsley L, Mugarza JA, Wilding JP, Calverley PM: Cardiovascular and metabolic effects of CPAP in obese males with OSA. Eur Respir J 2007;29:720–727.

234 Comondore VR, Cheema R, Fox J, Butt A, John Mancini GB, Fleetham JA, Ryan CF, Chan S, Ayas NT: The impact of CPAP on cardiovascular biomarkers in minimally symptomatic patients with obstructive sleep apnea: a pilot feasibility randomized crossover trial. Lung 2009;187:17–22.

235 Patruno V, Aiolfi S, Costantino G, Murgia R, Selmi C, Malliani A, Montano N: Fixed and autoadjusting continuous positive airway pressure treatments are not similar in reducing cardiovascular risk factors in patients with obstructive sleep apnea. Chest 2007;131:1393–1399.
236 Shoelson SE, Lee J, Goldfine AB: Inflammation and insulin resistance. J Clin Invest 2006;116:1793–1801.
237 Tilg H, Moschen AR: Inflammatory mechanisms in the regulation of insulin resistance. Mol Med 2008;14:222–231.
238 Williams A, Scharf SM: Obstructive sleep apnea, cardiovascular disease, and inflammation – is NF-kappaB the key? Sleep Breath 2007;11:69–76.
239 Ramasamy R, Yan SF, Schmidt AM: The RAGE axis and endothelial dysfunction: maladaptive roles in the diabetic vasculature and beyond. Trends Cardiovasc Med 2005;15:237–243.
240 Koyama H, Yamamoto H, Nishizawa Y: RAGE and soluble RAGE: potential therapeutic targets for cardiovascular diseases. Mol Med 2007;13:625–635.
241 Yan SF, D'Agati V, Schmidt AM, Ramasamy R: Receptor for advanced glycation endproducts (RAGE): a formidable force in the pathogenesis of the cardiovascular complications of diabetes and aging. Curr Mol Med 2007;7:699–710.
242 Meerwaldt R, Links T, Zeebregts C, Tio R, Hillebrands JL, Smit A: The clinical relevance of assessing advanced glycation endproducts accumulation in diabetes. Cardiovasc Diabetol 2008;7:29.
243 Tan KC, Chow WS, Lam JC, Lam B, Bucala R, Betteridge J, Ip MS: Advanced glycation endproducts in nondiabetic patients with obstructive sleep apnea. Sleep 2006;29:329–333.
244 Veasey S: Obstructive sleep apnea: rapidly AGE-ing us all. Sleep 2006;29:280–281.
245 Oltmanns KM, Gehring H, Rudolf S, Schultes B, Rook S, Schweiger U, Born J, Fehm HL, Peters A: Hypoxia causes glucose intolerance in humans. Am J Respir Crit Care Med 2004;169:1231–1237.
246 Louis M, Punjabi NM: Effects of acute intermittent hypoxia on glucose metabolism in awake healthy volunteers. J Appl Physiol 2009;106:1538–1544.
247 Iiyori N, Alonso LC, Li J, Sanders MH, Garcia-Ocana A, O'Doherty RM, Polotsky VY, O'Donnell CP: Intermittent hypoxia causes insulin resistance in lean mice independent of autonomic activity. Am J Respir Crit Care Med 2007;175:851–857.
248 Jun J, Polotsky VY: Sleep disordered breathing and metabolic effects: evidence from animal models. Sleep Med Clin 2007;2:263–277.
249 Paquot N, Schneiter P, Jequier E, Tappy L: Effects of glucocorticoids and sympathomimetic agents on basal and insulin-stimulated glucose metabolism. Clin Physiol 1995;15:231–240.
250 Navegantes LC, Sjostrand M, Gudbjornsdottir S, Strindberg L, Elam M, Lonnroth P: Regulation and counterregulation of lipolysis in vivo: different roles of sympathetic activation and insulin. J Clin Endocrinol Metab 2003;88:5515–5520.
251 Grassi G, Arenare F, Quarti-Trevano F, Seravalle G, Mancia G: Heart rate, sympathetic cardiovascular influences, and the metabolic syndrome. Prog Cardiovasc Dis 2009;52:31–37.
252 Bloch-Damti A, Bashan N: Proposed mechanisms for the induction of insulin resistance by oxidative stress. Antioxid Redox Signal 2005;7:1553–1567.
253 Robertson RP: Oxidative stress and impaired insulin secretion in type 2 diabetes. Curr Opin Pharmacol 2006;6:615–619.
254 Mullington JM, Haack M, Toth M, Serrador JM, Meier-Ewert HK: Cardiovascular, inflammatory, and metabolic consequences of sleep deprivation. Prog Cardiovasc Dis 2009;51:294–302.
255 Tuomilehto H, Peltonen M, Partinen M, Seppa J, Saaristo T, Korpi-Hyovalti E, Oksa H, Puolijoki H, Saltevo J, Vanhala M, Tuomilehto J: Sleep duration is associated with an increased risk for the prevalence of type 2 diabetes in middle-aged women – the FIN-D2D survey. Sleep Med 2008;9:221–227.
256 Hayashino Y, Fukuhara S, Suzukamo Y, Okamura T, Tanaka T, Ueshima H: Relation between sleep quality and quantity, quality of life, and risk of developing diabetes in healthy workers in Japan: the High-Risk and Population Strategy for Occupational Health Promotion (HIPOP-OHP) Study. BMC Public Health 2007;7:129.
257 Cappuccio FP, D'Elia L, Strazzullo P, Miller MA: Quantity and quality of sleep and incidence of type 2 diabetes: a systematic review and meta-analysis. Diabetes Care 2010;33:414–420.
258 Xu Q, Song Y, Hollenbeck A, Blair A, Schatzkin A, Chen H: Day napping and short night sleeping are associated with higher risk of diabetes in older adults. Diabetes Care 2010;33:78–83.
259 Bergman RN, Ader M, Huecking K, Van Citters G: Accurate assessment of beta-cell function: the hyperbolic correction. Diabetes 2002;51(suppl 1):S212–S220.
260 Prigeon RL, Kahn SE, Porte D Jr: Changes in insulin sensitivity, glucose effectiveness, and B-cell function in regularly exercising subjects. Metabolism 1995;44:1259–1263.
261 Resnick HE, Redline S, Shahar E, Gilpin A, Newman A, Walter R, Ewy GA, Howard BV, Punjabi NM: Diabetes and sleep disturbances: findings from the Sleep Heart Health Study. Diabetes Care 2003;26:702–709.
262 West SD, Nicoll DJ, Stradling JR: Prevalence of obstructive sleep apnoea in men with type 2 diabetes. Thorax 2006;61:945–950.

263 Aronsohn RS, Whitmore H, Van Cauter E, Tasali E: Impact of untreated obstructive sleep apnea on glucose control in type 2 diabetes. Am J Respir Crit Care Med 2010;181:507–513.
264 Mondini S, Guilleminault C: Abnormal breathing patterns during sleep in diabetes. Ann Neurol 1985;17:391–395.
265 Ficker JH, Dertinger SH, Siegfried W, Konig HJ, Pentz M, Sailer D, Katalinic A, Hahn EG: Obstructive sleep apnoea and diabetes mellitus: the role of cardiovascular autonomic neuropathy. Eur Respir J 1998;11:14–19.
266 Tasali E, Mokhlesi B, Van Cauter E: Obstructive sleep apnea and type 2 diabetes: interacting epidemics. Chest 2008;133:496–506.
267 Li J, Thorne LN, Punjabi NM, Sun CK, Schwartz AR, Smith PL, Marino RL, Rodriguez A, Hubbard WC, O'Donnell CP, Polotsky VY: Intermittent hypoxia induces hyperlipidemia in lean mice. Circ Res 2005;97:698–706.
268 Li J, Savransky V, Nanayakkara A, Smith PL, O'Donnell CP, Polotsky VY: Hyperlipidemia and lipid peroxidation are dependent on the severity of chronic intermittent hypoxia. J Appl Physiol 2007; 102:557–563.
269 Savransky V, Bevans S, Nanayakkara A, Li J, Smith PL, Torbenson MS, Polotsky VY: Chronic intermittent hypoxia causes hepatitis in a mouse model of diet-induced fatty liver. Am J Physiol Gastrointest Liver Physiol 2007;293:G871–G877.
270 Savransky V, Jun J, Li J, Nanayakkara A, Fonti S, Moser AB, Steele KE, Schweitzer MA, Patil SP, Bhanot S, Schwartz AR, Polotsky VY: Dyslipidemia and atherosclerosis induced by chronic intermittent hypoxia are attenuated by deficiency of stearoyl coenzyme A desaturase. Circ Res 2008;103:1173–1180.
271 Jun J, Polotsky VY: Metabolic consequences of sleep-disordered breathing. ILAR J 2009;50:289–306.
272 Drager LF, Jun J, Polotsky VY: Obstructive sleep apnea and dyslipidemia: implications for atherosclerosis. Curr Opin Endocrinol Diabetes Obes 2010;17:161–165.
273 Börgel J, Sanner BM, Bittlinsky A, Keskin F, Bartels NK, Buechner N, Huesing A, Rump LC, Mügge A: Obstructive sleep apnoea and its therapy influence high-density lipoprotein cholesterol serum levels. Eur Respir J 2006;27:121–127.
274 Roche F, Sforza E, Pichot V, Maudoux D, Garcin A, Celle S, Picard-Kossovsky M, Gaspoz JM, Barthelemy JC: Obstructive sleep apnoea/hypopnea influences high-density lipoprotein cholesterol in the elderly. Sleep Med 2009;10:882–886.
275 Czerniawska J, Bielen P, Plywaczewski R, Czystowska M, Korzybski D, Sliwinski P, Gorecka D: Metabolic abnormalities in obstructive sleep apnea patients. Pneumonol Alergol Pol 2008;76:340–347.
276 Tan KC, Chow WS, Lam JC, Lam B, Wong WK, Tam S, Ip MS: HDL dysfunction in obstructive sleep apnea. Atherosclerosis 2006;184:377–382.
277 Steiropoulos P, Tsara V, Nena E, Fitili C, Kataropoulou M, Froudarakis M, Christaki P, Bouros D: Effect of continuous positive airway pressure treatment on serum cardiovascular risk factors in patients with obstructive sleep apnea-hypopnea syndrome. Chest 2007;132:843–851.
278 Robinson GV, Pepperell JC, Segal HC, Davies RJ, Stradling JR: Circulating cardiovascular risk factors in obstructive sleep apnoea: data from randomised controlled trials. Thorax 2004;59:777–782.
279 Drager LF, Bortolotto LA, Figueiredo AC, Krieger EM, Lorenzi GF: Effects of continuous positive airway pressure on early signs of atherosclerosis in obstructive sleep apnea. Am J Respir Crit Care Med 2007;176:706–712.
280 Baguet JP, Nadra M, Barone-Rochette G, Ormezzano O, Pierre H, Pepin JL: Early cardiovascular abnormalities in newly diagnosed obstructive sleep apnea. Vasc Health Risk Manag 2009;5:1063–1073.
281 Wilcox I, McNamara SG, Collins FL, Grunstein RR, Sullivan CE: 'Syndrome Z': the interaction of sleep apnoea, vascular risk factors and heart disease. Thorax 1998;53(suppl 3):S25–S28.
282 Vgontzas AN, Bixler EO, Chrousos GP: Sleep apnea is a manifestation of the metabolic syndrome. Sleep Med Rev 2005;9:211–224.
283 Nieto FJ, Peppard PE, Young TB: Sleep disordered breathing and metabolic syndrome. WMJ 2009;108: 263–265.
284 Nock NL, Li L, Larkin EK, Patel SR, Redline S: Empirical evidence for 'syndrome Z': a hierarchical 5-factor model of the metabolic syndrome incorporating sleep disturbance measures. Sleep 2009;32: 615–622.
285 Eckel RH, Grundy SM, Zimmet PZ: The metabolic syndrome. Lancet 2005;365:1415–1428.
286 Wolk R, Somers VK: Sleep and the metabolic syndrome. Exp Physiol 2007;92:67–78.
287 Lam JC, Ip MS: Obstructive sleep apnea and the metabolic syndrome. Expert Rev Respir Med 2009;3:177–186.

288 Alberti KG, Eckel RH, Grundy SM, Zimmet PZ, Cleeman JI, Donato KA, Fruchart JC, James WP, Loria CM, Smith SC Jr: Harmonizing the metabolic syndrome: a joint interim statement of the International Diabetes Federation Task Force on Epidemiology and Prevention, National Heart, Lung and Blood Institute, American Heart Association, World Heart Federation, International Atherosclerosis Society and International Association for the Study of Obesity. Circulation 2009;120:1640–1645.

289 Alberti KG, Zimmet P, Shaw J: The metabolic syndrome – a new worldwide definition. Lancet 2005;366:1059–1062.

290 Gale EA: Should we dump the metabolic syndrome? Yes. BMJ 2008;336:640.

291 Kahn R: Metabolic syndrome – what is the clinical usefulness? Lancet 2008;371:1892–1893.

292 Sattar N, McConnachie A, Shaper AG, Blauw GJ, Buckley BM, de Craen AJ, Ford I, Forouhi NG, Freeman DJ, Jukema JW, Lennon L, Macfarlane PW, Murphy MB, Packard CJ, Stott DJ, Westendorp RG, Whincup PH, Shepherd J, Wannamethee SG: Can metabolic syndrome usefully predict cardiovascular disease and diabetes? Outcome data from two prospective studies. Lancet 2008;371:1927–1935.

293 Alberti KG, Zimmet PZ: Definition, diagnosis and classification of diabetes mellitus and its complications. 1. Diagnosis and classification of diabetes mellitus: provisional report of a WHO consultation. Diabet Med 1998;15:539–553.

294 Third report of the National Cholesterol Education Program (NCEP) expert panel on detection, evaluation, and treatment of high blood cholesterol in adults (Adult Treatment Panel III): final report. Circulation 2002;106:3143–3421.

295 Grundy SM, Cleeman JI, Daniels SR, Donato KA, Eckel RH, Franklin BA, Gordon DJ, Krauss RM, Savage PJ, Smith SC Jr, Spertus JA, Costa F: Diagnosis and management of the metabolic syndrome: an American Heart Association/National Heart, Lung, and Blood Institute Scientific Statement. Circulation 2005;112:2735–2752.

296 Ford ES, Giles WH, Dietz WH: Prevalence of the metabolic syndrome among US adults: findings from the third National Health and Nutrition Examination Survey. JAMA 2002;287:356–359.

297 Cameron AJ, Shaw JE, Zimmet PZ: The metabolic syndrome: prevalence in worldwide populations. Endocrinol Metab Clin North Am 2004;33:351–375.

298 Ford ES: Prevalence of the metabolic syndrome defined by the International Diabetes Federation among adults in the US. Diabetes Care 2005;28:2745–2749.

299 Hu G, Qiao Q, Tuomilehto J, Balkau B, Borch-Johnsen K, Pyorala K: Prevalence of the metabolic syndrome and its relation to all-cause and cardiovascular mortality in nondiabetic European men and women. Arch Intern Med 2004;164:1066–1076.

300 Gruber A, Horwood F, Sithole J, Ali NJ, Idris I: Obstructive sleep apnoea is independently associated with the metabolic syndrome but not insulin resistance state. Cardiovasc Diabetol 2006;5:22.

301 Sasanabe R, Banno K, Otake K, Hasegawa R, Usui K, Morita M, Shiomi T: Metabolic syndrome in Japanese patients with obstructive sleep apnea syndrome. Hypertens Res 2006;29:315–322.

302 Parish JM, Adam T, Facchiano L: Relationship of metabolic syndrome and obstructive sleep apnea. J Clin Sleep Med 2007;3:467–472.

303 Chin K, Oga T, Takahashi K, Takegami M, Nakayama-Ashida Y, Wakamura T, Sumi K, Nakamura T, Horita S, Oka Y, Minami I, Fukuhara S, Kadotani H: Associations between obstructive sleep apnea, metabolic syndrome, and sleep duration, as measured with an actigraph, in an urban male working population in Japan. Sleep 2010;33:89–95.

304 Drager LF, Bortolotto LA, Maki-Nunes C, Trombetta IC, Alves MJ, Fraga RF, Negrao CE, Krieger EM, Lorenzi-Filho G: The incremental role of obstructive sleep apnoea on markers of atherosclerosis in patients with metabolic syndrome. Atherosclerosis 2010;208:490–495.

305 Drager LF, Bortolotto LA, Maki-Nunes C, Trombetta IC, Negrao CE, Krieger EM, Lorenzi-Filho G: Atherosclerosis in obstructive sleep apnoea: it does not matter whether patients are sleepy or not. Atherosclerosis 2010;211:30–31.

306 Saletu M, Sauter C, Lalouschek W, Saletu B, Kapfhammer G, Benesch T, Zeitlhofer J: Is excessive daytime sleepiness a predictor of carotid atherosclerosis in sleep apnea? Atherosclerosis 2008;196:810–816.

307 Mota PC, Drummond M, Winck JC, Santos AC, Almeida J, Marques JA: APAP impact on metabolic syndrome in obstructive sleep apnea patients. Sleep Breath 2010, E-pub ahead of print.

308 Ip MS, Lam B, Lauder IJ, Tsang KW, Chung KF, Mok YW, Lam WK: A community study of sleep-disordered breathing in middle-aged Chinese men in Hong Kong. Chest 2001;119:62–69.

309 Netzer NC, Stoohs RA, Netzer CM, Clark K, Strohl KP: Using the Berlin Questionnaire to identify patients at risk for the sleep apnea syndrome. Ann Intern Med 1999;131:485–491.

310 Drager LF, Genta PR, Pedrosa RP, Nerbass FB, Gonzaga CC, Krieger EM, Lorenzi-Filho G: Characteristics and predictors of obstructive sleep apnea in patients with systemic hypertension. Am J Cardiol 2010;105:1135–1139.

311 Dixon JB, Bhathal PS, O'Brien PE: Nonalcoholic fatty liver disease: predictors of nonalcoholic steatohepatitis and liver fibrosis in the severely obese. Gastroenterology 2001;121:91–100.

312 Kim CH, Younossi ZM: Nonalcoholic fatty liver disease: a manifestation of the metabolic syndrome. Cleve Clin J Med 2008;75:721–728.

313 Shifflet A, Wu GY: Non-alcoholic steatohepatitis: an overview. J Formos Med Assoc 2009;108:4–12.

314 Vanni E, Bugianesi E, Kotronen A, De Minicis S, Yki-Jarvinen H, Svegliati-Baroni G: From the metabolic syndrome to NAFLD or vice versa? Dig Liver Dis 2010;42:320–330.

315 Ahmed MH, Byrne CD: Obstructive sleep apnea syndrome and fatty liver: association or causal link? World J Gastroenterol 2010;16:4243–4252.

316 Tian JL, Zhang Y, Chen BY: Sleep apnea hypopnea syndrome and liver injury. Chin Med J (Engl) 2010;123:89–94.

317 Tanné F, Gagnadoux F, Chazouilleres O, Fleury B, Wendum D, Lasnier E, Lebeau B, Poupon R, Serfaty L: Chronic liver injury during obstructive sleep apnea. Hepatology 2005;41:1290–1296.

318 Kallwitz ER, Herdegen J, Madura J, Jakate S, Cotler SJ: Liver enzymes and histology in obese patients with obstructive sleep apnea. J Clin Gastroenterol 2007;41:918–921.

319 Savransky V, Nanayakkara A, Vivero A, Li J, Bevans S, Smith PL, Torbenson MS, Polotsky VY: Chronic intermittent hypoxia predisposes to liver injury. Hepatology 2007;45:1007–1013.

320 Kohler M, Pepperell JC, Davies RJ, Stradling JR: Continuous positive airway pressure and liver enzymes in obstructive sleep apnoea: data from a randomized controlled trial. Respiration 2009;78: 141–146.

321 Day CP, James OF: Steatohepatitis: a tale of two 'hits'? Gastroenterology 1998;114:842–845.

322 Day CP, Saksena S: Non-alcoholic steatohepatitis: definitions and pathogenesis. J Gastroenterol Hepatol 2002;17(suppl 3):S377–S384.

323 Browning JD, Horton JD: Molecular mediators of hepatic steatosis and liver injury. J Clin Invest 2004; 114:147–152.

324 Diehl AM: Lessons from animal models of NASH. Hepatol Res 2005;33:138–144.

325 Clark JM, Diehl AM: Nonalcoholic fatty liver disease: an underrecognized cause of cryptogenic cirrhosis. JAMA 2003;289:3000–3004.

326 Clark JM, Diehl AM: Defining nonalcoholic fatty liver disease: implications for epidemiologic studies. Gastroenterology 2003;124:248–250.

327 Day CP: Natural history of NAFLD: remarkably benign in the absence of cirrhosis. Gastroenterology 2005;129:375–378.

328 McCullough AJ: Pathophysiology of nonalcoholic steatohepatitis. J Clin Gastroenterol 2006;40(suppl 1):S17–S29.

329 Chin K, Nakamura T, Takahashi K, Sumi K, Ogawa Y, Masuzaki H, Muro S, Hattori N, Matsumoto H, Niimi A, Chiba T, Nakao K, Mishima M, Ohi M: Effects of obstructive sleep apnea syndrome on serum aminotransferase levels in obese patients. Am J Med 2003;114:370–376.

330 Jouet P, Sabate JM, Maillard D, Msika S, Mechler C, Ledoux S, Harnois F, Coffin B: Relationship between obstructive sleep apnea and liver abnormalities in morbidly obese patients: a prospective study. Obes Surg 2007;17:478–485.

331 Norman D, Bardwell WA, Arosemena F, Nelesen R, Mills PJ, Loredo JS, Lavine JE, Dimsdale JE: Serum aminotransferase levels are associated with markers of hypoxia in patients with obstructive sleep apnea. Sleep 2008;31:121–126.

332 Tatsumi K, Saibara T: Effects of obstructive sleep apnea syndrome on hepatic steatosis and nonalcoholic steatohepatitis. Hepatol Res 2005;33:100–104.

333 Mishra P, Nugent C, Afendy A, Bai C, Bhatia P, Afendy M, Fang Y, Elariny H, Goodman Z, Younossi ZM: Apnoeic-hypopnoeic episodes during obstructive sleep apnoea are associated with histological nonalcoholic steatohepatitis. Liver Int 2008;28:1080–1086.

334 Rashid S, Watanabe T, Sakaue T, Lewis GF: Mechanisms of HDL lowering in insulin resistant, hypertriglyceridemic states: the combined effect of HDL triglyceride enrichment and elevated hepatic lipase activity. Clin Biochem 2003;36:421–429.

335 Taskinen MR: Type 2 diabetes as a lipid disorder. Curr Mol Med 2005;5:297–308.

336 Savransky V, Nanayakkara A, Li J, Bevans S, Smith PL, Rodriguez A, Polotsky VY: Chronic intermittent hypoxia induces atherosclerosis. Am J Respir Crit Care Med 2007;175:1290–1297.

337 Cusi K: Role of insulin resistance and lipotoxicity in non-alcoholic steatohepatitis. Clin Liver Dis 2009; 13:545–563.

338 Edens MA, Kuipers F, Stolk RP: Non-alcoholic fatty liver disease is associated with cardiovascular disease risk markers. Obes Rev 2009;10:412–419.

339 Lizardi-Cervera J, Aguilar-Zapata D: Nonalcoholic fatty liver disease and its association with cardiovascular disease. Ann Hepatol 2009;8(suppl 1): S40–S43.

340 Montecucco F, Mach F: Does non-alcoholic fatty liver disease (NAFLD) increase cardiovascular risk? Endocr Metab Immune Disord Drug Targets 2008;8: 301–307.
341 Malhotra A, Loscalzo J: Sleep and cardiovascular disease: an overview. Prog Cardiovasc Dis 2009;51: 279–284.
342 Douketis JD, Paradis G, Keller H, Martineau C: Canadian guidelines for body weight classification in adults: application in clinical practice to screen for overweight and obesity and to assess disease risk. CMAJ 2005;172:995–998.
343 Arens R, Marcus CL: Pathophysiology of upper airway obstruction: a developmental perspective. Sleep 2004;27:997–1019.
344 Baeuerle PA, Baichwal VR: NF-kappa B as a frequent target for immunosuppressive and anti-inflammatory molecules. Adv Immunol 1997;65: 111–137.
345 Ghosh S, May MJ, Kopp EB: NF-kappa B and Rel proteins: evolutionarily conserved mediators of immune responses. Annu Rev Immunol 1998;16: 225–260.
346 Karin M, Ben-Neriah Y: Phosphorylation meets ubiquitination: the control of NF-[kappa]B activity. Annu Rev Immunol 2000;18:621–663.
347 Carmody RJ, Chen YH: Nuclear factor-kappaB: activation and regulation during Toll-like receptor signaling. Cell Mol Immunol 2007;4:31–41.
348 Kleiner DE, Brunt EM, Van Natta M, Behling C, Contos MJ, Cummings OW, Ferrell LD, Liu YC, Torbenson MS, Unalp-Arida A, Yeh M, McCullough AJ, Sanyal AJ: Design and validation of a histological scoring system for nonalcoholic fatty liver disease. Hepatology 2005;41:1313–1321.
349 Appropriate body-mass index for Asian populations and its implications for policy and intervention strategies. Lancet 2004;363:157–163.
350 Obesity: preventing and managing the global epidemic. Report of a WHO consultation. World Health Organ Tech Rep Ser 2000;894:1–253.
351 Clinical guidelines on the identification, evaluation, and treatment of overweight and obesity in adults – the evidence report. National Institutes of Health. Obes Res 1998;6(suppl 2):51S–209S.
352 Health Canada: Canadian Guidelines for Body Weight Classification in Adults. Ottawa, Health Canada, 2003, publication ID No 4645.
353 Khan NA, McAlister FA, Rabkin SW, Padwal R, Feldman RD, Campbell NR, Leiter LA, Lewanczuk RZ, Schiffrin EL, Hill MD, Arnold M, Moe G, Campbell TS, Herbert C, Milot A, Stone JA, Burgess E, Hemmelgarn B, Jones C, Larochelle P, Ogilvie RI, Houlden R, Herman RJ, Hamet P, Fodor G, Carruthers G, Culleton B, Dechamplain J, Pylypchuk G, Logan AG, Gledhill N, Petrella R, Tobe S, Touyz RM: The 2006 Canadian Hypertension Education Program recommendations for the management of hypertension- II. Therapy. Can J Cardiol 2006;22: 583–593.
354 Graham I, Atar D, Borch-Johnsen K, Boysen G, Burell G, Cifkova R, Dallongeville J, De Backer G, Ebrahim S, Gjelsvik B, Herrmann-Lingen C, Hoes A, Humphries S, Knapton M, Perk J, Priori SG, Pyorala K, Reiner Z, Ruilope L, Sans-Menendez S, Op Reimer WS, Weissberg P, Wood D, Yarnell J, Zamorano JL: European guidelines on cardiovascular disease prevention in clinical practice: executive summary. Atherosclerosis 2007;194:1–45.
355 Hara K, Matsushita Y, Horikoshi M, Yoshiike N, Yokoyama T, Tanaka H, Kadowaki T: A proposal for the cutoff point of waist circumference for the diagnosis of metabolic syndrome in the Japanese population. Diabetes Care 2006;29:1123–1124.
356 Oka R, Kobayashi J, Yagi K, Tanii H, Miyamoto S, Asano A, Hagishita T, Mori M, Moriuchi T, Kobayashi M, Katsuda S, Kawashiri MA, Nohara A, Takeda Y, Mabuchi H, Yamagishi M: Reassessment of the cutoff values of waist circumference and visceral fat area for identifying Japanese subjects at risk for the metabolic syndrome. Diabetes Res Clin Pract 2008;79:474–481.
357 New criteria for 'obesity disease' in Japan. Circ J 2002;66:987–992.

Endothelial Dysfunction in Adults with Obstructive Sleep Apnea

4

Chapter 4

Endothelial Dysfunction in Adults with Obstructive Sleep Apnea

Abstract

Vascular endothelial dysfunction refers to a loss of normal homeostatic functions in the blood vessels. It is characterized by reduced vasodilation and enhanced vasoconstriction functions and chronic prothrombotic and inflammatory activity. There is convincing evidence for endothelial dysfunction in obstructive sleep apnea (OSA): OSA is associated with alterations in vascular structures and their elastic properties, increased circulating cell-derived microparticles, reduced endothelial repair capacity, and vascular reactivity. These alterations may be related to the reduced availability of nitric oxide, which has major vasoprotective effects including vasodilation, inhibition of platelet adhesion and aggregation, inhibition of leukocyte-endothelial adhesion and inhibition of smooth muscle cell proliferation. It is unknown whether endothelial dysfunction in OSA is due to alterations in vasoconstriction mechanisms related to angiotensin II or endothelin 1. In OSA, endothelial dysfunction may be related to chronic intermittent hypoxia and to sleep loss and fragmentation. These conditions may increase the levels of various markers of inflammation and oxidative stress, as well as those of increased procoagulant and thrombotic activity. In addition, they may produce an imbalance of vasomotor function. Endothelial dysfunction contributes to the development of atherosclerosis and cardiovascular disorders associated with OSA. However, other diseases that are also associated with endothelial dysfunction are OSA comorbidities, e.g. obesity, insulin resistance, smoking habits and cardiovascular diseases such as hypertension and coronary artery disease. This makes it difficult to demonstrate a causal link between OSA and endothelial dysfunction; nevertheless, evidence for such a link has been produced by therapeutic studies. The administration of continuous positive airway pressure may reverse changes associated with endothelial dysfunction and, therefore, may decrease the risk of cardiovascular disease in OSA patients.

The vascular endothelium has a central role in maintaining normal vascular structure and function. It releases vasodilator mediators, e.g. nitric oxide (NO), and vasoconstrictor mediators, e.g. angiotensin (Ang) II and endothelin 1 (ET-1) that regulate not only vascular tone, but also the recruitment and activity of inflammatory cells, vascular permeability and fluid balance, and angiogenesis [1].

Endothelial dysfunction occurs when the effects of vasoconstrictor mediators override those of vasodilator mediators, causing damage to the arterial wall. It is characterized by reduced vasodilation, enhanced vasoconstriction functions, and chronic prothrombotic and inflammatory activity [1]. Endothelial dysfunction is an early marker of vascular abnormality that contributes to the development of atherosclerosis (a condition considered to be an inflammatory disorder), occurring early in its course, and it is predictive for the progression of future atherosclerotic disease [2]. Endothelial dysfunction is also involved in the development of vascular complications related to dyslipidemia, diabetes and cardiovascular diseases such as hypertension, coronary artery disease and chronic heart failure [1, 3–5].

Obstructive sleep apnea (OSA) is recognized as a risk factor for cardiovascular disorders including hypertension, coronary disease and stroke [6–8]. The increased prevalence of cardiovascular disorders associated with OSA has been attributed to the early development of atherosclerosis [7, 9]. Several studies (described below) suggest that endothelial dysfunction is present in OSA patients [9–12]; therefore, it has been hypothesized that endothelial dysfunction may be a potential mechanism by which OSA patients develop atherosclerosis and cardiovascular diseases. However, endothelial dysfunction has also been reported in OSA comorbidities such as cardiovascular disorders and diabetes; therefore, it is difficult to determine whether it is OSA and/or these other conditions that contribute to the endothelial dysfunction associated with OSA.

1 Obstructive Sleep Apnea May Alter Vascular Structure

1.1 *Arterial Structure and Elastic Properties*

Carotid artery intima-media thickness, carotid artery diameter and the elastic properties of the large arteries are markers of atherosclerosis [7, 13]. Abnormal values for these markers are associated with an increased risk of cardiovascular morbidity and mortality. For example, increased carotid artery intima-media thickness predicts the occurrence of carotid plaques and stroke, and increased arterial stiffness is an independent risk marker for premature coronary artery disease and cardiovascular mortality [14, 15].

Alterations in arterial structural and elastic property measures have been reported in OSA [16–34]. An increase in carotid intima-media thickness and the occurrence of atheromatous plaques have been observed in otherwise healthy OSA patients [19–21, 25]. Increases in the thickness of the intima and media and the occurrence of plaques were best predicted by the severity of oxygen desaturation in otherwise healthy OSA patients [19]. It is suggested that these changes may be an early cardiovascular consequence in OSA patients. In a small number of OSA patients (n = 19), those with moderate-to-severe OSA (n = 12) had a greater coronary atherosclerotic volume than patients with mild OSA [35]; the apnea-hypopnea index (AHI), the frequency of apnea and hypopnea events per hour of sleep, was positively correlated with the volume of coronary atherosclerotic plaques. Sleep fragmentation, assessed with the total arousal index and the respiratory arousal index, the frequency (per hour of sleep) of arousals and arousals related to respiratory events, respectively, was significantly associated with the volume of coronary atherosclerotic plaques [35]. Middle-aged patients with

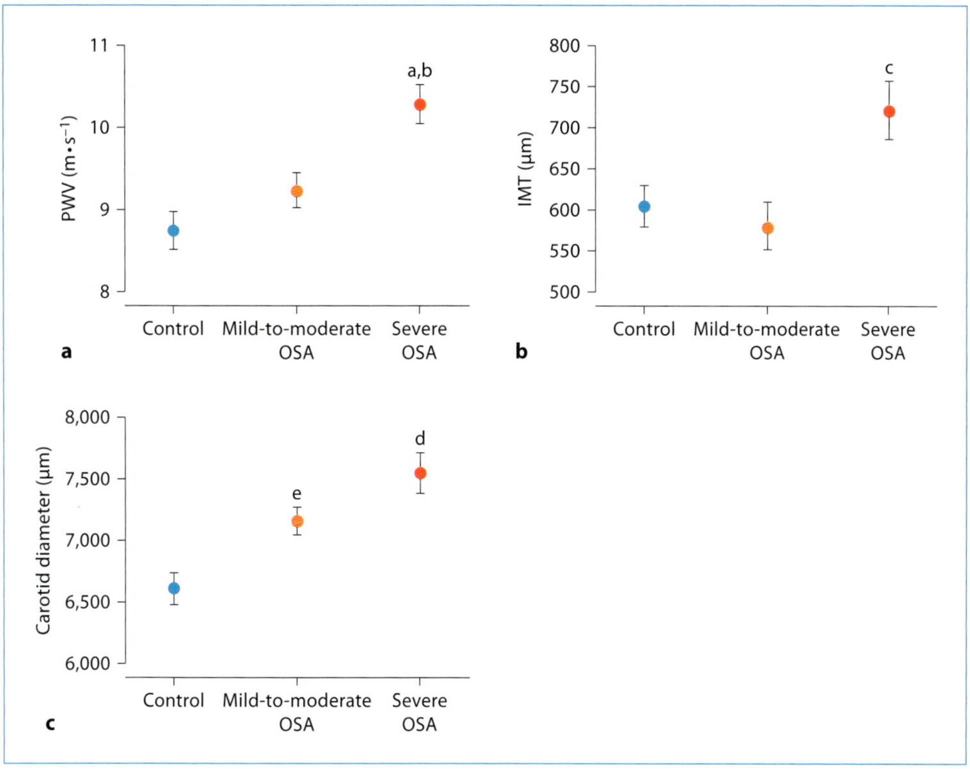

Fig. 1. Early endothelial dysfunction in OSA. Pulse wave velocity (PWV, **a**), intima-media thickness (IMT, **b**) and carotid diameter (**c**) values in healthy subjects (n = 12) and patients with mild-to-moderate (n = 15) and severe (n = 15) OSA. [a] $p < 0.001$, severe OSA compared with controls; [b] $p < 0.01$, severe OSA compared with mild-to-moderate OSA; [c] $p < 0.05$, severe OSA compared with controls and mild-to-moderate OSA; [d] $p < 0.0001$, severe OSA compared with controls; [e] $p < 0.05$, mild-to-moderate OSA compared with control subjects. Values are means ± SEM. After Drager et al. [20]. Reprinted with permission of the American Thoracic Society. © American Thoracic Society.

severe OSA and without overt cardiovascular disease had a significant increase in carotid artery intima-media thickness, carotid artery diameter and pulse wave velocity (a noninvasive measure that determines the elastic properties of the large arteries), compared with healthy control subjects matched for age, sex and body mass index (BMI). The degree of abnormality correlated with the severity of OSA (fig. 1) [20, 25]. Similar findings have been reported in other studies [16–18, 21, 24, 28]. The association of OSA and hypertension may have additive effects on these early markers of carotid atherosclerosis (fig. 2) [33].

The effects of continuous positive airway pressure (CPAP) administration on vascular structures and their elastic properties have been assessed. Compared with subtherapeutic CPAP, 4 weeks of effective CPAP treatment significantly reduced arterial stiffness in 102 patients with moderate to severe OSA ($p = 0.001$) [28]. A 4-month treatment with CPAP decreased intima-media thickness and pulse wave

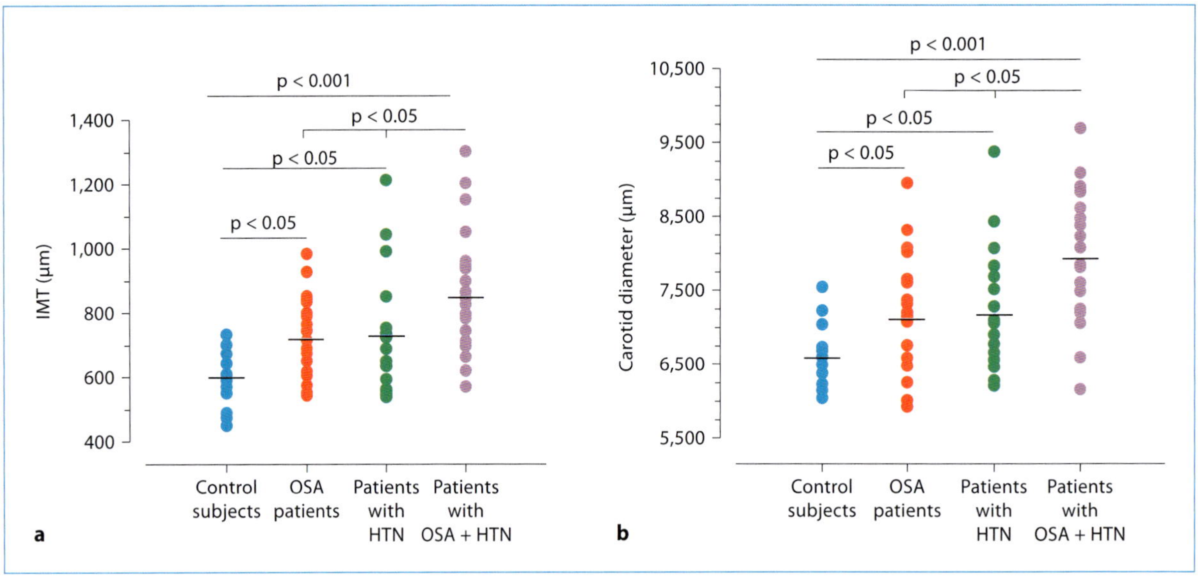

Fig. 2. Additive effect of OSA and hypertension (HTN) on early markers of carotid atherosclerosis. Participants (n = 94), free of smoking and diabetes mellitus, were divided into 4 groups: controls (n = 22), OSA (n = 25), HTN (n = 20) and OSA + HTN (n = 27). Carotid measurements included the thickness and diameter of the intima and media (IMT). Compared with controls, IMT (**a**) and carotid diameter (**b**) were similarly increased in the OSA and HTN groups, with a further significant increase in OSA + HTN patients. Short horizontal lines are means. After Drager et al. [33], with permission.

velocity (fig. 3) [36]. Significant decreases in pulse wave velocity have also been observed in OSA patients after 6 months of CPAP treatment [37].

Overall, these findings suggest that OSA may adversely affect arterial structures, while CPAP therapy may reduce these alterations.

1.2 Cell Apoptosis and Endothelial Repair Capacity

Microparticles are membrane vesicles released from many different cell types, including platelets, leukocytes, and vascular endothelial and smooth muscle cells [38]. Two mechanisms can result in their formation: cell activation and apoptosis (programmed cell death). They predict subclinical atherosclerosis [39] and cardiovascular risk [40], and are involved in a number of the damaging consequences of atherosclerosis, including endothelial dysfunction, coagulation, inflammation and remodeling, calcification and plaque rupture [41, 42].

Circulating cell-derived microparticles have been assessed in OSA patients, as they may be an additional cause of the predisposition of OSA patients to develop premature vascular disease [43–48]. The role of circulating apoptotic endothelial cells, i.e. CD146+ cells expressing annexin V (CD146+ cells are considered to be endothelial cell markers, although their specificity has been questioned; annexin V+ expression

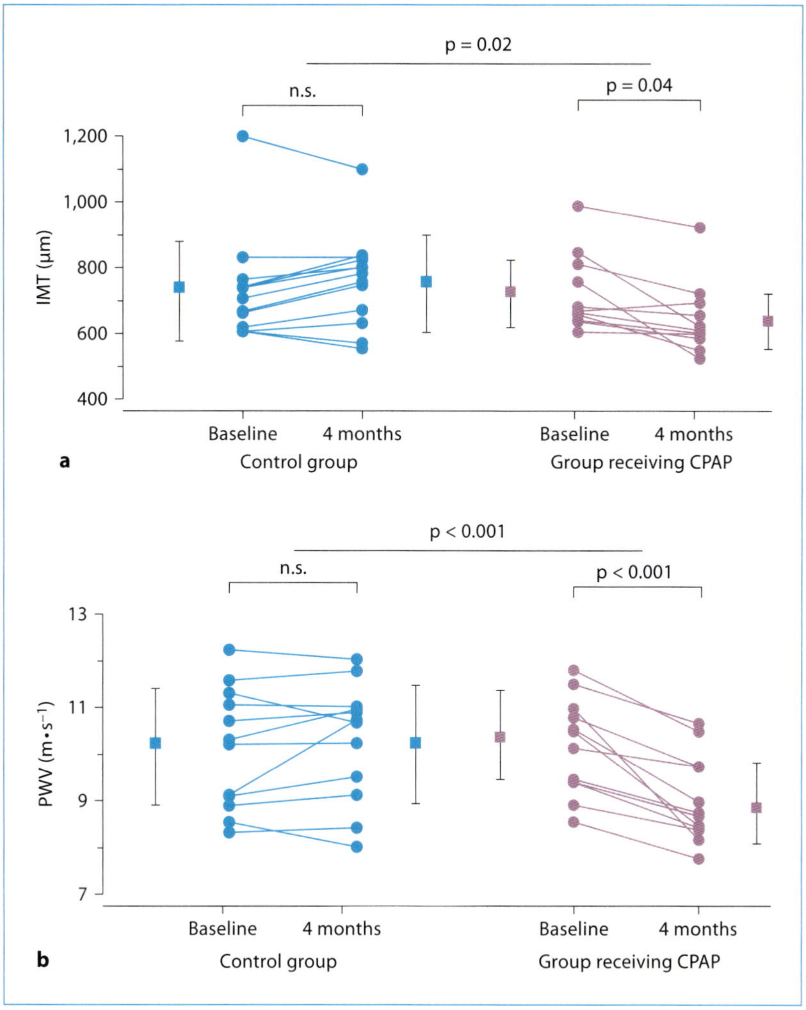

Fig. 3. Reduction in intima-media thickness (IMT) and pulse wave velocity (PWV) in OSA patients randomly assigned to receive CPAP for 4 months or no treatment (control group). **a** IMT significantly decreased in the group that received CPAP therapy ($p = 0.04$). In the control group, the IMT from baseline to 4 months was similar. The differences between the groups remained significant ($p = 0.02$). **b** PWV significantly decreased in all 12 subjects treated with CPAP ($p < 0.001$). In the control group, PWV from baseline to 4 months was similar. The differences between the groups were significant ($p < 0.001$). n.s. = Not significant. Short horizontal lines and bars are means ± SD. After Drager et al. [36]. Reprinted with permission of the American Thoracic Society. © American Thoracic Society.

differentiates apoptotic cells from dead cells) [49, 50] has been assessed in OSA patients [43, 44]. OSA patients have a higher density of circulating apoptotic endothelial cells than non-OSA subjects, and CPAP therapy reduced this increased density (fig. 4) [43, 44]. The levels of endothelial microparticles were higher in untreated nonobese otherwise healthy OSA patients than in nonsmoking healthy subjects matched for

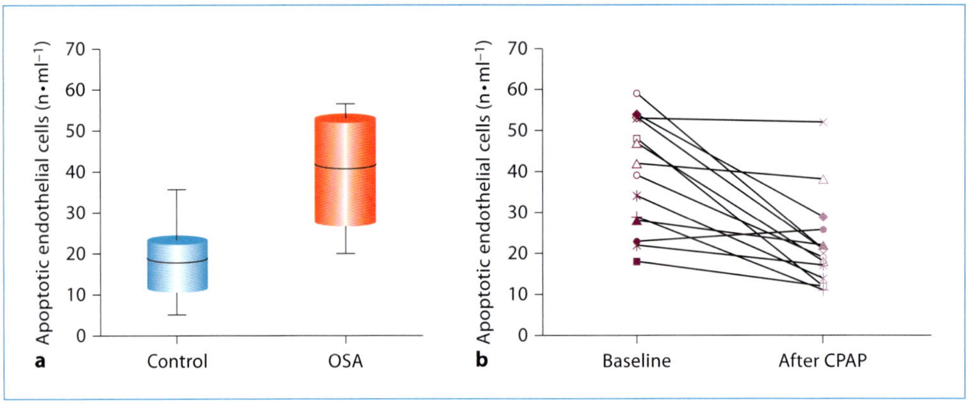

Fig. 4. Apoptotic endothelial cells in OSA. **a** Box-and-whisker plot of circulating apoptotic endothelial cells per volume of blood (per milliliter) in healthy control subjects (n = 10) and OSA patients (n = 14). The boxes represent values within the interquartile range, and the whiskers represent the data range; lines across the boxes represent the median values. **b** Plot of circulating apoptotic endothelial cell levels in the same 14 OSA patients at baseline and after 8 weeks of CPAP therapy ($p < 0.001$). OSA patients appear to have increased numbers of these cells, which decrease after CPAP therapy. After El Solh et al. [43]. Reprinted with permission of the American Thoracic Society. © American Thoracic Society.

age, gender and BMI [47]. Four weeks of CPAP therapy in a small number of patients (n = 8) tended to reduce the levels of endothelial microparticles, but this reduction was not significant.

Polymorphonuclear leukocytes contribute to the inflammatory processes associated with atherogenesis and the development of acute coronary syndrome lesions [51]. Polymorphonuclear leukocyte apoptosis is a critical injury-limiting mechanism that restricts their potential deleterious effect [45]. In contrast, delayed polymorphonuclear leukocyte apoptosis may increase these effects [52], and delayed neutrophil apoptosis has been observed in OSA patients [45]. When platelet-, leukocyte- and endothelial cell-derived microparticles were assessed in patients with minimally symptomatic OSA (n = 57) and closely matched control subjects without OSA (n = 15) [46], minimally symptomatic OSA patients had higher levels of platelet- and leukocyte-derived microparticles than the matched control subjects (fig. 5). However, the levels of endothelial cell-derived microparticles were similar in both groups. It is suggested that these OSA patients may have an increased cardiovascular risk, despite being minimally symptomatic.

Endothelial dysfunction can also result from a reduction in the endothelial repair capacity of bone marrow-derived endothelial progenitor cells [9, 53]. Reduced levels of bone marrow-derived endothelial progenitor cells are a marker of cardiovascular risk [54–56]. Endothelial progenitor cell levels are lower in otherwise healthy OSA patients than in control subjects, while the levels are significantly increased in patients who adhered to CPAP for >4 h • day^{-1} [47, 53]. In addition, endothelial cell progenitor

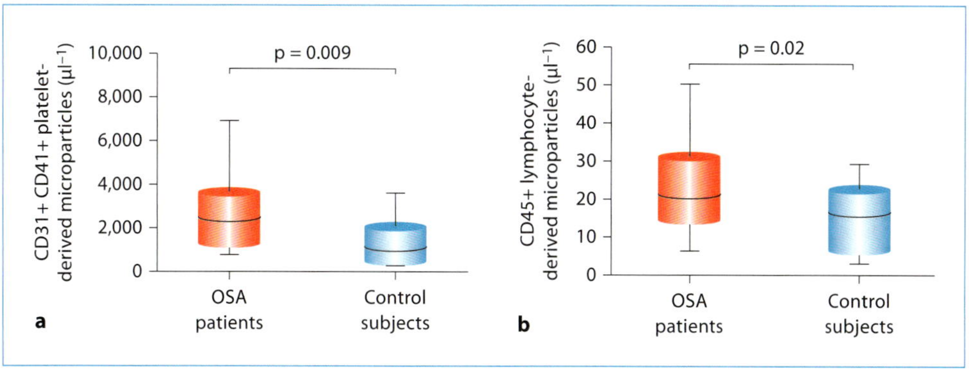

Fig. 5. Circulating cell-derived microparticles in patients with minimally symptomatic OSA. **a** CD31+ CD41+ platelet-derived microparticle levels were significantly higher in patients with minimally symptomatic OSA than in the control group without OSA. **b** CD45+ lymphocyte-derived microparticle levels were significantly higher in patients with minimally symptomatic OSA than in the control group without OSA. Box-and-whisker plots represent medians, interquartile ranges, and the 10th and 90th percentiles. Platelet and lymphocyte microparticles were assessed using monoclonal antibodies. After Ayers et al. [46], with permission. © European Respiratory Society.

and endothelial microparticle levels are inversely correlated [47]; similarly, reduced levels of endothelial progenitor cells have been observed in OSA patients [57], but this finding has not been replicated [58]. A reduced endothelial repair capacity may exacerbate endothelium dysfunction in OSA, as endothelial cells critically contribute to the homeostasis of vascular function [9, 47].

Overall, these findings suggest that OSA may be associated with increased levels of circulating cell-derived microparticles and a reduced endothelial cell repair capacity. CPAP therapy may counterbalance these alterations.

2 Obstructive Sleep Apnea May Adversely Affect Endothelial Regulation of the Peripheral Vasomotor Tone

2.1 *Alterations in Nitric-Oxide-Dependent Vasodilator Mechanisms*

2.1.1 Vascular Reactivity

Flow-mediated dilation (FMD) in the brachial artery or other conduit vessels reflects endothelial function and is mainly mediated by endothelial NO production [59]. FMD measures the change in the diameter of the brachial artery after a brief period of forearm ischemia, such as that induced by the inflation and release of a pneumatic tourniquet placed on the forearm. A decrease in FMD was observed in otherwise healthy patients with untreated OSA (n = 28), and this was reversed by CPAP treatment [60]. Analysis of brachial artery FMD among older participants in the baseline

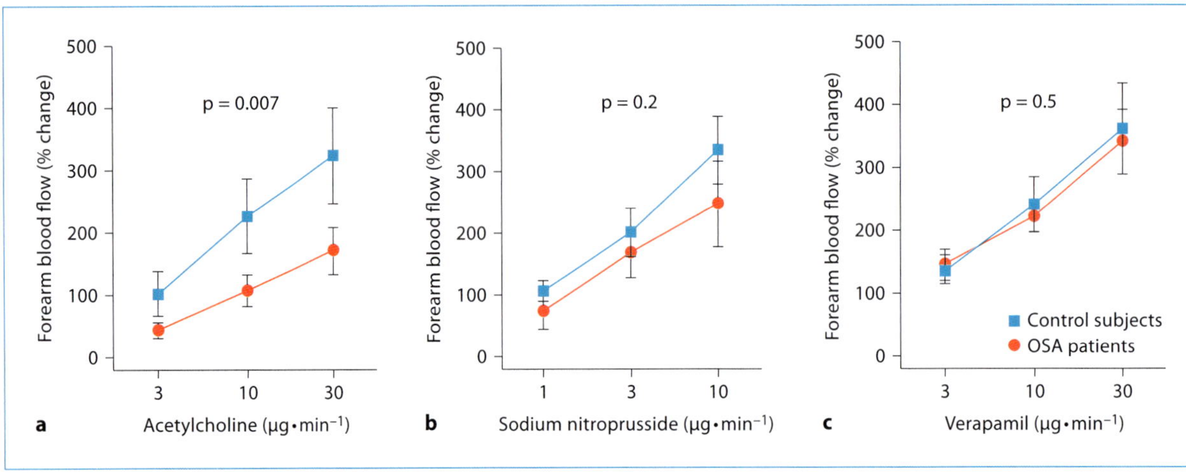

Fig. 6. Forearm blood flow responses to intra-arterial infusions of acetylcholine, sodium nitroprusside and verapamil in OSA patients (n = 8) and obese control subjects (n = 9). **a** Acetylcholine infusion induced a dose-dependent increase in forearm blood flow in both groups. The percent change in forearm blood flow was significantly reduced in the OSA patients compared with the control subjects ($p < 0.007$). **b**, **c** Administration of increasing doses of sodium nitroprusside (**b**) and verapamil (**c**) increased forearm blood flow in both groups, but there was no significant difference between the groups ($p = 0.2$ and $p = 0.5$, respectively). It is suggested that OSA patients have impaired resistance vessel endothelium-dependent vasodilation. Results are expressed as the percentage change in forearm blood flow. Data are the mean ± SEM. After Kato et al. [62], with permission.

examination of the Sleep Heart Health/Cardiovascular Health Study cohort (n = 1,037, aged ≥68 years, 56% female) [16] indicated that sleep apnea measures were associated with the baseline diameter of the brachial artery and the percentage of FMD. These associations remained significant, but weakened, after adjustment for other cardiovascular risk factors, particularly BMI.

Compared with control subjects, vascular reactivity in OSA patients was significantly altered following the administration of acetylcholine (an endothelium-dependent vasodilator that stimulates the endothelial release of NO) [61–63]. On the other hand, vascular reactivity in OSA patients was not significantly different from control subjects when endothelium-independent vasodilators such as sodium nitroprusside (an exogenous NO donor) or verapamil (a calcium channel blocker) were used (fig. 6) [62]. A 3-month CPAP treatment in otherwise healthy OSA patients improved endothelium-dependent vascular reactivity, but not endothelium-independent vasodilation, indicating the increased availability of NO (fig. 7) [63]. Overall, these findings suggest that OSA patients have an impairment of resistance vessel endothelium-dependent vasodilation. Similar findings have been reported by other authors [64].

The use of a mandibular repositioning device is an alternative treatment for patients with mild-to-moderate OSA that improves endothelial dysfunction in OSA [65]. The effects of 1 year of treatment with a mandibular repositioning device on

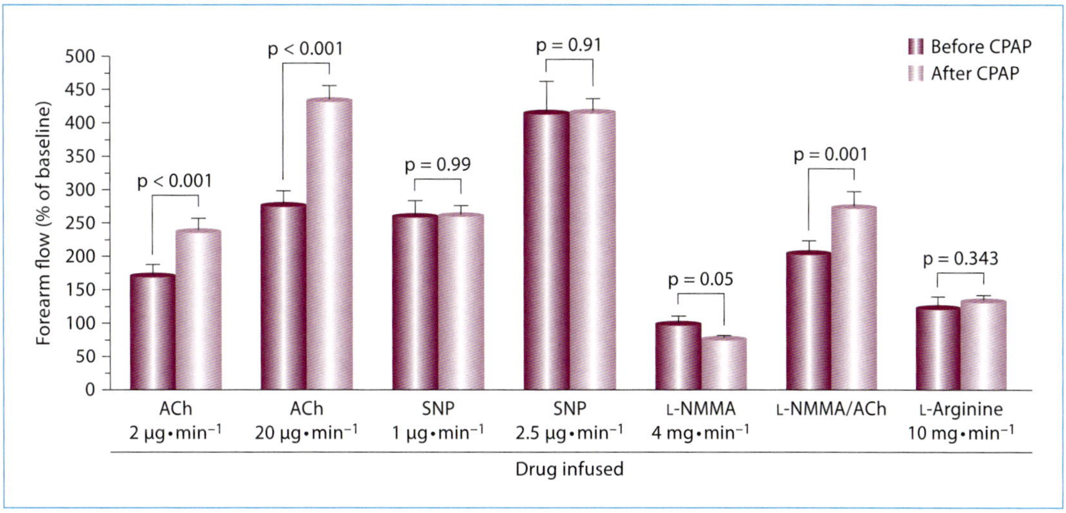

Fig. 7. Effect of 3-month CPAP treatment on endothelium-dependent and endothelium-independent vascular reactivity. Forearm blood flow response to intra-arterial infusions of acetylcholine (ACh), sodium nitroprusside (SNP), N^G-monomethyl-L-arginine (L-NMMA, an NO antagonist) and L-arginine (the NO synthase substrate for NO production) were measured in 10 patients with moderate-to-severe OSA. The response to ACh alone or ACh with L-NMMA was greater after CPAP than before ($p \le 0.001$). The improvement in vasodilation observed after ACh was only partially inhibited by coinfusion of L-NMMA (L-NMMA/ACh), indicating that NO endothelium-dependent pathways and non-NO pathways were enhanced. The vasoconstrictor response to L-NMMA was significantly greater after CPAP than before ($p = 0.05$), consistent with the enhanced release of NO from the vascular endothelium. The SNP responses were unchanged with CPAP. This is consistent with improved endothelial, but not smooth muscle, vasodilator function. After Lattimore et al. [63], with permission.

vascular reactivity were assessed by peripheral tonometry in nonobese OSA patients (n = 12, mean AHI 29.7), untreated OSA patients (n = 6) and control subjects without OSA (n = 10) [66]. Despite partial efficacy (mean AHI 19.6), treatment with the device was associated with a significant improvement in vascular reactivity. Other authors have reported similar findings [67].

In summary, there is increasing evidence suggesting that OSA decreases vasodilator mechanisms. In addition, these alterations may be improved by treatment of OSA.

2.1.2 Nitric Oxide Availability

NO (fig. 8) has major vasoprotective effects, including vasodilation and inhibition of platelet adhesion and aggregation, leukocyte-endothelial adhesion and smooth muscle cell proliferation [2, 68]. An important cause of endothelial dysfunction is the reduction in the bioactivity of endothelium-derived NO, as observed in diabetes, hypertension, smoking and atherosclerosis [2, 5, 68–70]. NO bioavailability is reduced in OSA patients and increased after CPAP treatment [71, 72]. Circulating NO and its derivatives (nitrate and nitrite, NOx) were assessed in 21 obese OSA patients before

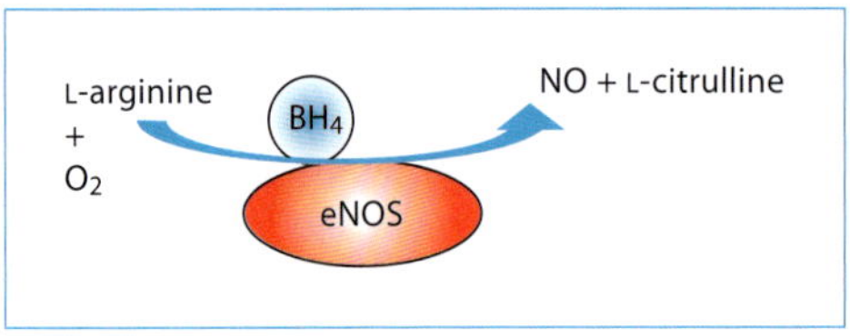

Fig. 8. NO production by NO synthase. Under physiological conditions, endothelial NO synthase (eNOS) produces NO from L-arginine, with citrulline formed as a by-product. Functional eNOS requires dimerization and the presence of the substrate L-arginine and the essential cofactor tetrahydro-L-biopterin (BH_4), a potent naturally occurring reducing agent [68]. After Yang and Ming [2], with permission of Marshfield Clinic. © 2006 Marshfield Clinic.

(baseline levels) and after 2 nights and 5.5 months of CPAP administration [72]. Age-matched, healthy volunteers (n = 13) and patients without OSA (n = 18), but with a similar spectrum of comorbidities, served as controls (control groups 1 and 2, respectively). Baseline NOx levels were significantly lower in OSA patients than in both control groups ($p < 0.01$ for each comparison). NOx concentrations increased after 2 nights of CPAP treatment and remained constant until follow-up ($p < 0.01$ compared with the levels before CPAP). A prospective randomized, placebo-controlled study assessed the plasma concentrations of total nitrate and NOx in middle-aged, newly diagnosed males with OSA and no other known comorbidities (n = 31) and healthy control subjects (n = 15) of the same age, gender and BMI [73]. OSA patients were randomized to sham CPAP and effective CPAP application for 12 weeks. NOx levels were significantly lower in OSA patients than in healthy subjects at baseline, and they were significantly increased after effective CPAP therapy, but not after sham CPAP (fig. 9) [73]. The endothelial NO synthase (eNOS) 296 polymorphism of the NO synthase (NOS) gene was associated with the occurrence of OSA, but not its severity, where a Glu/Asp variant was more frequent and a Glu/Glu variant was less frequent in OSA patients than in control subjects [74].

Oxidative reactions may play a prominent role in the impaired NO bioactivity observed in OSA patients, e.g. the reaction of NO with superoxide ions ($O_2^{-\bullet}$), to form peroxynitrite ($ONOO^-$). The reduced production of NO may also be related to the production of $O_2^-\bullet$ instead of NO by NOS. This is termed NO uncoupling and can occur under specific circumstances, such as when the concentrations of substrates or cofactors are compromised [2, 68, 75]. Uncoupling has been reported in conditions such as atherosclerosis, diabetes mellitus, hypertension and chronic smoking [68, 75, 76]. Asymmetric dimethyl arginine (ADMA) competes with L-arginine, the substrate of eNOS. High ADMA concentrations inhibit the synthesis of NO by eNOS by reducing the concentration of L-arginine available to be metabolized. This may uncouple the enzyme and could enhance oxidative stress [68, 77]. When the plasma levels of ADMA, NO metabolites and FMD were measured in the brachial artery before and at 1 and 4 weeks after CPAP therapy in 10 male OSA patients [78], FMD

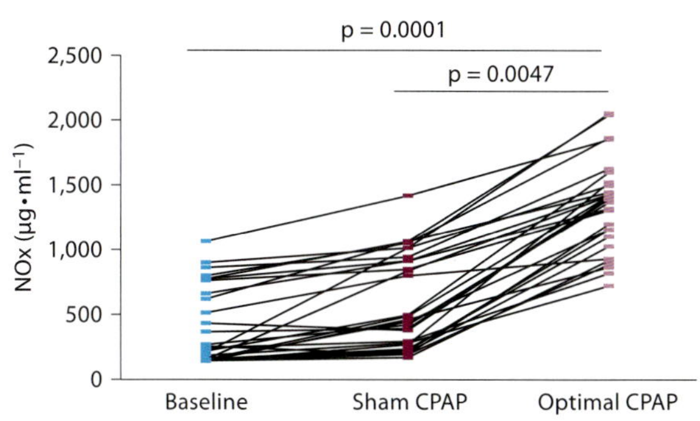

Fig. 9. Individual plasma NOx concentrations at baseline, after sham CPAP and optimal CPAP in OSA patients. Compared with sham CPAP, optimal CPAP therapy significantly increased the plasma NOx concentrations from baseline in OSA patients. This suggests that OSA is associated with a decrease in NO bioavailability that is normalized by CPAP therapy. After Alonso-Fernandez et al. [73], with permission.

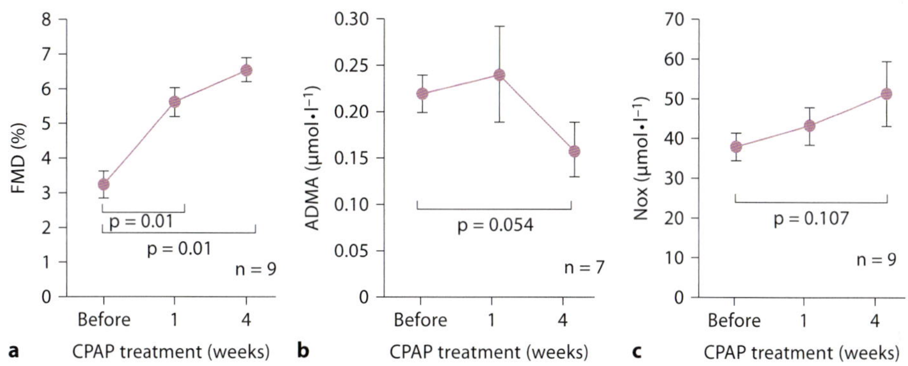

Fig. 10. Endothelium-dependent vasodilation of the brachial artery and ADMA and NOx plasma levels before and 1 and 4 weeks after CPAP therapy in 10 male OSA patients. Endothelium-dependent vasodilation was obtained by inducing forearm ischemia using a blood pressure cuff tourniquet set at 250 mm Hg for 5 min. Subsequent rapid deflation of the tourniquet resulted in FMD. The percent change in arterial diameter from baseline (**a**), plasma ADMA concentrations (**b**) and NOx metabolites (**c**) were assessed before and 1 and 4 weeks after CPAP therapy. All values are presented as means ± SEM. After Ohike et al. [78], with permission.

levels were significantly improved after 1 and 4 weeks of CPAP therapy, whereas the plasma NOx concentrations tended to increase. The plasma ADMA concentrations decreased inversely to percent FMD and NOx at 4 weeks (fig. 10). It is suggested that CPAP reduces the concentration of ADMA, thereby enhancing the production of NO and leading to an improvement of endothelium-dependent vasodilation. However, the relationship between the decrease in NO availability and ADMA levels in OSA remains to be clarified [79, 80].

Patients with OSA have reduced baseline expression levels of eNOS and activated eNOS (eNOS phosphorylated at serine 1177) by 59 and 94%, respectively, than observed in control subjects, and their levels were significantly increased in patients who adhered to CPAP ≥4 h daily (fig. 11) [53]. The levels of nitrotyrosine (a marker of nitrosative stress) and the expression of cyclooxygenase 2 and inducible NOS (markers of endothelial inflammation) were higher in OSA patients than in control subjects, and their levels were significantly decreased in patients who adhered to CPAP ≥4 h daily. Baseline FMD and endothelial progenitor cell levels were lower in OSA patients than in control subjects, and both were significantly increased in patients who adhered to CPAP ≥4 h daily. When brachial artery FMD and forearm subcutaneous biopsies were assessed in control subjects and before and after 12 weeks of CPAP therapy in OSA patients free of cardiovascular risk factors, FMD was significantly lower in OSA patients than in control subjects at baseline ($p = 0.02$) and significantly increased after CPAP treatment ($p = 0.04$) [81]. Patients with OSA had higher microcirculatory peroxynitrite deposits in the microvascular walls than control subjects. CPAP treatment decreased the deposition of microcirculatory peroxynitrite and the transcription of eNOS in microvascular endothelial cells. This study showed that OSA patients with low cardiovascular risk status had endothelial dysfunction and provided direct evidence of increased oxidant production in the microcirculation using subcutaneous biopsies, both of which were improved with treatment. Discrepancies in the expression of eNOS between these 2 studies have been related to technical differences [81]. These data suggest that reduced NO production was associated with lower eNOS expression or eNOS uncoupling. However, both studies suggest that OSA affects the vascular endothelium by promoting oxidative stress while decreasing NO availability, while effective CPAP therapy was associated with the improvement of these alterations.

Overall, it is suggested that OSA reduces the availability of endothelial NO, and that CPAP administration may increase NO bioavailability.

2.2 *Alterations in Vasoconstriction Mechanisms*

2.2.1 Downregulation of Vascular Sympathoadrenergic Receptors

Alterations of vasoconstriction function in OSA may be related to changes in the autonomic nervous system [11], including an increase in sympathetic nerve activity and an impairment of the baroreflex [82–84]. It has also been associated with the downregulation of vascular sympathoadrenergic receptors [85]. The response to sympathetic agonist stimulation is diminished if receptors have previously been continually stimulated [86], such as the downregulation of vascular sympathoadrenergic receptors (also termed refractoriness or desensitization) in OSA patients [85, 87–89].

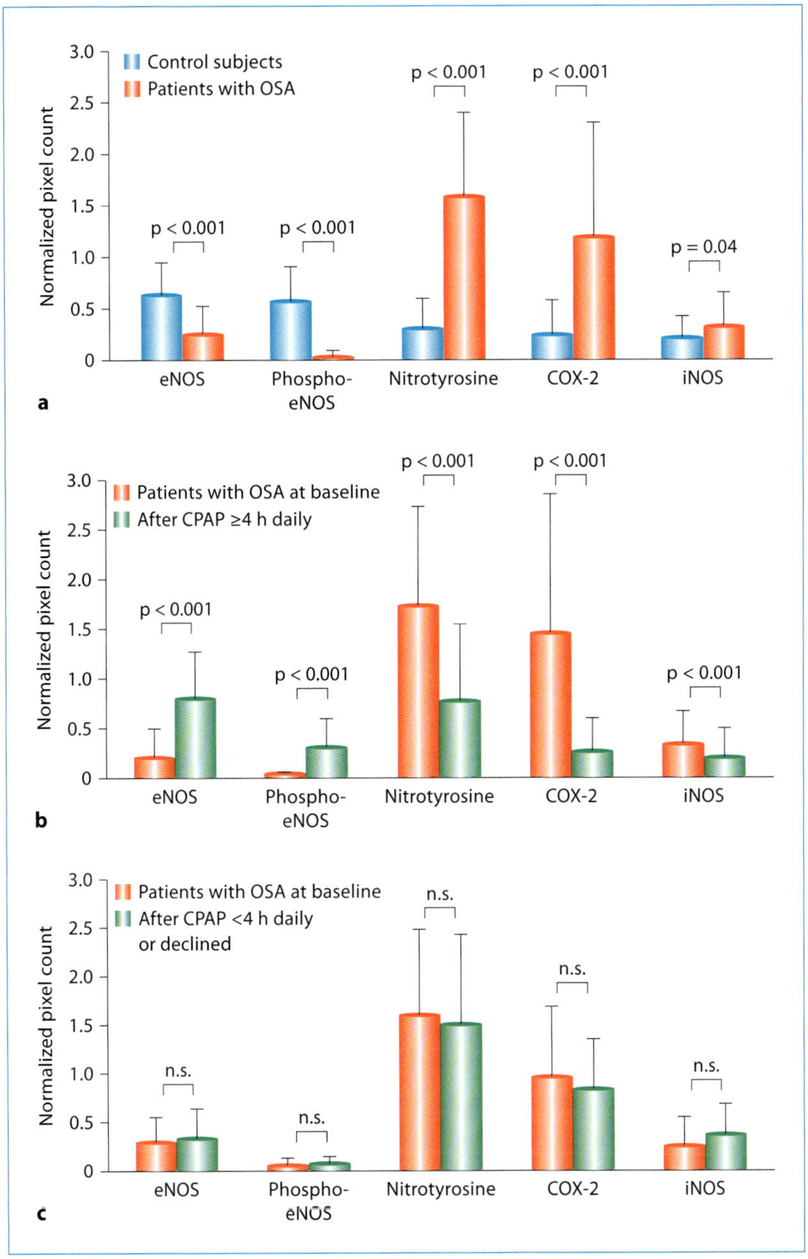

Fig. 11. Expression of protein markers for oxidative stress (tyrosine) and inflammation, i.e. cyclooxygenase 2 (COX-2), inducible NOS (iNOS), in freshly harvested venous endothelial cells at baseline and after CPAP therapy. **a** Expression of eNOS, phosphorylated (phospho-) eNOS, nitrotyrosine, COX-2 and iNOS in harvested venous endothelial cells. The baseline expression of eNOS and phospho-eNOS was lower in OSA patients (n = 30) than in control subjects (n = 15), whereas the expression of nitrotyrosine, COX-2 and iNOS was increased. **b** When patients adhered to CPAP ≥4 h daily (n = 14), the expression of eNOS and phospho-eNOS was significantly increased, whereas the expression of nitrotyrosine, COX-2 and iNOS was significantly decreased. **c** Protein expression did not change when patients used CPAP <4 h daily or refused CPAP therapy (n = 16). n.s. = Not significant. Data are means ± SD. After Jelic et al. [53], with permission.

2.2.2 Endothelin 1

ET-1 is a 21-amino-acid peptide mainly produced by endothelial cells and, to some extent, by vascular smooth muscle cells [90–92]. Reactive oxygen species (ROS), hypoxia, Ang II, vasopressin, cytokines, thrombin and shear stress enhance the production of ET-1, while NO, prostacyclin and atrial natriuretic peptide inhibit its synthesis and release. ET-1 contributes to vascular tone regulation and to the regulation of endothelial and smooth muscle cell proliferation. It has proinflammatory properties involving the activation of the nuclear factor κB (NF-κB) pathway and the production of ROS (fig. 12), and it contributes to endothelial dysfunction and atherosclerosis through these pathways [90, 93].

Conflicting results have been reported for ET-1 levels in OSA patients. This is linked to a methodological bias in the ET-1 assessment methods, the involvement of unmatched groups of participants and the presence of comorbidities (coexisting cardiovascular disorders may influence plasma ET-1 levels) [94–100]. Morbidly obese patients with severe OSA have higher ET-1 levels than less obese control subjects, which is significantly lowered by effective CPAP treatment (the presence of comorbidities other than obesity was not specified) [94]. Higher levels of ET-1 were observed in a small number of normotensive OSA patients (n = 9) than in control subjects (n = 66) [101]. Higher ET-1 levels were also observed in normotensive patients with OSA (n = 41) than in control subjects with lower BMI and lower systolic blood pressure (n = 41) [98], while higher nighttime plasma levels of ET-1 were observed in OSA patients (n = 32) than in healthy controls (n = 19), and the mean nocturnal level of ET-1 was significantly correlated with OSA severity assessed with the AHI [99]. OSA patients also had a significantly higher blood pressure than healthy controls. In contrast, ET-1 plasma levels were found to be similar in otherwise healthy OSA patients [95] or in hypertensive OSA patients [96] compared with control subjects. The levels of big ET-1, a precursor peptide cleaved by the ET-converting enzyme to form ET-1, are considerably raised in untreated OSA patients and drop to normal levels after long-term CPAP treatment in compliant patients [97]. However, ET-1 concentrations remained within the normal range and did not change after CPAP therapy. It was suggested that big ET-1 may be a more appropriate marker of endothelial alterations than ET-1 because of its longer half-life, i.e. 23 min versus 40–70 s, respectively [97, 102]. However, as ET-1 is mostly released abluminally from endothelial cells, the levels of circulating ET-1 or its precursors may not accurately reflect its production [103]. In other words, normal plasma ET-1 levels do not exclude its increased vascular production in OSA patients.

ET-1 acts through 2 distinct types of receptors: endothelin receptor type A (ET_A) and type B (ET_B) [92]. Activation of ET_A and ET_B on vascular smooth muscle cells results in vasoconstriction. Conversely, vascular endothelial cells exclusively express the ET_B subtype and mediate vasodilation via NO and prostacyclin. As ET-1 is mostly released abluminally from endothelial cells, the resultant effect of ET-1 on vascular tone in normal physiological conditions is vasoconstriction. ET-1 and ET_A gene

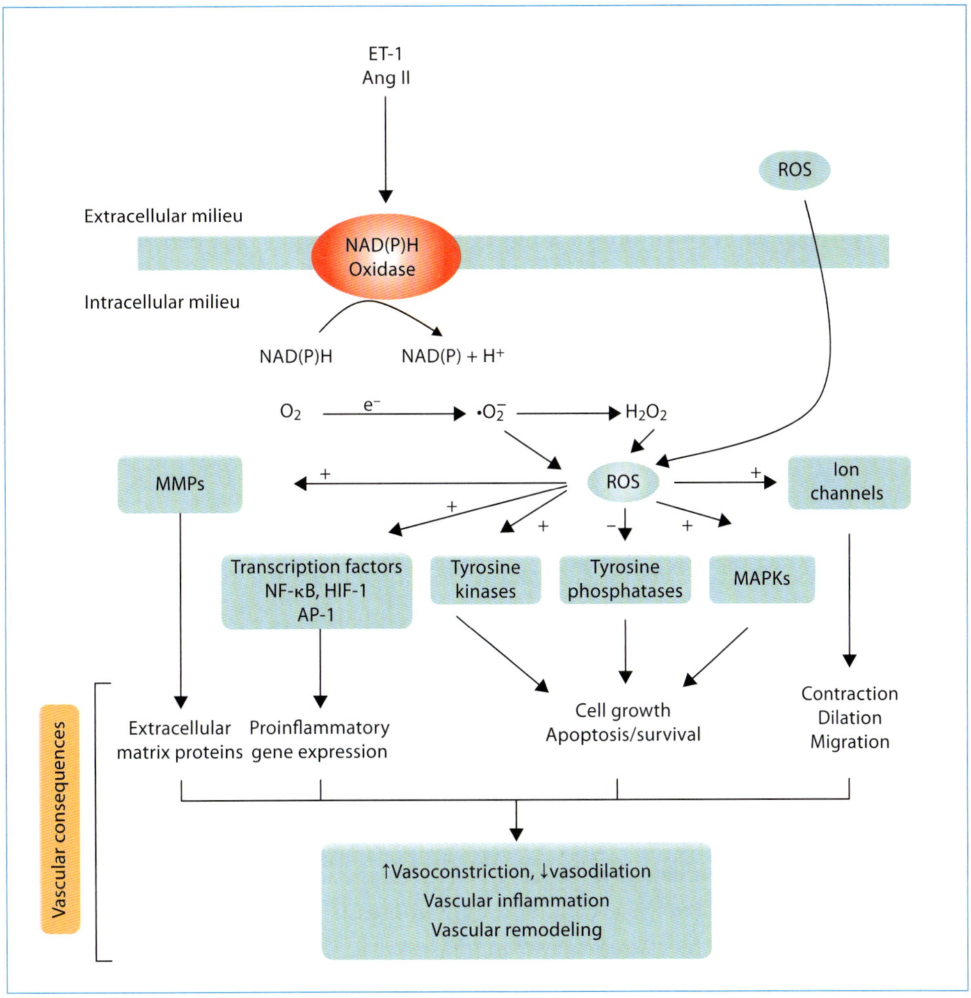

Fig. 12. ET-1, Ang II and redox-dependent signaling pathways in vascular smooth muscle cells. ET-1 and Ang II stimulate the production of intracellular ROS, primarily through the activation of nicotinamide adenine dinucleotide (phosphate) oxidase [NAD(P)H oxidase]. In addition, ROS produced in the extracellular milieu can enter cells by diffusion or through ion channels. Major targets of ROS in vascular smooth muscle cells include matrix metalloproteinases (MMPs), transcription factors, tyrosine kinases, tyrosine phosphatases, mitogen-activated protein kinases (MAPKs) and ion channels. The alterations produced by the activation or inhibition of these targets by excess ROS may contribute to vascular remodeling, vascular inflammation and endothelial dysfunction. HIF-1 = Hypoxia-inducible factor 1; AP-1 = activator protein 1; + = stimulatory effect; – = inhibitory effect. After Touyz [163], with permission.

polymorphisms have been assessed in OSA, where the ET-1 variant Lys198Asn (G/T) genotype was examined in patients with mild-to-severe OSA (n = 364) and control subjects (n = 57) [104]. The Lys198Asn genotype was significantly associated with the AHI, with a median AHI of 30 for the GG genotype, 27 for the GT genotype and

59 for the TT genotype ($p < 0.05$). A strong association was observed between the AHI and the Lys198Asn polymorphism in 191 obese patients ($p = 0.005$), but not in 173 nonobese patients. A strong association was observed between the BMI and OSA severity assessed with the AHI, but the increase in the AHI per unit of BMI was approximately 1.3 times greater in homozygous carriers of the mutant allele than in other carrier groups. It is suggested that the Lys198Asn polymorphism is associated with the severity of OSA in obese subjects. In a comparison between patients (393 Caucasian OSA patients, AHI >5 and daytime sleepiness) and control subjects with healthy sleep (n = 58), carriers of the mutant ET_A G231A allele had a significantly lower AHI ($p = 0.03$, odds ratio 0.53, 95% confidence interval 0.3–0.94) [105]. These findings need to be confirmed in a larger number of participants with well-defined phenotypes.

2.2.3 Angiotensin II

2.2.3.1 Ang II Production and Receptors. Ang II is a hormone produced by the renin-angiotensin system [106, 107]. Classically, the renin-angiotensin system consists of renin, which is released from the kidney juxtaglomerular cells, that cleaves liver-derived angiotensinogen to produce Ang I. Ang I is then converted to Ang II by angiotensin-converting enzyme (ACE) 1, mainly within the pulmonary circulation, but also within other tissues (e.g. in other arteries) [108]. These tissues are able to take up circulatory prorenin and renin through specific receptors, resulting in local angiotensin synthesis. This local Ang II production represents at least 40% of its total production in humans, and seems more closely related to vascular inflammatory responses than does circulating Ang II.

Ang II has vasoconstrictor effects and contributes to vascular tone regulation. It is a major mediator of oxidative stress, increases vascular permeability and thrombotic activity, and promotes the infiltration of leukocytes and tissue remodeling [109]. Most of the Ang-II-induced cardiovascular effects and Ang-II-induced vascular inflammation are mediated via the Ang II type 1 receptor. ACE inhibitors and Ang II antagonists have been shown to improve endothelial function in hypertensive patients [110].

2.2.3.2 ACE and Ang II in OSA. The gene encoding ACE1 is located on the long arm of chromosome 17 (17q23), and the level of circulating ACE1 is genetically determined [111]. Approximately 20% of the identified gene polymorphisms are located in the coding region and approximately 50% of these are missense mutations [112]. The presence (insertion, I) or absence (deletion, D) of a 287-bp sequence in intron 16 has been related to the circulating levels of ACE1. Mean ACE activity in DD carriers is approximately twice that observed in II carriers [111]. Analysis of the relationship between the ACE I/D polymorphism and OSA has provided conflicting results. Although an early study suggested that the D allele may be a risk factor for OSA [113], subsequent studies have not replicated this finding [114–116]. The ACE D allele may protect against hypertension, but whether this occurs only in severe OSA or also in

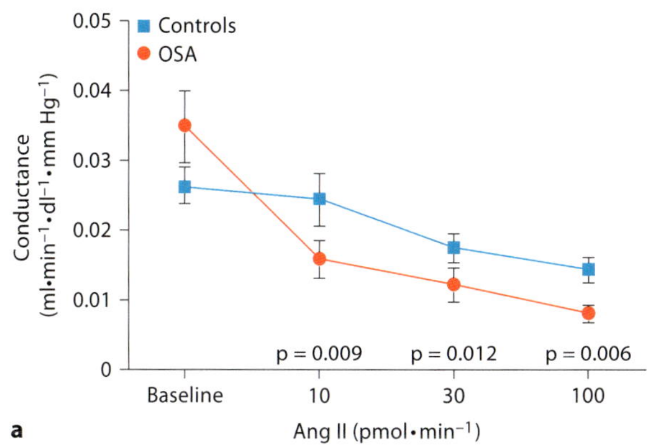

Fig. 13. Vasoconstrictor sensitivity to Ang II. Vasoconstrictor sensitivity of the forearm vasculature was studied in 10 OSA patients and 10 healthy controls who were free of regular medication, arterial hypertension, diabetes mellitus and dyslipidemia. Using 3 dosage steps, Ang II was infused into the brachial artery. Baseline forearm vascular conductance did not differ significantly between the 2 groups. During infusion, the mean conductance was 39.6% lower ($p < 0.002$) in the OSA patients than in the control subjects, suggesting enhanced vasoconstrictor sensitivity in the forearm vasculature in OSA. The p values refer to between-group comparisons with correction for baseline conductance. After Kraiczi et al. [119], with permission.

mild-to-moderate OSA is controversial [115, 116]. The I allele was associated with hypertension in patients with mild-to-moderate OSA ($p < 0.01$), but not in those with severe OSA [117], while the ACE I/D polymorphism was not associated with the severity of apnea in normotensive patients. It is suggested that the homozygous ACE I allele protects against severe OSA in hypertensive OSA males.

Patients with OSA (n = 24) had significantly increased blood pressure, Ang II and aldosterone compared with control subjects (n = 18); however, the increased levels of Ang II may have resulted from either the hypertension or the OSA [96]. CPAP treatment decreased daytime blood pressure, and this correlated with a decrease in the plasma concentration of Ang II. Higher levels of Ang II were observed in OSA patients than in control subjects, and these levels decreased after 12 weeks of CPAP therapy [118]. Enhanced vasoconstrictor sensitivity to an intra-arterial infusion of Ang II in the forearm vasculature has also been observed in OSA patients (fig. 13) [119].

In contrast, serial nocturnal plasma levels of Ang II and renin were similar in OSA patients (n = 32) and healthy controls (n = 19) [99], while there were no significant differences in mean serum ACE levels and the frequency of ACE gene polymorphisms in untreated OSA patients (n = 26), sleepy snorers (n = 26) and healthy controls (n = 26) [120]. Serum ACE levels did not change after 6 months of CPAP therapy.

In summary, it remains to be elucidated whether alterations in the renin-angiotensin system occur in OSA.

3 Potential Mechanisms Leading to Endothelial Dysfunction in Obstructive Sleep Apnea

3.1 *Chronic Intermittent Hypoxia/Reoxygenation*

Strong evidence indicates the potential role of chronic intermittent hypoxia in the development of endothelial dysfunction in OSA [7–9, 121]. OSA severity, assessed with oxygen desaturation indices or the AHI, has been associated with a decrease in endothelium-dependent vasodilation in the forearm [16, 62, 122, 123]; however, oxygen desaturation indices better predicted endothelial dysfunction than the AHI [8]. For example, an important role has been demonstrated for hypoxemia as a potential intermediate mechanism leading to endothelial dysfunction in OSA [123], where vascular function was compared in 2 groups of patients with OSA: 27 desaturators (2 major symptoms of OSA, AHI >15, >20 of 4% desaturations • h^{-1}) or 19 nondesaturators (2 major symptoms of OSA, AHI >15, 5 of 3% desaturations • h^{-1} and no 4% desaturations • h^{-1}).Vascular function was assessed by forearm venous occlusion plethysmography during the intra-arterial infusion of endothelium-dependent vasodilators (acetylcholine and substance P) and an endothelium-independent vasodilator (sodium nitroprusside). Compared with the nondesaturator group, patients with OSA and desaturations showed reduced vasodilation to all agonists (fig. 14; $p = 0.007$ for all). The impaired endothelium-dependent and endothelium-independent vasodilation was improved by CPAP therapy. It is suggested that patients with OSA and frequent nocturnal desaturations have impaired endothelium-dependent and endothelium-independent vasodilation that is proportional to hypoxemia and is improved by CPAP therapy. Other researchers have observed that oxygen desaturation indices were a significant determinant of alterations in carotid-femoral pulse wave velocity and brachial artery FMD in OSA patients [124].

3.2 *Oxidative Stress*

A link between endothelial dysfunction in OSA and increased oxidative stress has been observed [125, 126] that was reduced after CPAP administration [53, 81, 125]. Antioxidant treatments have been used to assess the link between oxidative stress and alterations in vascular reactivity in OSA, where FMD of the brachial artery was measured before and after the intravenous injection of 0.5 g vitamin C in otherwise healthy, untreated OSA patients (n = 10) and age- and sex-matched control subjects without sleep-disordered breathing (n = 10) [127]. Baseline FMD was significantly reduced in the OSA patients when compared with control subjects. After the intravenous injection of 0.5 g vitamin C, vasoreactivity increased in OSA patients to a level comparable to that observed in the control group, whereas it remained unchanged

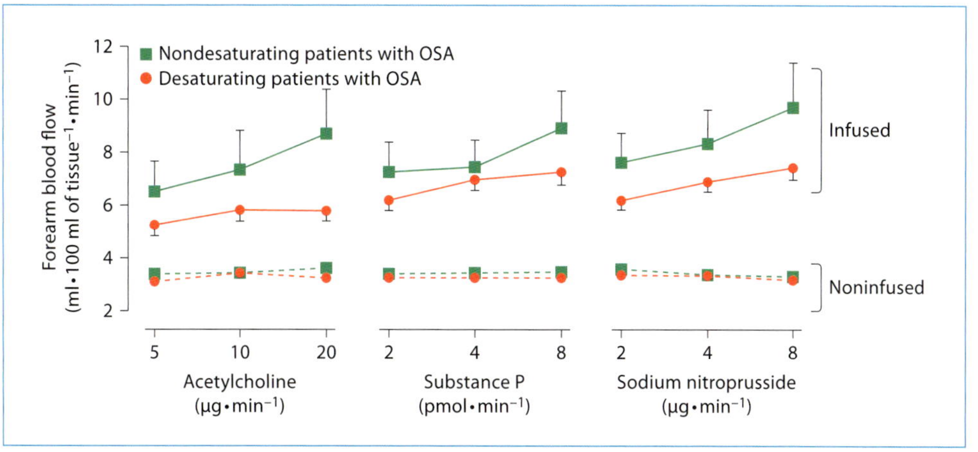

Fig. 14. Patients with OSA and frequent desaturations have impaired endothelium-dependent and endothelium-independent vasodilation that is proportional to hypoxemia. Infused (solid line) and noninfused (broken line) forearm blood flow in desaturating (closed symbols) and nondesaturating (open symbols) OSA patients during the intrabrachial artery infusion of acetylcholine, substance P and sodium nitroprusside. All dose responses in the infused arm were significant ($p < 0.001$). There were significant differences between the desaturating and nondesaturating patients (ANOVA) for acetylcholine ($p < 0.001$), substance P ($p = 0.007$) and sodium nitroprusside ($p < 0.001$). Values are the mean with 95% confidence intervals. After Cross et al. [123], with permission.

in the control subjects. The effects of the administration of allopurinol, a xanthine oxidase inhibitor (300 mg daily for 2 weeks), on vasoreactivity and the plasma levels of malondialdehyde, a marker of oxidative stress, were assessed in a randomized double-blind placebo-controlled crossover study in OSA patients (n = 12) [128]. Compared with placebo, allopurinol caused a significant increase in FMD and a significant decrease in plasma malondialdehyde levels. Overall, these findings support the hypothesis that oxidative stress is responsible for the alterations in vascular reactivity observed in OSA.

3.3 *Adipokines*

Visceral adipocytes express and release bioactive substances (adipokines) with inflammatory or protective properties [129–133]. Inflammatory adipokines contribute to the development and progression of endothelial dysfunction and include cytokines such as tumor necrosis factor (TNF) α and leptin [134, 135]. TNF-α may trigger inflammatory signaling cascades in the vascular endothelium and increase the production of ROS, the expression of cell adhesion molecules and leukocyte-endothelium interactions, which contribute to the development of endothelial dysfunction [136, 137]. NF-κB signaling is activated by chronic intermittent hypoxia and contributes to TNF-α expression by increasing its production [137, 138]. Leptin contributes to the development of endothelial dysfunction by several mechanisms including the activation of the sympathetic nervous system and the possible cross talk between insulin and leptin in the modulation of vascular tone and NO production [135, 139]. Conversely, adiponectin, another adipokine, may have a protective vascular effect and antiatherogenic properties [140–142]. For example, in endothelial cells, adiponectin increases NO production and attenuates inflammatory reactions at various levels including the expression of adhesion molecules and the activation of NF-κB [140, 141].

OSA is currently considered as an inflammatory condition associated with alterations in adipokine levels and insulin resistance [for reviews on these subjects, see chapters 2 and 3, this vol., pp. 43–66 and 67–137], which may all lead to endothelial dysfunction. Whether these mechanisms contribute to the development of endothelial dysfunction in OSA remains to be elucidated.

3.4 *Hypercoagulability*

Endothelial dysfunction is associated with a hypercoagulability state [136]. OSA is associated with increased procoagulant and thrombotic activity [for a review on this subject, see chapter 2, this vol., pp. 43–66]. It remains to be determined whether the hypercoagulability observed in OSA is an intermediate mechanism leading to endothelial dysfunction.

3.5 *Sleep Loss and Fragmentation*

Sleep loss and fragmentation may contribute to the development of endothelial dysfunction in OSA; however, this remains to be demonstrated. It is important to distinguish sleep deprivation per se from sleep fragmentation that is secondary to sleep apnea because the former can occur without the coexistence of sleep apnea. Experimental and clinical studies have suggested that short sleep duration may lead to the development of endothelial dysfunction and an increase in endothelial cell activation and circulating levels of inflammatory markers [143–145]. Flow-mediated vasodilation, which is endothelium-dependent vasodilation, was decreased in 30 healthy male college students after chronic sleep deprivation [144], while acute exposure to 40 h of total sleep deprivation in healthy subjects increased microvascular reactivity and the levels of circulating inflammatory markers [146]. Acute total sleep deprivation has also been associated with increased circulating levels of soluble intercellular adhesion molecule 1 and E-selectin [147], TNF-α, interleukin 1β, interleukin 1 receptor antagonist and interleukin 6 [147–149]. Chronic short sleep duration was associated with an increase in intima-media thickness in the 2,437 participants of the Study of Health in Pomerania (Germany) [150]. This association remained significant after adjustment for potential confounding factors including age, sex, lifestyle indicators, socioeconomic determinants, cardiovascular diseases (hypertension and myocardial infarction), and biological variables (lipid profile and diabetes).

Overall, these findings suggest that acute and chronic short sleep deprivation could trigger endothelial dysfunction [9, 12, 151]. Several mechanisms may link sleep loss and fragmentation with the development of endothelial dysfunction in OSA [152], including insulin resistance and increased weight, increased sympathetic activity and inflammation, and increased coagulant and thrombotic activity [152–155]. However, it remains to be determined whether this occurs in association with the sleep loss and fragmentation related to OSA.

3.6 *Confounders and the Development of Endothelial Dysfunction in Obstructive Sleep Apnea*

OSA comorbidities, such as obesity and diabetes mellitus, can also increase the risk of endothelial dysfunction [10, 156], making it difficult to interpret a potential causal link between OSA and endothelial dysfunction. Patients with and without OSA whose BMI ranged from normal to obese were assessed to determine whether the endothelial alterations that are commonly attributed to obesity were in fact related to OSA [157]. OSA patients had decreased brachial artery FMD and lower expression levels of eNOS and phosphorylated eNOS in freshly harvested endothelial cells. Regardless of central adiposity, OSA patients had increased expression levels of NF-κB (a marker of vascular inflammation) and nitrotyrosine in harvested endothelial cells compared with OSA-free subjects. Higher BMI or central obesity in OSA patients and in OSA-free subjects did not affect brachial artery FMD or the expression of eNOS, phosphorylated eNOS, nitrotyrosine and NF-κB. After 4 weeks of CPAP therapy, FMD and the expression levels of eNOS and phosphorylated eNOS were significantly increased, whereas the expression levels of nitrotyrosine and nuclear NF-κB were significantly decreased in OSA patients who adhered to CPAP ≥4 h daily. It was suggested that untreated OSA, rather than obesity, is a major determinant of vascular endothelial dysfunction in obese patients. This study emphasized the importance of the systematic identification and effective treatment of OSA in obese patients for the accurate assessment and treatment of vascular risk in this condition. Similar findings have been reported regarding the role of hypertension in the development of endothelial dysfunction in OSA patients, where the association of OSA and hypertension may have additive effects on early markers of carotid atherosclerosis (see above, fig. 2) [33].

Overall, confounders such as obesity and hypertension may have detrimental effects by increasing the risk for endothelial dysfunction and, thus, its cardiovascular consequences in OSA patients. On the other hand, OSA may be considered as a cardiovascular risk factor per se and needs to be accurately assessed in patients with such confounders (it is of note that some authors have suggested that OSA should be included in the definition of metabolic syndrome) [158–160].

4 Conclusion

Increasing evidence indicates that endothelial dysfunction occurs in OSA and that it may be an intermediate mechanism that leads to increased cardiovascular risk in

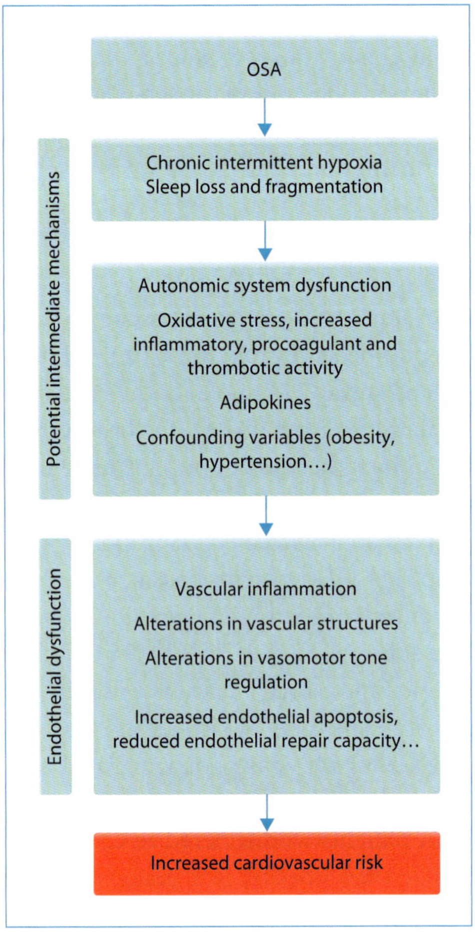

Fig. 15. Potential mechanisms linking OSA, endothelial dysfunction, atherosclerosis and cardiovascular risk. Chronic intermittent hypoxia and sleep loss and fragmentation associated with OSA may increase: sympathetic nervous system activation; oxidative stress, resulting in reduced NO bioavailability and decreased NO-dependent vasodilation; vasoconstrictor mediator release and enhanced vasoconstrictor activity; activity of transcription factors, e.g. NF-κB, resulting in the increased production of proinflammatory cytokines, chemokines and adhesion molecules. These activated pathways could contribute to the development of endothelial dysfunction, atherosclerosis and cardiovascular disorders associated with OSA.

OSA patients. The mechanisms that promote endothelial dysfunction include recurrent intermittent hypoxia and, possibly, sleep loss and fragmentation associated with repetitive obstructive respiratory events occurring during sleep. These events may reduce vasodilation/enhance vasoconstriction functions in association with increased endothelial cell apoptosis and chronic prothrombotic and inflammatory activity. The combined effect of these factors may cause damage to the arterial wall (fig. 15) [9–11]. Other diseases and lifestyle factors, which have been reported to have some link to endothelial dysfunction, such as obesity, insulin resistance, smoking habits or cardiovascular diseases, are also OSA comorbidities. However, evidence for a causal relationship between OSA and endothelial dysfunction has been demonstrated in therapeutic studies. CPAP treatment may improve the changes associated with endothelial dysfunction, and may therefore decrease the cardiovascular risk in OSA.

Animal studies are necessary to assess functional vascular remodeling, e.g. alterations in vasodilator and vasoconstrictor function, and structural vascular remodeling, e.g. the development of preatherosclerotic lesions and atherosclerosis associated with chronic intermittent hypoxia [for reviews on this subject, see 161, 162]. Further studies are needed to identify: (1) early markers of endothelial dysfunction associated with OSA that may be used in clinical practice and (2) clinical profiles of patients at greater risk of endothelial dysfunction in whom an evaluation for OSA may be routinely recommended. Genetic studies may help to identify these patient subpopulations.

5 References

1 Hirata Y, Nagata D, Suzuki E, Nishimatsu H, Suzuki J, Nagai R: Diagnosis and treatment of endothelial dysfunction in cardiovascular disease. Int Heart J 2010;51:1–6.

2 Yang Z, Ming XF: Recent advances in understanding endothelial dysfunction in atherosclerosis. Clin Med Res 2006;4:53–65.

3 Grover-Paez F, Zavalza-Gomez AB: Endothelial dysfunction and cardiovascular risk factors. Diabetes Res Clin Pract 2009;84:1–10.

4 Vanhoutte PM: Endothelial dysfunction: the first step toward coronary arteriosclerosis. Circ J 2009;73: 595–601.

5 Versari D, Daghini E, Virdis A, Ghiadoni L, Taddei S: Endothelial dysfunction as a target for prevention of cardiovascular disease. Diabetes Care 2009; 32(suppl 2):S314–S321.

6 McNicholas WT, Bonsigore MR: Sleep apnoea as an independent risk factor for cardiovascular disease: current evidence, basic mechanisms and research priorities. Eur Respir J 2007;29:156–178.

7 Levy P, Pepin JL, Arnaud C, Baguet JP, Dematteis M, Mach F: Obstructive sleep apnea and atherosclerosis. Prog Cardiovasc Dis 2009;51:400–410.

8 Dempsey JA, Veasey SC, Morgan BJ, O'Donnell CP: Pathophysiology of sleep apnea. Physiol Rev 2010; 90:47–112.

9 Atkeson A, Yeh SY, Malhotra A, Jelic S: Endothelial function in obstructive sleep apnea. Prog Cardiovasc Dis 2009;51:351–362.

10 Budhiraja R, Parthasarathy S, Quan SF: Endothelial dysfunction in obstructive sleep apnea. J Clin Sleep Med 2007;3:409–415.

11 Foster GE, Poulin MJ, Hanly PJ: Intermittent hypoxia and vascular function: implications for obstructive sleep apnoea. Exp Physiol 2007;92:51–65.

12 Atkeson A, Jelic S: Mechanisms of endothelial dysfunction in obstructive sleep apnea. Vasc Health Risk Manag 2008;4:1327–1335.

13 Stamatelopoulos K, Karatzi K, Sidossis LS: Noninvasive methods for assessing early markers of atherosclerosis: the role of body composition and nutrition. Curr Opin Clin Nutr Metab Care 2009;12: 467–473.

14 Simon A, Chironi G: The relationship between carotid intima-media thickness and coronary atherosclerosis revisited. Eur Heart J 2007;28:2049–2050.

15 Simon A, Megnien JL, Chironi G: The value of carotid intima-media thickness for predicting cardiovascular risk. Arterioscler Thromb Vasc Biol 2010;30:182–185.

16 Nieto FJ, Herrington DM, Redline S, Benjamin EJ, Robbins JA: Sleep apnea and markers of vascular endothelial function in a large community sample of older adults. Am J Respir Crit Care Med 2004;169: 354–360.

17 Suzuki T, Nakano H, Maekawa J, Okamoto Y, Ohnishi Y, Yamauchi M, Kimura H: Obstructive sleep apnea and carotid-artery intima-media thickness. Sleep 2004;27:129–133.

18 Altin R, Ozdemir H, Mahmutyazicioglu K, Kart L, Uzun L, Ozer T, Savranlar A, Aydin M: Evaluation of carotid artery wall thickness with high-resolution sonography in obstructive sleep apnea syndrome. J Clin Ultrasound 2005;33:80–86.

19 Baguet JP, Hammer L, Levy P, Pierre H, Launois S, Mallion JM, Pepin JL: The severity of oxygen desaturation is predictive of carotid wall thickening and plaque occurrence. Chest 2005;128:3407–3412.

20 Drager LF, Bortolotto LA, Lorenzi MC, Figueiredo AC, Krieger EM, Lorenzi-Filho G: Early signs of atherosclerosis in obstructive sleep apnea. Am J Respir Crit Care Med 2005;172:613–618.

21 Minoguchi K, Yokoe T, Tazaki T, Minoguchi H, Tanaka A, Oda N, Okada S, Ohta S, Naito H, Adachi M: Increased carotid intima-media thickness and serum inflammatory markers in obstructive sleep apnea. Am J Respir Crit Care Med 2005;172:625–630.

22 Phillips C, Hedner J, Berend N, Grunstein R: Diurnal and obstructive sleep apnea influences on arterial stiffness and central blood pressure in men. Sleep 2005;28:604–609.
23 Schulz R, Seeger W, Fegbeutel C, Husken H, Bodeker RH, Tillmanns H, Grebe M: Changes in extracranial arteries in obstructive sleep apnoea. Eur Respir J 2005;25:69–74.
24 Saletu M, Nosiska D, Kapfhammer G, Lalouschek W, Saletu B, Benesch T, Zeitlhofer J: Structural and serum surrogate markers of cerebrovascular disease in obstructive sleep apnea (OSA): association of mild OSA with early atherosclerosis. J Neurol 2006; 253:746–752.
25 Drager LF, Bortolotto LA, Figueiredo AC, Silva BC, Krieger EM, Lorenzi-Filho G: Obstructive sleep apnea, hypertension, and their interaction on arterial stiffness and heart remodeling. Chest 2007;131: 1379–1386.
26 Tsioufis C, Thomopoulos K, Dimitriadis K, Amfilochiou A, Tousoulis D, Alchanatis M, Stefanadis C, Kallikazaros I: The incremental effect of obstructive sleep apnoea syndrome on arterial stiffness in newly diagnosed essential hypertensive subjects. J Hypertens 2007;25:141–146.
27 Baguet JP, Levy P, Barone-Rochette G, Tamisier R, Pierre H, Peeters M, Mallion JM, Pepin JL: Masked hypertension in obstructive sleep apnea syndrome. J Hypertens 2008;26:885–892.
28 Kohler M, Craig S, Nicoll D, Leeson P, Davies RJ, Stradling JR: Endothelial function and arterial stiffness in minimally symptomatic obstructive sleep apnea. Am J Respir Crit Care Med 2008;178: 984–988.
29 Protogerou AD, Laaban JP, Czernichow S, Kostopoulos C, Lekakis J, Safar ME, Blacher J: Structural and functional arterial properties in patients with obstructive sleep apnoea syndrome and cardiovascular comorbidities. J Hum Hypertens 2008;22:415–422.
30 Wattanakit K, Boland L, Punjabi NM, Shahar E: Relation of sleep-disordered breathing to carotid plaque and intima-media thickness. Atherosclerosis 2008;197:125–131.
31 Baguet JP, Nadra M, Barone-Rochette G, Ormezzano O, Pierre H, Pepin JL: Early cardiovascular abnormalities in newly diagnosed obstructive sleep apnea. Vasc Health Risk Manag 2009;5:1063–1073.
32 Chung S, Yoon IY, Shin YK, Lee CH, Kim JW, Ahn HJ: Endothelial dysfunction and inflammatory reactions of elderly and middle-aged men with obstructive sleep apnea syndrome. Sleep Breath 2009;13:11–17.
33 Drager LF, Bortolotto LA, Krieger EM, Lorenzi-Filho G: Additive effects of obstructive sleep apnea and hypertension on early markers of carotid atherosclerosis. Hypertension 2009;53:64–69.
34 Drager LF, Bortolotto LA, Maki-Nunes C, Trombetta IC, Alves MJ, Fraga RF, Negrao CE, Krieger EM, Lorenzi-Filho G: The incremental role of obstructive sleep apnoea on markers of atherosclerosis in patients with metabolic syndrome. Atherosclerosis 2010;208:490–495.
35 Turmel J, Series F, Boulet LP, Poirier P, Tardif JC, Rodes-Cabeau J, Larose E, Bertrand OF: Relationship between atherosclerosis and the sleep apnea syndrome: an intravascular ultrasound study. Int J Cardiol 2009;132:203–209.
36 Drager LF, Bortolotto LA, Figueiredo AC, Krieger EM, Lorenzi GF: Effects of continuous positive airway pressure on early signs of atherosclerosis in obstructive sleep apnea. Am J Respir Crit Care Med 2007;176:706–712.
37 Saito T, Sugiyama S, Asai K, Yasutake M, Mizuno K: Effects of long-term treatment for obstructive sleep apnea on pulse wave velocity. Hypertens Res 2010; 33:844–849.
38 Van Wijk MJ, Van Bavel E, Sturk A, Nieuwland R: Microparticles in cardiovascular diseases. Cardiovasc Res 2003;59:277–287.
39 Chironi G, Simon A, Hugel B, Del Pino M, Gariepy J, Freyssinet JM, Tedgui A: Circulating leukocyte-derived microparticles predict subclinical atherosclerosis burden in asymptomatic subjects. Arterioscler Thromb Vasc Biol 2006;26:2775–2780.
40 Boulanger CM, Amabile N, Tedgui A: Circulating microparticles: a potential prognostic marker for atherosclerotic vascular disease. Hypertension 2006; 48:180–186.
41 Nomura S: Dynamic role of microparticles in type 2 diabetes mellitus. Curr Diabetes Rev 2009;5:245–251.
42 Sabatier F, Camoin-Jau L, Anfosso F, Sampol J, Dignat-George F: Circulating endothelial cells, microparticles and progenitors: key players towards the definition of vascular competence. J Cell Mol Med 2009;13:454–471.
43 El Solh AA, Akinnusi ME, Baddoura FH, Mankowski CR: Endothelial cell apoptosis in obstructive sleep apnea: a link to endothelial dysfunction. Am J Respir Crit Care Med 2007;175: 1186–1191.
44 El Solh AA, Akinnusi ME, Berim IG, Peter AM, Paasch LL, Szarpa KR: Hemostatic implications of endothelial cell apoptosis in obstructive sleep apnea. Sleep Breath 2008;12:331–337.

45 Dyugovskaya L, Polyakov A, Lavie P, Lavie L: Delayed neutrophil apoptosis in patients with sleep apnea. Am J Respir Crit Care Med 2008;177:544–554.
46 Ayers L, Ferry B, Craig S, Nicoll D, Stradling JR, Kohler M: Circulating cell-derived microparticles in patients with minimally symptomatic obstructive sleep apnoea. Eur Respir J 2009;33:574–580.
47 Jelic S, Lederer DJ, Adams T, Padeletti M, Colombo PC, Factor P, Le Jemtel TH: Endothelial repair capacity and apoptosis are inversely related in obstructive sleep apnea. Vasc Health Risk Manag 2009;5:909–920.
48 Priou P, Gagnadoux F, Tesse A, Mastronardi ML, Agouni A, Meslier N, Racineux JL, Martinez MC, Trzepizur W, Andriantsitohaina R: Endothelial dysfunction and circulating microparticles from patients with obstructive sleep apnea. Am J Pathol 2010;177:974–983.
49 Goon PK, Watson T, Lip GY: Circulating endothelial cells in obstructive sleep apnea: an important methodological lesson. Am J Respir Crit Care Med 2007;175:1346, author reply 1347.
50 Tzouvelekis A, Kotsianidis I, Steiropoulos P, Bouros D: Role of CD146 in detection of apoptotic circulating endothelial cells in obstructive sleep apnea. Am J Respir Crit Care Med 2007;175:1346–1347, author reply 1347.
51 Zidar N, Jeruc J, Balazic J, Stajer D: Neutrophils in human myocardial infarction with rupture of the free wall. Cardiovasc Pathol 2005;14:247–250.
52 Maianski NA, Maianski AN, Kuijpers TW, Roos D: Apoptosis of neutrophils. Acta Haematol 2004;111: 56–66.
53 Jelic S, Padeletti M, Kawut SM, Higgins C, Canfield SM, Onat D, Colombo PC, Basner RC, Factor P, Le Jemtel TH: Inflammation, oxidative stress, and repair capacity of the vascular endothelium in obstructive sleep apnea. Circulation 2008;117:2270–2278.
54 Werner N, Kosiol S, Schiegl T, Ahlers P, Walenta K, Link A, Bohm M, Nickenig G: Circulating endothelial progenitor cells and cardiovascular outcomes. N Engl J Med 2005;353:999–1007.
55 Werner N, Wassmann S, Ahlers P, Schiegl T, Kosiol S, Link A, Walenta K, Nickenig G: Endothelial progenitor cells correlate with endothelial function in patients with coronary artery disease. Basic Res Cardiol 2007;102:565–571.
56 Sirker AA, Astroulakis ZM, Hill JM: Vascular progenitor cells and translational research: the role of endothelial and smooth muscle progenitor cells in endogenous arterial remodelling in the adult. Clin Sci (Lond) 2009;116:283–299.
57 De la Pena M, Barcelo A, Barbe F, Pierola J, Pons J, Rimbau E, Ayllon O, Agusti AG: Endothelial function and circulating endothelial progenitor cells in patients with sleep apnea syndrome. Respiration 2008;76:28–32.
58 Martin K, Stanchina M, Kouttab N, Harrington EO, Rounds S: Circulating endothelial cells and endothelial progenitor cells in obstructive sleep apnea. Lung 2008;186:145–150.
59 Corretti MC, Anderson TJ, Benjamin EJ, Celermajer D, Charbonneau F, Creager MA, Deanfield J, Drexler H, Gerhard-Herman M, Herrington D: Guidelines for the ultrasound assessment of endothelial-dependent flow-mediated vasodilation of the brachial artery: a report of the International Brachial Artery Reactivity Task Force. J Am Coll Cardiol 2002;39:257–265.
60 Ip MS, Tse HF, Lam B, Tsang KW, Lam WK: Endothelial function in obstructive sleep apnea and response to treatment. Am J Respir Crit Care Med 2004;169:348–353.
61 Carlson JT, Rangemark C, Hedner JA: Attenuated endothelium-dependent vascular relaxation in patients with sleep apnoea. J Hypertens 1996;14:577–584.
62 Kato M, Roberts-Thomson P, Phillips BG, Haynes WG, Winnicki M, Accurso V, Somers VK: Impairment of endothelium-dependent vasodilation of resistance vessels in patients with obstructive sleep apnea. Circulation 2000;102:2607–2610.
63 Lattimore JL, Wilcox I, Skilton M, Langenfeld M, Celermajer DS: Treatment of obstructive sleep apnoea leads to improved microvascular endothelial function in the systemic circulation. Thorax 2006;61:491–495.
64 Bayram NA, Ciftci B, Keles T, Durmaz T, Turhan S, Bozkurt E, Peker Y: Endothelial function in normotensive men with obstructive sleep apnea before and 6 months after CPAP treatment. Sleep 2009;32:1257–1263.
65 Kushida CA, Morgenthaler TI, Littner MR, Alessi CA, Bailey D, Coleman J Jr, Friedman L, Hirshkowitz M, Kapen S, Kramer M, Lee-Chiong T, Owens J, Pancer JP: Practice parameters for the treatment of snoring and obstructive sleep apnea with oral appliances: an update for 2005. Sleep 2006;29:240–243.
66 Itzhaki S, Dorchin H, Clark G, Lavie L, Lavie P, Pillar G: The effects of 1-year treatment with a herbst mandibular advancement splint on obstructive sleep apnea, oxidative stress, and endothelial function. Chest 2007;131:740–749.

67 Trzepizur W, Gagnadoux F, Abraham P, Rousseau P, Meslier N, Saumet JL, Racineux JL: Microvascular endothelial function in obstructive sleep apnea: impact of continuous positive airway pressure and mandibular advancement. Sleep Med 2009;10:746–752.

68 Forstermann U, Munzel T: Endothelial nitric oxide synthase in vascular disease: from marvel to menace. Circulation 2006;113:1708–1714.

69 Lerman A, Zeiher AM: Endothelial function: cardiac events. Circulation 2005;111:363–368.

70 Versari D, Daghini E, Virdis A, Ghiadoni L, Taddei S: Endothelium-dependent contractions and endothelial dysfunction in human hypertension. Br J Pharmacol 2009;157:527–536.

71 Ip MS, Lam B, Chan LY, Zheng L, Tsang KW, Fung PC, Lam WK: Circulating nitric oxide is suppressed in obstructive sleep apnea and is reversed by nasal continuous positive airway pressure. Am J Respir Crit Care Med 2000;162:2166–2171.

72 Schulz R, Schmidt D, Blum A, Lopes-Ribeiro X, Lucke C, Mayer K, Olschewski H, Seeger W, Grimminger F. Decreased plasma levels of nitric oxide derivatives in obstructive sleep apnoea: response to CPAP therapy. Thorax 2000;55:1046–1051.

73 Alonso-Fernandez A, Garcia-Rio F, Arias MA, Hernanz A, de la Pena M, Pierola J, Barcelo A, Lopez-Collazo E, Agusti A. Effects of CPAP on oxidative stress and nitrate efficiency in sleep apnoea: a randomised trial. Thorax 2009;64:581–586.

74 Bayazit YA, Yilmaz M, Erdal E, Ciftci TU, Ceylan A, Kokturk O, Celenk F, Kemaloglu YK: Role of nitric oxide synthase gene intron 4 and exon 7 polymorphisms in obstructive sleep apnea syndrome. Eur Arch Otorhinolaryngol 2009;266:449–454.

75 Szabo C: Role of nitrosative stress in the pathogenesis of diabetic vascular dysfunction. Br J Pharmacol 2009;156:713–727.

76 Muller G, Morawietz H. Nitric oxide, NAD(P)H oxidase, and atherosclerosis. Antioxid Redox Signal 2009;11:1711–1731.

77 Sydow K, Munzel T: ADMA and oxidative stress. Atheroscler Suppl 2003;4:41–51.

78 Ohike Y, Kozaki K, Iijima K, Eto M, Kojima T, Ohga E, Santa T, Imai K, Hashimoto M, Yoshizumi M, Ouchi Y: Amelioration of vascular endothelial dysfunction in obstructive sleep apnea syndrome by nasal continuous positive airway pressure – possible involvement of nitric oxide and asymmetric NG, NG-dimethylarginine. Circ J 2005;69:221–226.

79 Ozkan Y, Firat H, Simsek B, Torun M, Yardim-Akaydin S: Circulating nitric oxide (NO), asymmetric dimethylarginine (ADMA), homocysteine, and oxidative status in obstructive sleep apnea-hypopnea syndrome (OSAHS). Sleep Breath 2008; 12:149–154.

80 Barcelo A, de la Pena M, Ayllon O, Vega-Agapito MV, Pierola J, Perez G, Gonzalez C, Alonso A, Agusti AG: Increased plasma levels of asymmetric dimethylarginine and soluble CD40 ligand in patients with sleep apnea. Respiration 2009;77:85–90.

81 Patt BT, Jarjoura D, Haddad DN, Sen CK, Roy S, Flavahan NA, Khayat RN: Endothelial dysfunction in the microcirculation of patients with obstructive sleep apnea. Am J Respir Crit Care Med 2010;182: 1540–1545.

82 Cortelli P, Parchi P, Sforza E, Contin M, Pierangeli G, Barletta G, Lugaresi E: Cardiovascular autonomic dysfunction in normotensive awake subjects with obstructive sleep apnoea syndrome. Clin Auton Res 1994;4:57–62.

83 Lai CJ, Yang CC, Hsu YY, Lin YN, Kuo TB: Enhanced sympathetic outflow and decreased baroreflex sensitivity are associated with intermittent hypoxia-induced systemic hypertension in conscious rats. J Appl Physiol 2006;100:1974–1982.

84 Sverrisdottir YB, Jansson LM, Hagg U, Gan LM: Muscle sympathetic nerve activity is related to a surrogate marker of endothelial function in healthy individuals. PLoS One 2010;5:e9257.

85 Grote L, Kraiczi H, Hedner J: Reduced alpha- and beta(2)-adrenergic vascular response in patients with obstructive sleep apnea. Am J Respir Crit Care Med 2000;162:1480–1487.

86 Hayes MJ, Qing F, Rhodes CG, Rahman SU, Ind PW, Sriskandan S, Jones T, Hughes JM: In vivo quantification of human pulmonary beta-adrenoceptors: effect of beta-agonist therapy. Am J Respir Crit Care Med 1996;154:1277–1283.

87 Mills PJ, Dimsdale JE, Coy TV, Ancoli-Israel S, Clausen JL, Nelesen RA: Beta 2-adrenergic receptor characteristics in sleep apnea patients. Sleep 1995; 18:39–42.

88 Nelesen RA, Dimsdale JE, Mills PJ, Clausen JL, Ziegler MG, Ancoli-Israel S: Altered cardiac contractility in sleep apnea. Sleep 1996;19:139–144.

89 Mills PJ, Dimsdale JE, Ancoli-Israel S, Clausen J, Loredo JS: The effects of hypoxia and sleep apnea on isoproterenol sensitivity. Sleep 1998;21:731–735.

90 Dhaun N, Goddard J, Webb DJ: The endothelin system and its antagonism in chronic kidney disease. J Am Soc Nephrol 2006;17:943–955.

91 Marasciulo FL, Montagnani M, Potenza MA. Endothelin-1: the yin and yang on vascular function. Curr Med Chem 2006;13:1655–1665.

92 Watts SW: Endothelin receptors: what's new and what do we need to know? Am J Physiol Regul Integr Comp Physiol 2010;298:R254–R260.
93 Schorlemmer A, Matter ML, Shohet RV: Cardioprotective signaling by endothelin. Trends Cardiovasc Med 2008;18:233–239.
94 Phillips BG, Narkiewicz K, Pesek CA, Haynes WG, Dyken ME, Somers VK: Effects of obstructive sleep apnea on endothelin-1 and blood pressure. J Hypertens 1999;17:61–66.
95 Grimpen F, Kanne P, Schulz E, Hagenah G, Hasenfuss G, Andreas S: Endothelin-1 plasma levels are not elevated in patients with obstructive sleep apnoea. Eur Respir J 2000;15:320–325.
96 Møller DS, Lind P, Strunge B, Pedersen EB: Abnormal vasoactive hormones and 24-hour blood pressure in obstructive sleep apnea. Am J Hypertens 2003;16:274–280.
97 Jordan W, Reinbacher A, Cohrs S, Grunewald RW, Mayer G, Ruther E, Rodenbeck A: Obstructive sleep apnea: plasma endothelin-1 precursor but not endothelin-1 levels are elevated and decline with nasal continuous positive airway pressure. Peptides 2005;26:1654–1660.
98 Zamarron-Sanz C, Ricoy-Galbaldon J, Gude-Sampedro F, Riveiro-Riveiro A: Plasma levels of vascular endothelial markers in obstructive sleep apnea. Arch Med Res 2006;37:552–555.
99 Gjørup PH, Sadauskiene L, Wessels J, Nyvad O, Strunge B, Pedersen EB: Abnormally increased endothelin-1 in plasma during the night in obstructive sleep apnea: relation to blood pressure and severity of disease. Am J Hypertens 2007;20:44–52.
100 Gjørup PH, Wessels J, Pedersen EB: Abnormally increased nitric oxide synthesis and increased endothelin-1 in plasma in patients with obstructive sleep apnoea. Scand J Clin Lab Invest 2008;68:375–385.
101 Saarelainen S, Seppala E, Laasonen K, Hasan J: Circulating endothelin-1 in obstructive sleep apnea. Endothelium 1997;5:115–118.
102 Hemsen A, Ahlborg G, Ottosson-Seeberger A, Lundberg JM: Metabolism of big endothelin-1 (1–38) and (22–38) in the human circulation in relation to production of endothelin-1 (1–21). Regul Pept 1995;55:287–297.
103 Wagner OF, Christ G, Wojta J, Vierhapper H, Parzer S, Nowotny PJ, Schneider B, Waldhausl W, Binder BR: Polar secretion of endothelin-1 by cultured endothelial cells. J Biol Chem 1992;267:16066–16068.
104 Diefenbach K, Kretschmer K, Bauer S, Malzahn U, Penzel T, Roots I, Fietze I: Endothelin-1 gene variant Lys198Asn and plasma endothelin level in obstructive sleep apnea. Cardiology 2009;112:62–68.
105 Buck D, Diefenbach K, Penzel T, Malzahn U, Roots I, Fietze I: Genetic polymorphisms in endothelin-receptor-subtype-A-gene as susceptibility factor for obstructive sleep apnea syndrome. Sleep Med 2010; 11:213–217.
106 Cheng ZJ, Vapaatalo H, Mervaala E: Angiotensin II and vascular inflammation. Med Sci Monit 2005;11: RA194–RA205.
107 Probstfield JL, O'Brien KD: Progression of cardiovascular damage: the role of renin-angiotensin system blockade. Am J Cardiol 2010;105:10A–20A.
108 Bader M. Tissue renin-angiotensin-aldosterone systems: targets for pharmacological therapy. Annu Rev Pharmacol Toxicol 2010;50:439–465.
109 Dzau VJ: Theodore Cooper lecture: tissue angiotensin and pathobiology of vascular disease: a unifying hypothesis. Hypertension 2001;37:1047–1052.
110 Yavuz D, Koc M, Toprak A, Akpinar I, Velioglu A, Deyneli O, Haklar G, Akalin S: Effects of ACE inhibition and AT1-receptor antagonism on endothelial function and insulin sensitivity in essential hypertensive patients. J Renin Angiotensin Aldosterone Syst 2003;4:197–203.
111 Rigat B, Hubert C, Alhenc-Gelas F, Cambien F, Corvol P, Soubrier F: An insertion/deletion polymorphism in the angiotensin I-converting enzyme gene accounting for half the variance of serum enzyme levels. J Clin Invest 1990;86:1343–1346.
112 Sayed-Tabatabaei FA, Oostra BA, Isaacs A, van Duijn CM, Witteman JC: ACE polymorphisms. Circ Res 2006;98:1123–1133.
113 Xiao Y, Huang X, Qiu C, Zhu X, Liu Y: Angiotensin I-converting enzyme gene polymorphism in Chinese patients with obstructive sleep apnea syndrome. Chin Med J (Engl) 1999;112:701–704.
114 Barcelo A, Elorza MA, Barbe F, Santos C, Mayoralas LR, Agusti AG: Angiotensin converting enzyme in patients with sleep apnoea syndrome: plasma activity and gene polymorphisms. Eur Respir J 2001;17: 728–732.
115 Lin L, Finn L, Zhang J, Young T, Mignot E: Angiotensin-converting enzyme, sleep-disordered breathing, and hypertension. Am J Respir Crit Care Med 2004;170:1349–1353.
116 Patel SR, Emma KL, Mignot E, Lin L, Redline S: The association of angiotensin converting enzyme (ACE) polymorphisms with sleep apnea and hypertension. Sleep 2007;30:531–533.
117 Koyama RG, Drager LF, Lorenzi-Filho G, Cintra FD, Pereira AC, Poyares D, Krieger JE, Castro RM, Tufik S, de Mello MT, Pedrazzoli M: Reciprocal interactions of obstructive sleep apnea and hypertension associated with ACE I/D polymorphism in males. Sleep Med 2009;10:1107–1111.

118 Kizawa T, Nakamura Y, Takahashi S, Sakurai S, Yamauchi K, Inoue H: Pathogenic role of angiotensin II and oxidised LDL in obstructive sleep apnoea. Eur Respir J 2009;34:1390–1398.
119 Kraiczi H, Hedner J, Peker Y, Carlson J: Increased vasoconstrictor sensitivity in obstructive sleep apnea. J Appl Physiol 2000;89:493–498.
120 Benjamin JA, Moller M, Ebden P, Bartle I, Lewis KE: Serum angiotensin converting enzyme and the obstructive sleep apnea hypopnea syndrome. J Clin Sleep Med 2008;4:325–331.
121 Levy P, Pepin JL, Arnaud C, Tamisier R, Borel JC, Dematteis M, Godin-Ribuot D, Ribuot C: Intermittent hypoxia and sleep-disordered breathing: current concepts and perspectives. Eur Respir J 2008;32:1082–1095.
122 Kraiczi H, Caidahl K, Samuelsson A, Peker Y, Hedner J: Impairment of vascular endothelial function and left ventricular filling: association with the severity of apnea-induced hypoxemia during sleep. Chest 2001;119:1085–1091.
123 Cross MD, Mills NL, Al-Abri M, Riha R, Vennelle M, Mackay TW, Newby DE, Douglas NJ: Continuous positive airway pressure improves vascular function in obstructive sleep apnoea/hypopnoea syndrome: a randomised controlled trial. Thorax 2008;63:578–583.
124 Chung S, Yoon IY, Lee CH, Kim JW: The association of nocturnal hypoxemia with arterial stiffness and endothelial dysfunction in male patients with obstructive sleep apnea syndrome. Respiration 2010;79:363–369.
125 Jurado-Gamez B, Fernandez-Marin MC, Gomez-Chaparro JL, Munoz-Cabrera L, Lopez-Barea J, Perez-Jimenez F, Lopez-Miranda J. Relationship of oxidative stress and endothelial dysfunction in sleep apnoea. Eur Respir J 2011;37:873–879.
126 Monneret D, Pepin JL, Godin-Ribuot D, Ducros V, Baguet JP, Levy P, Faure P: Association of urinary 15-F2t-isoprostane level with oxygen desaturation and carotid intima-media thickness in nonobese sleep apnea patients. Free Radic Biol Med 2010;48:619–625.
127 Grebe M, Eisele HJ, Weissmann N, Schaefer C, Tillmanns H, Seeger W, Schulz R: Antioxidant vitamin C improves endothelial function in obstructive sleep apnea. Am J Respir Crit Care Med 2006;173:897–901.
128 El Solh AA, Saliba R, Bosinski T, Grant BJ, Berbary E, Miller N: Allopurinol improves endothelial function in sleep apnoea: a randomised controlled study. Eur Respir J 2006;27:997–1002.
129 Fried SK, Bunkin DA, Greenberg AS: Omental and subcutaneous adipose tissues of obese subjects release interleukin-6: depot difference and regulation by glucocorticoid. J Clin Endocrinol Metab 1998;83:847–850.
130 Hotamisligil GS: Mechanisms of TNF-alpha-induced insulin resistance. Exp Clin Endocrinol Diabetes 1999;107:119–125.
131 Weisberg SP, McCann D, Desai M, Rosenbaum M, Leibel RL, Ferrante AW Jr: Obesity is associated with macrophage accumulation in adipose tissue. J Clin Invest 2003;112:1796–1808.
132 Hopkins TA, Ouchi N, Shibata R, Walsh K: Adiponectin actions in the cardiovascular system. Cardiovasc Res 2007;74:11–18.
133 Trayhurn P, Wang B, Wood IS: Hypoxia in adipose tissue: a basis for the dysregulation of tissue function in obesity? Br J Nutr 2008;100:227–235.
134 Knudson JD, Dincer UD, Zhang C, Swafford AN Jr, Koshida R, Picchi A, Focardi M, Dick GM, Tune JD: Leptin receptors are expressed in coronary arteries, and hyperleptinemia causes significant coronary endothelial dysfunction. Am J Physiol Heart Circ Physiol 2005;289:H48–H56.
135 Knudson JD, Payne GA, Borbouse L, Tune JD: Leptin and mechanisms of endothelial dysfunction and cardiovascular disease. Curr Hypertens Rep 2008;10:434–439.
136 Goldberg RB: Cytokine and cytokine-like inflammation markers, endothelial dysfunction, and imbalanced coagulation in development of diabetes and its complications. J Clin Endocrinol Metab 2009;94:3171–3182.
137 Zhang H, Park Y, Wu J, Chen X, Lee S, Yang J, Dellsperger KC, Zhang C: Role of TNF-alpha in vascular dysfunction. Clin Sci (Lond) 2009;116:219–230.
138 Csiszar A, Wang M, Lakatta EG, Ungvari Z. Inflammation and endothelial dysfunction during aging: role of NF-kappaB. J Appl Physiol 2008;105:1333–1341.
139 Kim JA, Montagnani M, Koh KK, Quon MJ: Reciprocal relationships between insulin resistance and endothelial dysfunction: molecular and pathophysiological mechanisms. Circulation 2006;113:1888–1904.
140 Goldstein BJ, Scalia RG, Ma XL: Protective vascular and myocardial effects of adiponectin. Nat Clin Pract Cardiovasc Med 2009;6:27–35.
141 Gustafson B: Adipose tissue, inflammation and atherosclerosis. J Atheroscler Thromb 2010;17:332–341.
142 Han SH, Sakuma I, Shin EK, Koh KK: Antiatherosclerotic and anti-insulin resistance effects of adiponectin: basic and clinical studies. Prog Cardiovasc Dis 2009;52:126–140.

143 Amir O, Alroy S, Schliamser JE, Asmir I, Shiran A, Flugelman MY, Halon DA, Lewis BS: Brachial artery endothelial function in residents and fellows working night shifts. Am J Cardiol 2004;93:947–949.
144 Takase B, Akima T, Uehata A, Ohsuzu F, Kurita A: Effect of chronic stress and sleep deprivation on both flow-mediated dilation in the brachial artery and the intracellular magnesium level in humans. Clin Cardiol 2004;27:223–227.
145 Van Leeuwen WM, Lehto M, Karisola P, Lindholm H, Luukkonen R, Sallinen M, Harma M, Porkka-Heiskanen T, Alenius H: Sleep restriction increases the risk of developing cardiovascular diseases by augmenting proinflammatory responses through IL-17 and CRP. PLoS One 2009;4:e4589.
146 Sauvet F, Leftheriotis G, Gomez-Merino D, Langrume C, Drogou C, Van Beers P, Bourrilhon C, Florence G, Chennaoui M: Effect of acute sleep deprivation on vascular function in healthy subjects. J Appl Physiol 2010;108:68–75.
147 Frey DJ, Fleshner M, Wright KP Jr: The effects of 40 hours of total sleep deprivation on inflammatory markers in healthy young adults. Brain Behav Immun 2007;21:1050–1057.
148 Dinges DF, Douglas SD, Zaugg L, Campbell DE, McMann JM, Whitehouse WG, Orne EC, Kapoor SC, Icaza E, Orne MT: Leukocytosis and natural killer cell function parallel neurobehavioral fatigue induced by 64 hours of sleep deprivation. J Clin Invest 1994;93:1930–1939.
149 Vgontzas AN, Zoumakis E, Bixler EO, Lin HM, Follett H, Kales A, Chrousos GP: Adverse effects of modest sleep restriction on sleepiness, performance, and inflammatory cytokines. J Clin Endocrinol Metab 2004;89:2119–2126.
150 Wolff B, Volzke H, Schwahn C, Robinson D, Kessler C, John U: Relation of self-reported sleep duration with carotid intima-media thickness in a general population sample. Atherosclerosis 2008;196:727–732.
151 Mullington JM, Haack M, Toth M, Serrador JM, Meier-Ewert HK: Cardiovascular, inflammatory, and metabolic consequences of sleep deprivation. Prog Cardiovasc Dis 2009;51:294–302.
152 Patel SR: Sleep – an affair of the heart. Sleep 2009;32:289–290.
153 Knutson KL: Impact of sleep and sleep loss on glucose homeostasis and appetite regulation. Sleep Med Clin 2007;2:187–197.
154 Van Cauter E, Holmback U, Knutson K, Leproult R, Miller A, Nedeltcheva A, Pannain S, Penev P, Tasali E, Spiegel K: Impact of sleep and sleep loss on neuroendocrine and metabolic function. Horm Res 2007;67(suppl 1):2–9.
155 Al Lawati NM, Patel SR, Ayas NT: Epidemiology, risk factors, and consequences of obstructive sleep apnea and short sleep duration. Prog Cardiovasc Dis 2009;51:285–293.
156 Avogaro A, de Kreutzenberg SV, Fadini G: Endothelial dysfunction: causes and consequences in patients with diabetes mellitus. Diabetes Res Clin Pract 2008;82(suppl 2):S94–S101.
157 Jelic S, Lederer DJ, Adams T, Padeletti M, Colombo PC, Factor PH, Le Jemtel TH: Vascular inflammation in obesity and sleep apnea. Circulation 2010;121:1014–1021.
158 Vgontzas AN, Bixler EO, Chrousos GP: Sleep apnea is a manifestation of the metabolic syndrome. Sleep Med Rev 2005;9:211–224.
159 Nieto FJ, Peppard PE, Young TB: Sleep disordered breathing and metabolic syndrome. WMJ 2009;108:263–265.
160 Nock NL, Li L, Larkin EK, Patel SR, Redline S: Empirical evidence for 'syndrome Z': a hierarchical 5-factor model of the metabolic syndrome incorporating sleep disturbance measures. Sleep 2009;32:615–622.
161 Dematteis M, Godin-Ribuot D, Arnaud C, Ribuot C, Stanke-Labesque F, Pepin JL, Levy P: Cardiovascular consequences of sleep-disordered breathing: contribution of animal models to understanding the human disease. ILAR J 2009;50:262–281.
162 Kanagy NL: Vascular effects of intermittent hypoxia. ILAR J 2009;50:282–288.
163 Touyz RM: Recent advances in intracellular signalling in hypertension. Curr Opin Nephrol Hypertens 2003;12:165–174.

Hemodynamic and Autonomic Changes in Adults with Obstructive Sleep Apnea

5

Chapter 5

Hemodynamic and Autonomic Changes in Adults with Obstructive Sleep Apnea

Abstract

Obstructive sleep apnea (OSA) is characterized by repetitive episodes of complete or partial obstruction of the upper airway during sleep that lead to an increase in airway resistance and respiratory effort. This may produce oxygen desaturation, hypercapnia and central nervous system arousal that restore airflow. OSA is associated with hemodynamic changes that are related to alterations in the activity of the autonomic nervous system. During the course of an apnea, the heart rate may slow down, increase or remain stable. The blood pressure decreases at the start of the apnea and increases at its terminal portion. When ventilation resumes, heart rate, blood pressure and ventilation reach a peak accompanied by an abrupt reduction in left ventricular stroke volume. During the early phase of apnea, sympathetic nerve activity (SNA) is suppressed; it then increases constantly and reaches a peak at the end of apnea and on arousal. As soon as ventilation resumes, there is an abrupt inhibition of SNA in the peripheral blood vessels. The resumption of ventilation occurs in the context of peripheral vasoconstriction and increased peripheral resistance. This situation persists for several seconds after the SNA has ceased, due to the kinetics of norepinephrine uptake, release and washout at the neurovascular junction. Hypoxemia, hypercapnia, lung inflation and blood pressure are important factors that may modulate these autonomic changes. The alterations in the autonomic nervous system are carried over into wakefulness and may contribute to the development of the cardiovascular disorders associated with OSA, including sympathovagal imbalance accompanied with changes in the baroreflex and chemoreflex. The hemodynamic and autonomic dysfunction associated with OSA is improved following treatment with continuous positive airway pressure.

During the last 2 decades, clinicians and researchers have demonstrated that obstructive sleep apnea (OSA) is associated with acute and chronic hemodynamic and autonomic changes. These changes may contribute to the development and progression of the cardiovascular and metabolic disorders associated with OSA.

1 Control of Cardiovascular Function during Normal Sleep Stages

Sleep stage classification depends on the observation of electroencephalographic waves and patterns, electro-oculographic patterns, and mental or submental muscle tone, as recorded by electromyography [1, 2]. Sleep consists of rapid eye movement (REM) sleep and non-REM sleep. In 2007, the following terminology was recommended by the American Academy of Sleep Medicine for the different sleep stages: stage W (wakefulness), stages N1 (non-REM 1) and N2 (non-REM 2) being light sleep, stage N3 (non-REM 3) being deep sleep (often named slow-wave sleep) and stage R (REM sleep) [2]. The onset of sleep begins with the non-REM stages. After a few minutes of stage N1 sleep, stage N2 follows, and sleep deepens into stage N3. After 20–40 min of deep sleep, the 1st period of REM sleep begins, which lasts for 5–15 min. This sequence of sleep stages forms a sleep cycle with a normal duration of 80–110 min, and approximately 5 sleep cycles are observed in a normal night. The distribution of sleep stages within the sleep cycles gradually changes over the course of the night. Stage N3 sleep is present more often in the early sleep cycles than in the later ones; conversely, REM sleep is present more often in the later sleep cycles. Throughout the night, the total percentage of wakefulness is less than 5%. Normal sleep consists of approximately 20–25% REM and 75% non-REM, including 110–120 min of slow-wave sleep; however, the amount of REM sleep decreases with age. Light sleep represents 45–55% of the total sleep time. The total duration of sleep varies between 7.5 and 8.5 h in the majority of healthy subjects. Although the use of the American Academy of Sleep Medicine terminology is gradually becoming more widespread, the nomenclature of Rechtschaffen and Kales [1] is used to describe the sleep stages in this book as this nomenclature was used in most of the studies cited as references. Under this system, non-REM sleep is composed of 4 stages, with stages 1 and 2 being light sleep and stages 3 and 4 being deep sleep.

Hemodynamic changes during sleep depend on the sympathetic-parasympathetic balance [3]. Activity of the autonomic nervous system has been assessed by measurements of sympathetic nerve activity (SNA) using microneurography, which provides direct measurements of efferent SNA related to muscle blood vessels (muscle SNA, MSNA) [4], blood and urine catecholamine levels [5], and power spectral analysis of heart rate variability [6, 7].

Variables derived from heart rate variability analysis include the power of the high-frequency (HF) range, which is detected by spectral analysis of RR intervals. This reflects the parasympathetic modulation of the heart rate because sympathetic stimulation of the sinus node is substantially attenuated at frequencies above 0.15 Hz. The power of the low-frequency (LF) range may reflect cardiac sympathetic activity, although this is controversial [6]. The LF/HF ratio is an estimation of the sympathovagal balance: an increase in this ratio would indicate an increase in sympathetic activity and/or a reduction in vagal activity.

As non-REM sleep deepens, respiratory drive, minute ventilation, and arterial oxygen pressure (Pao_2) gradually decrease, whereas arterial carbon dioxide pressure ($Paco_2$) increases [8]. This is associated with a progressive increase in parasympathetic activity, whereas SNA decreases (the decrease in SNA in slow-wave sleep is often more than 50% of its wakefulness level; fig. 1, 2) [4, 7]. Heart rate, blood pressure and systemic vascular resistance also decrease (fig. 3) [4, 9–11]. The decrease

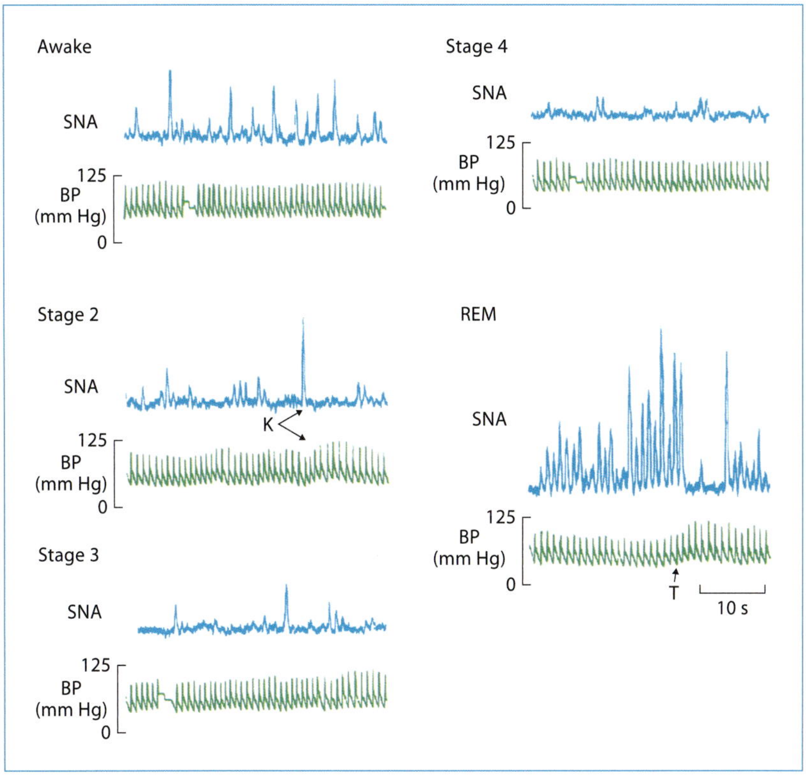

Fig. 1. Recordings of MSNA and mean blood pressure (BP) in a single healthy subject while awake and while in stage 2, 3, 4 and REM sleep. As non-REM sleep deepens (stages 2–4), SNA, BP and BP variability are gradually reduced. Arousal stimuli elicit K complexes on the electroencephalogram (not shown) that are accompanied by increases in SNA and BP (indicated by the arrows, stage 2 sleep). In contrast to the changes during non-REM sleep, heart rate, BP and BP variability increase during REM sleep, together with a profound increase in the frequency and amplitude of SNA. There is a frequent association between REM twitches (momentary periods of the restoration of muscle tone, denoted by T on the tracing) and the abrupt inhibition of sympathetic nerve discharges and BP increases. After Somers et al. [4], with permission. © 1993 Massachusetts Medical Society.

in heart rate appears to be mainly related to the increase in parasympathetic nerve activity, whereas the decrease in blood pressure appears to be primarily related to a reduction in the sympathetic vasomotor tone [12]. The normal respiratory sinus arrhythmia observed during non-REM sleep is due to a near sinusoidal modulation of heart rate variation. During inspiration, in order to adapt to the increase in venous return, the heart rate accelerates, resulting in an increase in cardiac output, while during expiration, the heart rate slows progressively [3]. Cardiac output has been reported to remain unchanged [9] or to decrease [10] during non-REM sleep.

REM sleep is characterized by unstable autonomic activity and cardiovascular function. The cardiac efferent vagal tone is generally suppressed [11], while MSNA in REM sleep is increased and may reach a similar or higher level to that observed

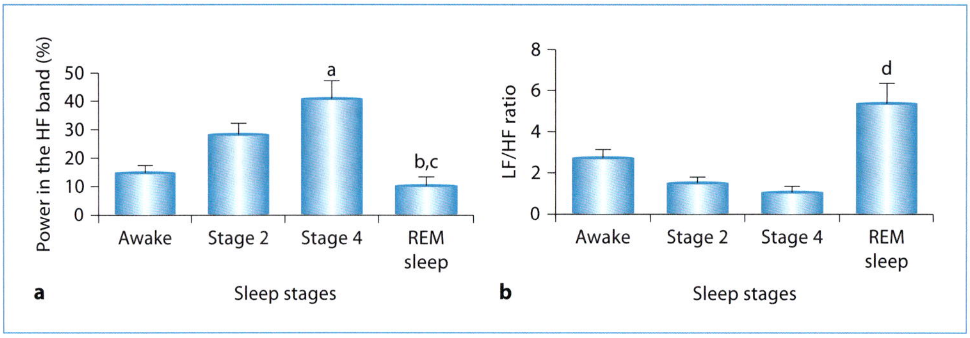

Fig. 2. Activity of the autonomic nervous system assessed by power spectral analysis of heart rate variability: percentage power in the HF band and LF/HF ratio across states of consciousness in 10 healthy male subjects. **a** As non-REM sleep deepens (stages 2–4), the percentage power of the HF band increases, whereas it decreases in REM sleep. This reflects the increase in cardiac vagal activity in non-REM sleep and its decrease in REM sleep. **b** As non-REM sleep deepens, the LF/HF ratio gradually decreases, whereas it increases during REM sleep. This reflects the decrease in cardiac sympathetic activity in non-REM sleep and its increase during REM sleep. [a] $p < 0.001$: significantly different from waking; [b] $p < 0.05$: significantly different from stage 2 sleep; [c] $p < 0.001$: significantly different from stage 4 sleep; [d] $p < 0.001$: significantly different from waking as well as stage 2 and stage 4 sleep. After Elsenbruch et al. [7], with permission.

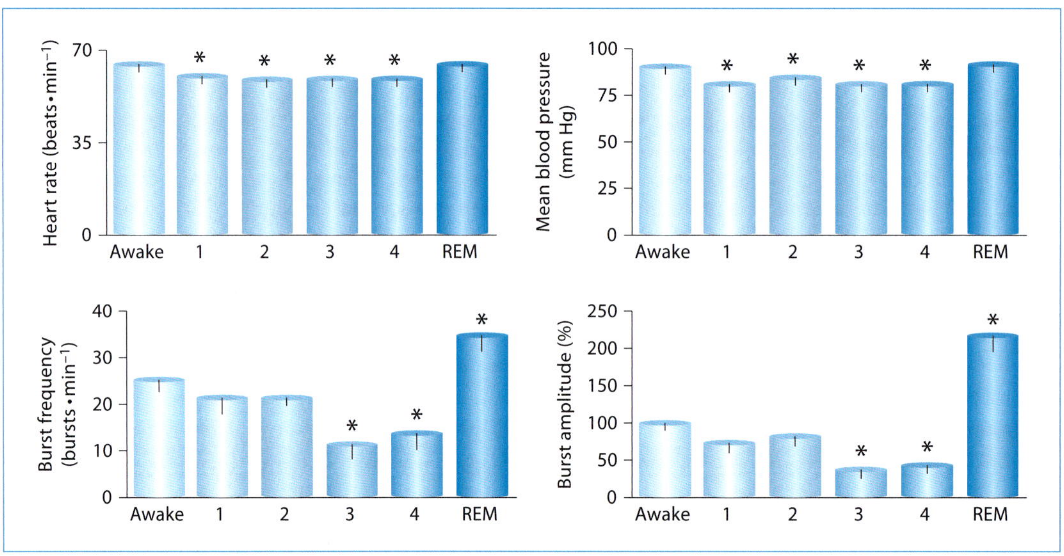

Fig. 3. Heart rate, mean blood pressure, and sympathetic burst frequency and amplitude during wakefulness in non-REM and REM sleep in healthy subjects. Heart rate and blood pressure were significantly lower during all stages of non-REM sleep than during wakefulness, and sympathetic burst activity was significantly lower during stages 3 and 4. During REM sleep, sympathetic burst activity increased significantly, but blood pressure and heart rate were similar to those recorded during wakefulness. * $p < 0.001$. Values are the mean ± SE. After Somers et al. [4], with permission. © 1993 Massachusetts Medical Society.

during wakefulness [4]. This increase in SNA is in fact initiated before the transition from non-REM to REM sleep [13]. Bursts of SNA are associated with transient increases in heart rate and arterial blood pressure that may also reach levels similar to those observed during wakefulness [4]. Breathing patterns may become highly irregular and can result in oxygen desaturation.

There are a limited number of publications focusing on the pulmonary hemodynamics of healthy subjects. During sleep, pulmonary arterial pressure has been shown to increase by 4–5 mm Hg in a small number of normal subjects, although there were no significant differences between the different stages of sleep [14, 15].

2 Hemodynamic and Autonomic Changes during the Apnea-Ventilation Resumption Cycle

OSA is characterized by repetitive episodes of complete or partial obstruction of the upper airway during sleep, leading to an increase in airway resistance and respiratory effort that may produce oxygen desaturation, hypercapnia and central nervous system arousal that restore airflow. OSA is associated with hemodynamic changes related to alterations in the activity of the autonomic nervous system.

2.1 *Hemodynamic Changes*

2.1.1 Heart Rate and Blood Pressure

During an apneic episode, the heart rate may slow down, increase or remain unchanged, depending on whether parasympathetic or sympathetic influences predominate [16]. Blood pressure decreases at the initial part of the apnea and increases at its terminal portion, while oxyhemoglobin saturation (Sao_2) decreases at the end of the apnea [17].

When ventilation resumes, the heart rate, blood pressure and ventilation reach a peak, accompanied by arousal and peak oxygen desaturation (fig. 4, 5) [18]. The recurrent rise in blood pressure may increase the mean nocturnal blood pressure; indeed, patients with isolated nocturnal hypertension and nonhypertensive or hypertensive patients who do not display the normal physiological reduction of 10–20% in nocturnal blood pressure ('nondippers') have been shown to be at risk for OSA [19–25]. Arterial pressure peak values in REM sleep are increased compared to those in non-REM sleep [26]. Arousals may contribute, via the activation of the sympathetic nervous system, to the surges in heart rate and blood pressure that occur during the ventilatory resumption phase (these surges are not suppressed by oxygen administration). However, postapneic surges in heart rate and blood pressure are not necessarily accompanied by arousal.

2.1.2 Peripheral Resistance

The resumption of ventilation occurs in the context of peripheral vasoconstriction and increased peripheral resistance (fig. 6). This situation persists for several seconds

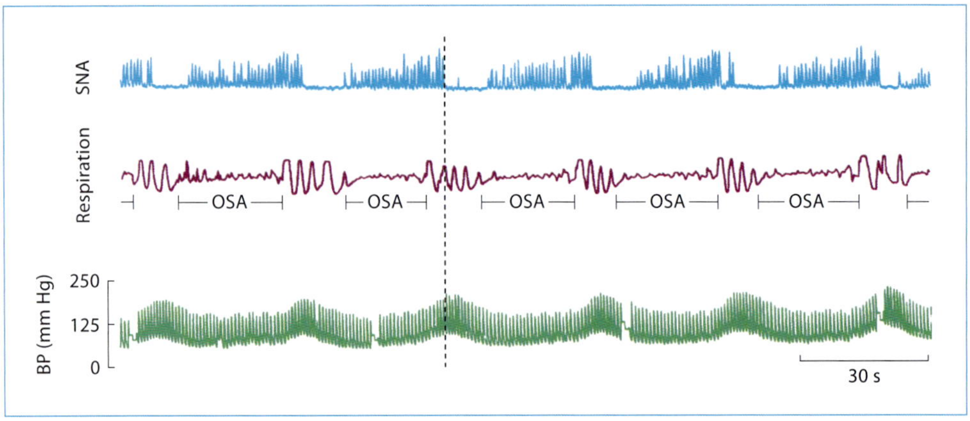

Fig. 4. SNA and blood pressure (BP) during the apnea-ventilation resumption cycle in non-REM sleep. Recordings of SNA, respiration and BP during 3 min of stage 2 sleep, showing incessant oscillations in BP and SNA in response to the occurrence of repetitive obstructive apneas. The vertical dashed line shows that ventilation resumption is accompanied by a surge in BP and an abrupt decrease in SNA. These oscillations occurred continuously during sleep and throughout all sleep stages. After Somers et al. [18], with permission.

after SNA has ceased, due to the kinetics of norepinephrine uptake, release and washout at the neurovascular junction [27–29].

2.1.3 Stroke Volume and Cardiac Output

The changes in ventricular stroke volume and cardiac output throughout the apnea-ventilation resumption cycle are described in figure 7 and table 1. Stroke volume and cardiac output have been assessed during apnea-ventilation resumption cycles [30], and the relationship between stroke volume and cardiac output and oxygen desaturation has been characterized in patients with severe OSA [31]. Using continuous isotopic assessment of the left ventricular volume, the ventricular counts are proportional to the ventricular volume, with the difference between end-diastolic and end-systolic volume being proportional to stroke volume. Most notably, a reduction in ventricular stroke volume was observed when ventilation resumed, which appears to be independent of O_2 saturation.

2.2 Autonomic Changes

During the early phase of apnea, SNA is suppressed [18]. It then increases constantly and reaches a peak at the end of apnea and on arousal. This increase in SNA critically contributes to the surges in heart rate and blood pressure that usually occur at the termination of apnea (fig. 4) [17, 18]. However, as soon as ventilation resumes, there is an abrupt inhibition of SNA to the peripheral blood vessels that is alleviated by the treatment of OSA with continuous positive airway pressure (CPAP; fig. 5) [18].

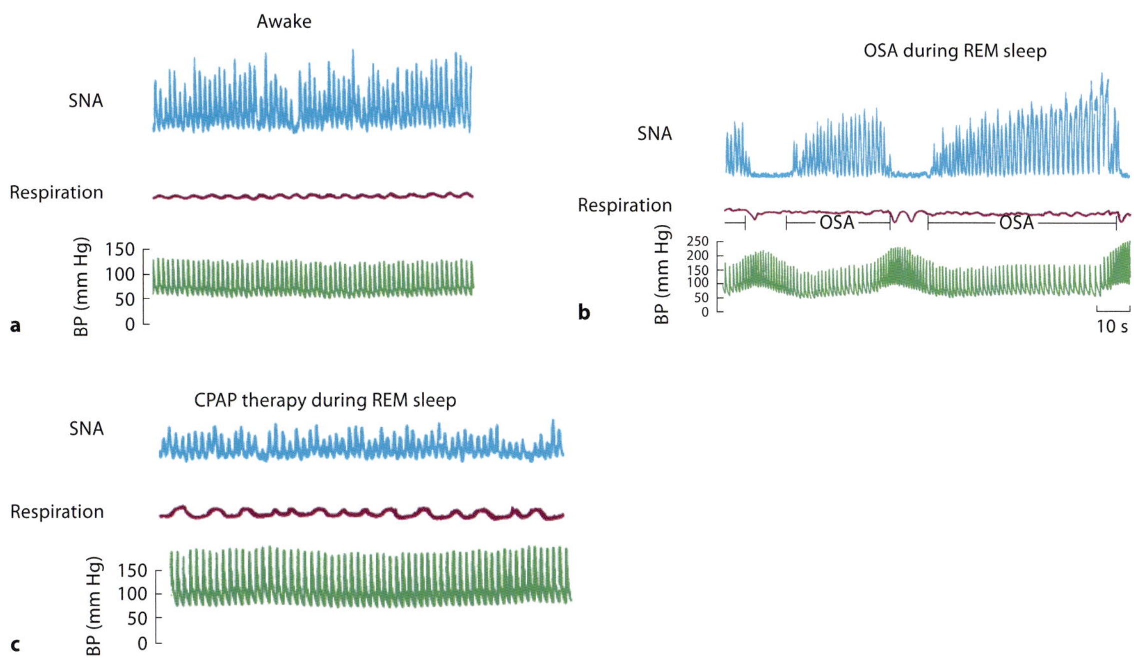

Fig. 5. SNA and blood pressure (BP) during the apnea-ventilation resumption cycle in REM sleep. Recordings of SNA, respiratory rate and intra-arterial BP in the same individual when awake (**a**), with OSA episodes during REM sleep (**b**) and with the elimination of OSA episodes by CPAP therapy during REM sleep (**c**). SNA was very high during wakefulness, but increased even further secondary to OSA during REM sleep. BP increased from 130/65 mm Hg when the individual was awake to 256/110 mm Hg at the end of the apneic episode. Elimination of apneic episodes by CPAP therapy resulted in the decrease in SNA and prevented BP surges during REM sleep. After Somers et al. [18], with permission.

The levels of PaO_2 and $PaCO_2$, lung inflation, and blood pressure are important factors that modulate these autonomic changes [32, 33]. In short, SNA may be increased by hypoxemia and hypercapnia, whereas it may be inhibited by lung inflation and the postapneic surge in blood pressure. However, there is a body of evidence demonstrating that chronic intermittent hypoxia is the main cause of these autonomic alterations [32] as described below.

2.2.1 Levels of PaO_2 and $PaCO_2$

Hypoxemia stimulates peripheral arterial chemoreceptors and causes an increase in efferent SNA and minute ventilation [34–37]. It may contribute to the increase in SNA associated with obstructive apneas [38–40]. Indeed, these surges of SNA have been significantly blunted by the administration of oxygen (fraction of inspired oxygen, $FIO_2 = 100\%$) [41]. Hypercapnia induces an increase in ventilation, heart rate, cardiac output and blood pressure. It has a direct vasodilator effect, but increases sympathetic

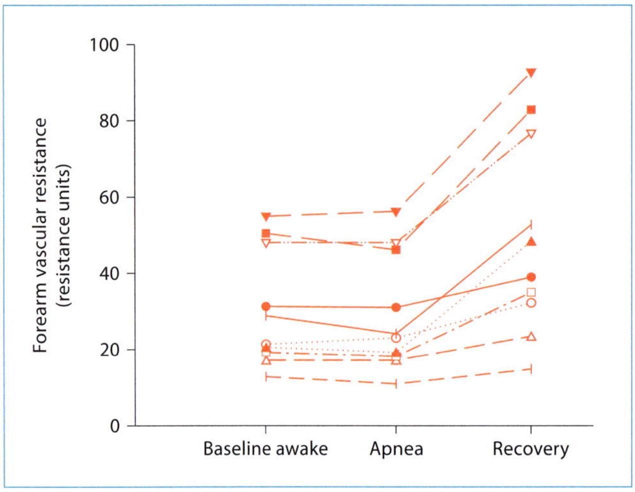

Fig. 6. Forearm vascular resistance at baseline (being awake), during spontaneous obstructive apnea and at recovery after apnea termination in 10 individuals. Forearm vascular resistance increased by 71% in the recovery period (from 29.3 ± 15.4 resistance units during apnea to 49.8 ± 26.5 resistance units during recovery, $p < 0.05$); all patients showed an increase in resistance. Resistance in the recovery period was significantly different from that in the baseline or apneic periods ($p < 0.05$), which were not significantly different from one another. Each symbol represents an individual subject. Values are the mean of at least 3 measurements. After Anand et al. [28], with permission.

vasoconstrictor activity [42]. When the effects of hypercapnia and hypoxia on MSNA and minute ventilation are compared: (1) hypercapnia is a potent stimulus of MSNA and minute ventilation; (2) during spontaneous breathing, hypercapnia has a greater effect on SNA and minute ventilation than hypoxia; (3) cessation of breathing has a marked potentiating effect on MSNA during hypoxia, but not during hypercapnia, and (4) combined hypoxia and hypercapnia have a synergistic effect on MSNA and minute ventilation [38]. It is suggested that the levels of $Paco_2$ may alter the sympathetic response to hypoxia and respiration [38, 43].

2.2.2 Lung Inflation

In normal subjects, lung inflation is associated with a decrease in sympathetic activity, an increase in heart rate that may be vagally mediated and a reflex inhibition of inspiratory neurons in the brainstem at high lung volumes (the Hering-Breuer reflex). During apneas, the lung inflation reflex may not exist, and this may contribute to an increase in SNA [18]. In contrast, the reflex may be exacerbated during ventilation resumption, when SNA is abruptly inhibited.

2.2.3 Blood Pressure

Stimulation of aortic arch and carotid sinus baroreceptors reflexively decreases sympathetic outflow and increases parasympathetic cardiac efferent activity [33].

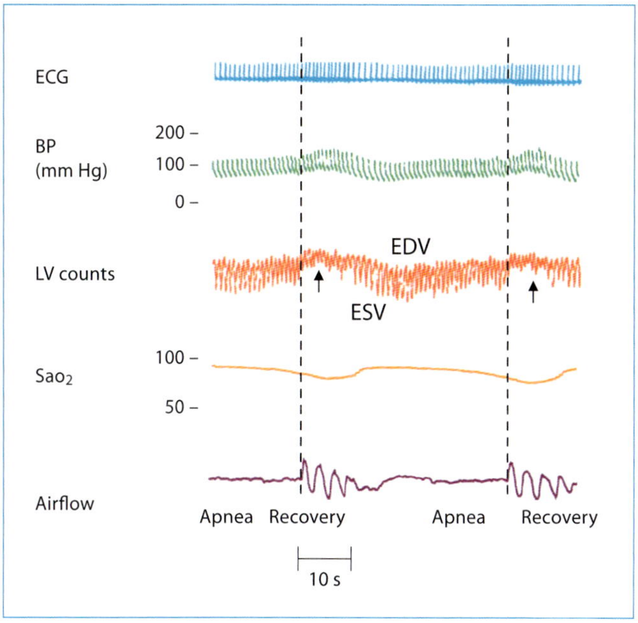

Fig. 7. Left ventricular stroke volume during the apnea-ventilation resumption cycle. Polygraph record of a patient with severe OSA and nocturnal O_2 desaturation displaying the electrocardiogram (ECG), systemic blood pressure (BP), continuous isotopic assessment of the left ventricular volume (LV counts), oximetry (Sao_2) and respiration (airflow). End-systolic volume (ESV) and end-diastolic volume (EDV) are noted. The vertical dashed lines help to distinguish the apneic phase from the ventilation resumption phase. Stroke volume is greatest at the beginning of apnea and decreases progressively throughout the apnea. There are a drastic increase in ESV, associated with the resumption of ventilation (arrow), and a further abrupt reduction in stroke volume (as EDV does not significantly change). After Garpestad et al. [30], with permission.

A compensatory relationship also exists between arterial blood pressure and ventilation: a reduction in arterial blood pressure increases the respiratory rate, whereas a transient elevation of arterial blood pressure results in a diminution or cessation of breathing efforts. The increase in blood pressure occurring during ventilation resumption may elicit a reduction in the ventilatory and sympathetic responses to chemoreflex stimulation by hypoxemia [39]. Respiration may also modulate the baroreceptors' influence on cardiac sympathovagal activity [44]. The modulatory role of respiration on the influence of baroreceptors on cardiac sympathovagal activity may be critical to the succession of apnea and ventilation resumption in OSA patients [33, 45].

2.3 Pulmonary Arterial Pressure Changes during the Apnea-Ventilation Resumption Cycle

The pulmonary artery pressure (PAP), measured relative to atmospheric pressure, shows wide variations throughout an apnea and reaches its highest level during the

Table 1. Hemodynamic alterations of intrathoracic cardiovascular structures during the apnea-ventilation resumption cycle

During the course of an obstructive apnea, the negative intrathoracic pressure swings due to repetitive inspiratory efforts elicit:
- ↑ transmural pressure of the intrathoracic cardiovascular structures
- ↑ inspiratory afterload of the left ventricle that impairs its emptying
- ↑ venous return and filling of the right ventricle that result in its distension and a left-forward shift in the interventricular septum

Ventilation resumption is associated with:
- ↓ negative intrathoracic pressure
- ↓ transmural pressure of intrathoracic cardiovascular structures
- ↓ left ventricle afterload
- ↓ stroke volume
- lung inflation, which provokes:
  - a mechanical distortion of the left ventricle
  - ↑ pulmonary vascular resistance
  - ↑ right ventricle afterload

Transmural pressure is the difference between the interior and exterior pressure of the structure in question. Cardiac output (i.e. stroke volume × heart rate) is either unchanged or increased [96, 97]. This uncertainty may be related to methodological bias, e.g. the use of different techniques, some of which have limited accuracy, and the level of increase in the heart rate. Although the heart rate increases at the termination of apnea, this may be insufficient to compensate for the decrease in left ventricular stroke volume, resulting in a decrease in cardiac output [30]. ↑ = Increase; ↓ = decrease.

resumption of ventilation [46, 47]. The measurement of PAP relative to intrathoracic pressure, i.e. transmural pressure (PAP_{tm}), assesses PAP independently of the interference exerted by intrathoracic pressure (i.e. PAP_{tm} = PAP – intrathoracic pressure) [46, 47]. In normal subjects, the intrathoracic pressure only changes by a small amount during the respiratory cycle, and PAP_{tm} remains close to the intravascular pressure. However, during obstructive apneas, intrathoracic pressure may become very negative (e.g. –40 mm Hg), and PAP_{tm} is much higher than intravascular pressure (i.e. PAP_{tm} = PAP + 40 mm Hg, if the intrathoracic pressure is –40 mm Hg). PAP_{tm} oscillations during the course of an obstructive apnea are greatly smoothed when compared to those of PAP measured relative to atmospheric pressure [46, 47]. PAP_{tm} slowly increases from the early or middle portion of an apnea and progressively reaches a peak at the resumption of ventilation [46, 48, 49]. The course of PAP_{tm} is, therefore, very different from that of peripheral arterial pressure, which surges at the resumption of ventilation. A significant but mild increase in systolic PAP_{tm} from a mean of 28 mm Hg at the initial part of the apnea to a mean of 38.6 mm Hg at the end of the apnea has been observed [49]. At the beginning of the resumption of ventilation, the increase in PAP may be due to the concomitant increase in heart rate and cardiac output [50].

Swings in the negative intrathoracic pressure due to repetitive inspiratory efforts cause an increased transmural pressure on the intrathoracic cardiovascular structures. This results in an increased inspiratory afterload of the left ventricle that impairs its emptying, and an increase in the venous return and filling of the right ventricle that results in its distension and a left-forward shift in the interventricular septum [51]. These alterations are associated with an increase in the pulmonary capillary wedge pressure [52] and an increase in pulmonary vascular resistance, which may both contribute to the increase in PAP in OSA during sleep [53].

Acute PAP changes during OSA correlate inversely with the degree of arterial hypoxemia [46, 48, 49]. PAP alterations related to Sao_2 fluctuations depend on the timing of the pulmonary vessel response to the hypoxic stimulus (the pulmonary vessel response is fully developed only after some minutes after exposure to hypoxia) [48]. When PAP_{tm} was compared during sequences of apneas in 2 groups of patients who either had a constant and small Sao_2 fall after each apneic event or marked Sao_2 falls [48], the highest PAP_{tm} values were associated with apnea sequences with deep and prolonged oxyhemoglobin desaturations, and that in this case, the PAP_{tm} became progressively higher without returning to baseline values. In contrast, when short and mild desaturations occurred, PAP_{tm} returned to a constant baseline value soon after each apnea, i.e. at the beginning of the following apnea (fig. 8) [48]. It is suggested that, in obstructive apneas, systolic PAP_{tm} shows rapid changes, which reflect esophageal pressure variations, and slower changes, which are likely to be caused by Sao_2. Such a relationship between the severity of oxygen desaturation and the increase in PAP_{tm} has also been observed by other authors [49]. However, when the effect of acute oxygen administration on PAP_{tm} is assessed, in spite of the marked attenuation in the falls and oscillations of Sao_2 observed in all patients, O_2 administration in the majority of cases affects neither the levels of PAP_{tm} nor the amplitude of its variations induced by obstructive apneas. This suggests that, besides the critical importance of the hypoxic stimulus, there may be other important mechanisms that alter pulmonary hemodynamics during the apnea-ventilation resumption cycle [54].

PAP appears to be higher in REM sleep than in non-REM sleep, even after adjusting for sleep stage differences in arterial desaturation [55]. This may be related to the greater severity of apneas during REM sleep than during non-REM sleep [48], or it may be due to neural mechanisms related to REM sleep [55]. Some studies have shown that PAP progressively increases throughout the night in sleep apnea patients [56, 57], but this is controversial [49]. In addition, pulmonary hemodynamics may also depend on hypercapnia and acidosis [58].

In summary, the mild-to-moderate increase in PAP_{tm} during the apnea-ventilation resumption cycle may be due to several factors, including intrathoracic pressure changes, Sao_2 fluctuations, variations in heart rate and cardiac output, the time of night and the sleep stage.

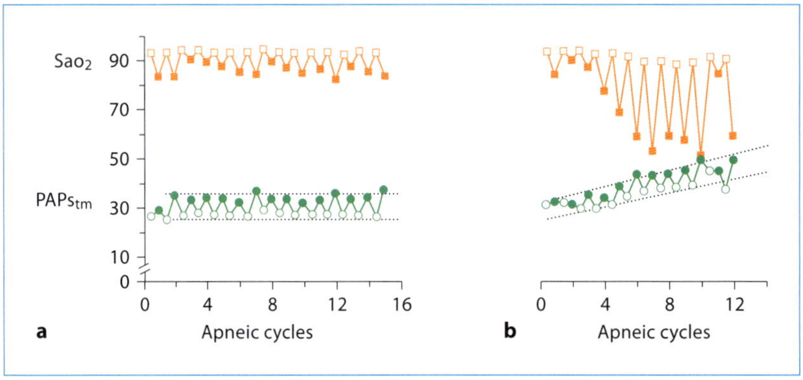

Fig. 8. Slow and fast changes in PAP_{tm} in OSA. This figure shows the highest and lowest values of SaO_2 and the simultaneous values for transmural systolic pulmonary artery pressure ($PAPs_{tm}$) recorded in a representative OSA patient [48]. Two recordings of consecutive apneic cycles are shown, with the start of the apnea marked by open symbols, and the end of the apnea marked by closed symbols. An apneic cycle was defined as the period including all of the occluded breathing efforts of an apnea, as well as the unoccluded breaths of the ventilatory period, which preceded another apnea. **a** Data recorded in a sequence of apneic cycles demonstrating more or less constant and mild SaO_2 swings. **b** Data recorded in a sequence of closely recurring apneas where the SaO_2, due to marked falls, shows large swings. In **a**, $PAPs_{tm}$ returns to a constant baseline level whenever SaO_2 rises. However, in **b**, the $PAPs_{tm}$ oscillations do not increase proportionately to the SaO_2 swings, but the lowest (early apnea) and highest (end apnea) values tend to increase progressively. It is suggested that $PAPs_{tm}$ is influenced by SaO_2, but does not vary at the same speed as SaO_2. Rapid changes in $PAPs_{tm}$ may reflect esophageal pressure variations, whereas slower changes are likely to be caused by hypoxia. After Marrone et al. [48], with permission. © European Respiratory Society.

3 Chronic Autonomic Cardiovascular Dysfunction

3.1 Daytime Sympathetic Overactivity

The increase in SNA observed during sleep in OSA patients is carried over into wakefulness, even under conditions of normoxia (fig. 9) [18, 59]. It is not known how or if the chronic intermittent hypoxic stimulus associated with the recurrent apnea-ventilation resumption cycles occurring during sleep contributes to this daytime increase in SNA. Studies of MSNA in various experimental hypoxic conditions in healthy subjects have shown that the increased MSNA response persists for several minutes or hours after the hypoxic stress has ceased [34–37, 60]. It is hypothesized that nighttime chronic intermittent hypoxia may contribute to the activation of the central nervous system and the increase in peripheral chemosensitivity that are carried over into wakefulness, resulting in sustained daytime sympathetic overactivity [32, 34, 61–63].

The daytime sympathetic overactivity observed in OSA occurs independently of obesity, a confounding condition that is also associated with sympathetic overactivity [64]. This was demonstrated by the analysis of MSNA in 86 middle-aged normotensive subjects. The subjects were classified into 4 groups (lean or obese, with or without

Fig. 9. Recordings of SNA during wakefulness in OSA patients and matched control subjects. The sympathetic burst frequency (bursts • min^{-1}) during wakefulness was significantly higher in OSA patients (n = 10) than in control subjects (n = 10) (means ± SE 59 ± 14 vs. 34 ± 3 bursts • min^{-1}, respectively; p < 0.001). After Somers et al. [18], with permission.

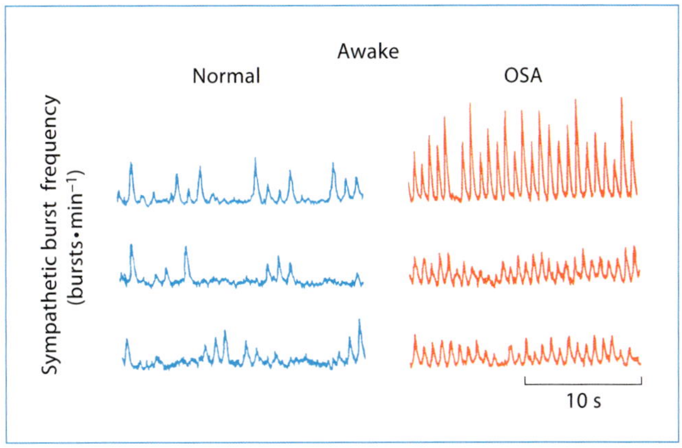

Fig. 10. Values of MSNA in lean subjects with (L+) or without (L–) OSA and in obese subjects with (O+) or without (O–) OSA. Data are shown as the mean ± SEM. * p < 0.05, ** p < 0.01. After Grassi et al. [64], with permission.

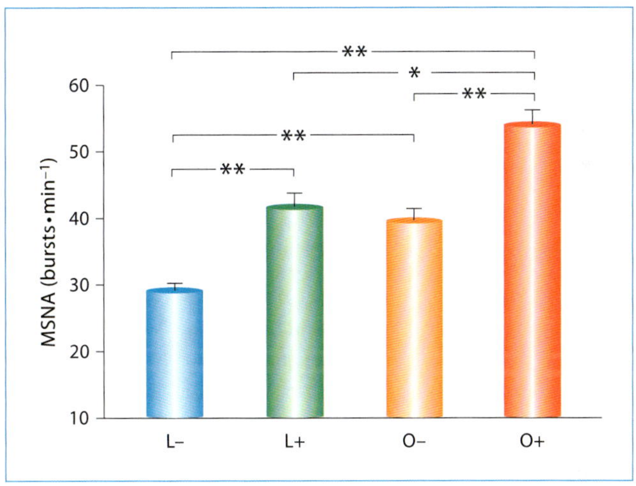

OSA) that were matched for age, gender and blood pressure values [64]. The 2 obese groups were matched for body mass index and waist-to-hip ratio, as were the 2 lean groups. Compared with the non-OSA lean group, MSNA showed a similar increase in the OSA lean group and in the non-OSA obese group (p < 0.01), while a further increase was detected in OSA subjects (p < 0.01; fig. 10). It is suggested that OSA exerts sympathostimulating effects independently of body weight, and that the sympathostimulation in OSA contributes to the overall adrenergic activation of the obese state. It is also suggested that the sympathetic activation observed in obese subjects occurs independently in OSA. These findings were also confirmed in metabolic syndrome patients with and without OSA compared with healthy control subjects without OSA [65]. MSNA was significantly higher in metabolic syndrome patients without OSA than in controls (61.9 ± 3.9 vs. 37.7 ± 4.1 bursts • 100 heartbeats^{-1}, respectively,

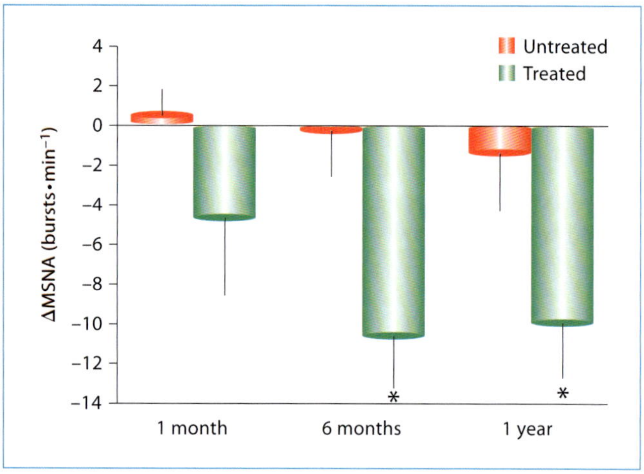

Fig. 11. Daytime changes of MSNA during repeated measurements in untreated OSA patients (n = 9) and in OSA patients treated with CPAP (n = 11). MSNA did not significantly change in untreated patients. In treated patients, MSNA significantly decreased after 6 months and 1 year of CPAP treatment. * $p < 0.05$ versus baseline. Data are means ± SEM. After Narkiewicz et al. [70], with permission.

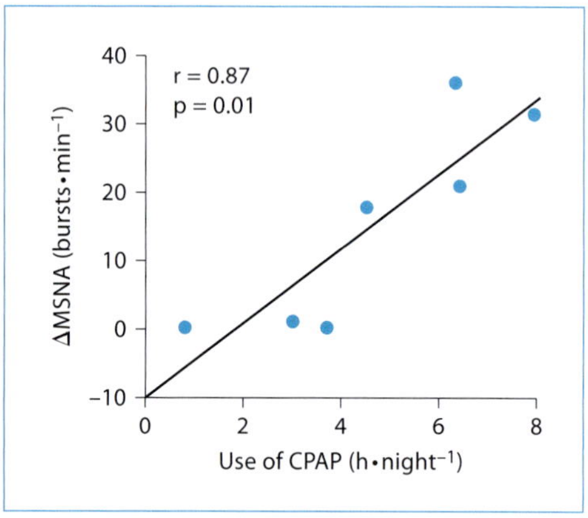

Fig. 12. Relationship between compliance level with CPAP administration and MSNA during wakefulness in OSA patients. MSNA was measured via peroneal microneurography in 7 patients with documented OSA before and at least 1 month after compliance-monitored nasal CPAP therapy. There was a direct linear correlation between the decrease in MSNA and the average hours of CPAP use per night. After Waradekar et al. [71]. Reprinted with permission of the American Thoracic Society. © American Thoracic Society.

$p < 0.01$); a further marked increase was detected in metabolic syndrome patients with OSA (77.1 ± 4.3 bursts • 100 heartbeats^{-1}, $p < 0.01$). Compared with controls, baroreflex control of the heart rate and MSNA was markedly impaired in metabolic syndrome patients with OSA; a further impairment in baroreflex-heart rate modulation was detected in metabolic syndrome patients with OSA. It is suggested that sympathetic activation of metabolic syndrome occurs independently of OSA, and OSA markedly potentiates the neuroadrenergic abnormalities associated with metabolic syndrome. Overall, autonomic alterations associated with OSA may increase the cardiovascular and metabolic risk of patients with confounders such as obesity, metabolic syndrome, systemic hypertension, heart failure and cardiac arrhythmias [66–69].

Prolonged CPAP administration reduces sympathetic overactivity (fig. 11) [70], with the degree of improvement varying directly with compliance level (fig. 12) [18, 71]; however, the level may not reach that of normal subjects [71].

3.2 Downregulation of Vascular Sympathoadrenergic Receptors

Alterations in vascular motor function are associated with the downregulation of vascular sympathoadrenergic receptors, a potential consequence of chronic sympathetic overactivity [72]. A reduced response to the intra-arterial infusion of α- and β-receptor agonists was observed in OSA patients when compared to normotensive control subjects [72]. Such a downregulation has also been observed in other studies [73–75].

3.3 Polymorphisms in α- and β-Adrenergic Receptor Genes

The Arg389Gly polymorphism of the β_1-adrenergic receptor has been associated with an increased risk of OSA in hypertensive men and with hypertension in subjects with mild OSA [76]. Also, in men, there was a dose-dependent increase in the apnea-hypopnea index, with the lowest level in Gly389Gly carriers and the highest level in Arg389Arg carriers. It is suggested that these findings may highlight the role of the sympathetic nervous system in OSA and hypertension. A lack of an association has been reported between polymorphisms of the β_2-adrenergic receptor gene and OSA and between α-adrenergic receptor genes and OSA [76, 77]. The presence of the arginine 64 allele of the β_3-adrenergic receptor gene was not associated with the presence of OSA, but it was associated with an increased tendency to develop obesity in those patients who suffer from OSA [78]. The role of these polymorphisms in the α- and β-adrenergic receptor genes remains to be elucidated.

3.4 Chemoreflex Changes

The sympathetic response to hypoxia is enhanced in OSA patients compared to control subjects, and this response is reduced by the administration of CPAP [40, 79–81]. MSNA responses to acute hypoxia (FIo_2 of 0.1, for 5 min) were determined in OSA patients (n = 24, mean apnea-hypopnea index $47 \bullet h^{-1}$) and in age- and weight-matched nonapneic control subjects (n = 14) [81]. Basal MSNA was higher in the OSA patients than in the control subjects ($p < 0.05$), and the MSNA responses to hypoxia were also markedly enhanced in OSA patients ($p < 0.001$; fig. 13). In OSA patients who were retested after 1–24 months of CPAP therapy (n – 11), basal MSNA ($p < 0.01$) and the responses of MSNA to hypoxia ($p < 0.01$) decreased significantly. It is suggested that the sympathetic responses to hypoxic chemoreflex stimulation are enhanced in OSA and may partially normalize following CPAP therapy.

3.5 Cardiac Vagal Dysfunction and Baroreflex Changes

Cardiac vagal regulation is comprised of a tonic and a dynamic component [82]. Spectral analysis of heart rate variability measurements can be used to assess vagal activity. The measurement of the baroreflex sensitivity (referred to as the baroreflex gain) assesses its responsiveness [83].

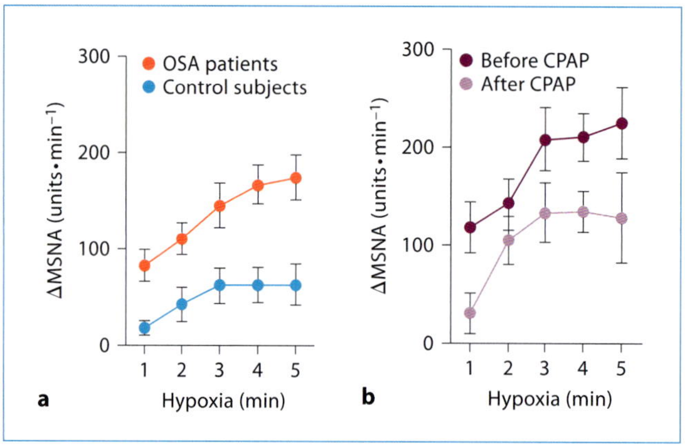

Fig. 13. Sympathetic responses to hypoxia (FIO_2 0.1 for 5 min) in OSA patients: effect of CPAP. **a** Effect of acute hypoxia on the changes of MSNA in OSA patients (n = 22) and control subjects (n = 12). Basal MSNA was higher in OSA patients than in control subjects ($p < 0.05$). The MSNA responses to hypoxia were markedly enhanced in OSA patients compared to control subjects ($p < 0.001$). **b** Effect of acute hypoxia on the changes of MSNA in OSA patients (n = 11) before and after treatment with CPAP. In OSA patients who were retested after 1–24 months of CPAP therapy (n = 11), basal MSNA and the responses of MSNA to hypoxia decreased significantly ($p < 0.01$). After Imadojemu et al. [81], with permission.

Fig. 14. HF component from the spectral analysis of RR intervals in OSA patients and control subjects during wakefulness. Mean HF power of RR interval variability was significantly lower in the moderate-to-severe OSA patients (n = 11) than in the control subjects (n = 12; * $p < 0.05$), but it was not significantly different between mild OSA patients (n = 13) and control subjects. The HF spectral component of the RR interval is expressed in normalized units (NU). Data are the mean ± SEM. After Narkiewicz et al. [84], with permission.

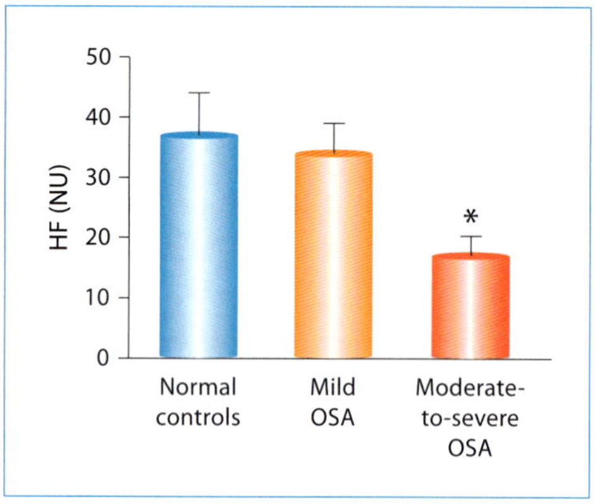

Daytime vagal activity is lower in OSA patients than in control subjects [84, 85]. For example, analysis of the HF component from the spectral analysis of RR intervals in patients with mild (n = 13) and moderate-to-severe (n = 11) OSA and in control subjects (n = 12) indicated that the HF component was significantly lower in the moderate-to-severe OSA patients than in the control subjects ($p < 0.05$), but it was not significantly different between mild OSA patients and control subjects (fig. 14) [84]. Daytime vagal activity increases with CPAP treatment, with the level of improvement depending on the level of adherence to CPAP treatment [86, 87].

The sensitivity of the baroreflex is reduced during sleep and wakefulness in OSA patients compared to control subjects [88, 89]. For example, this was observed in patients with mild-to-moderate OSA (n = 14), in patients with severe OSA (n = 14) and in non-OSA subjects (n = 10), carefully matched for age, body mass index and other relevant variables (fig. 15) [89]. Acute CPAP administration in patients with severe OSA (n = 18) slightly, but significantly, increases baroreflex sensitivity to the heart rate [90]. This was associated with a decrease in cardiovascular variability during sleep, a risk factor associated with a poor prognostic outcome [91, 92]. Similarly, an increase in baroreflex sensitivity, which was associated with a decrease in systolic blood pressure, was observed after a single night of CPAP treatment in patients with refractory hypertension and OSA (n = 11) [93]. A 4-week randomized controlled study of effective versus subtherapeutic CPAP administration in patients with moderate-to-severe OSA (n = 102) revealed that, in comparison to subtherapeutic CPAP administration, effective CPAP therapy was associated with a significant increase in daytime baroreflex sensitivity to blood pressure (from 7.1 ± 3.3 to 8.8 ± 4.2 ms • mm Hg^{-1}, respectively, $p < 0.001$) [94]. Compared to baseline, the increase in sensitivity following effective CPAP application averaged 24%. This was associated with a reduction in sympathetic activity and mean arterial blood pressure. Six months of CPAP therapy have also been shown to markedly increase the sensitivity of the baroreflex to heart rate [88].

Overall, these studies show that the alterations in cardiac vagal activity during sleep in OSA patients are carried over into wakefulness. They may be alleviated by CPAP therapy, the beneficial effect of which persists during wakefulness. Alterations in the sympathovagal balance and reduced baroreflex sensitivity have been associated with a poor prognosis in cardiac patients, including sudden death and ventricular fibrillation after myocardial infarction [91, 92]. These alterations in cardiac vagal activity may contribute to the development of cardiovascular pathologies associated with OSA.

3.6 *Relationship between Nighttime Chronic Intermittent Hypoxia and Daytime Autonomic and Blood Pressure Changes*

Healthy volunteers who were exposed to nocturnal intermittent hypoxia for 14 consecutive nights exhibited increased resting MSNA and reduced sympathetic baroreflex gain [60]. This was associated with a significant sustained daytime, but not nighttime, elevation in blood pressure after a single night of exposure (3 mm Hg for mean end-diastolic pressure) and further increased daytime pressures after 2 weeks of exposure (8 mm Hg systolic and 5 mm Hg diastolic). It is suggested that the sympathoactivation induced by intermittent hypoxia is likely to contribute to blood pressure elevation and may be derived from reduced baroreflex inhibition. In the same model, using healthy subjects, exposure to nocturnal intermittent hypoxia for 28 consecutive nights was associated with an increase in MSNA, diastolic blood pressure and vascular resistance [95]. These findings highlight the link between chronic intermittent hypoxia, sympathetic overactivity and increased blood pressure.

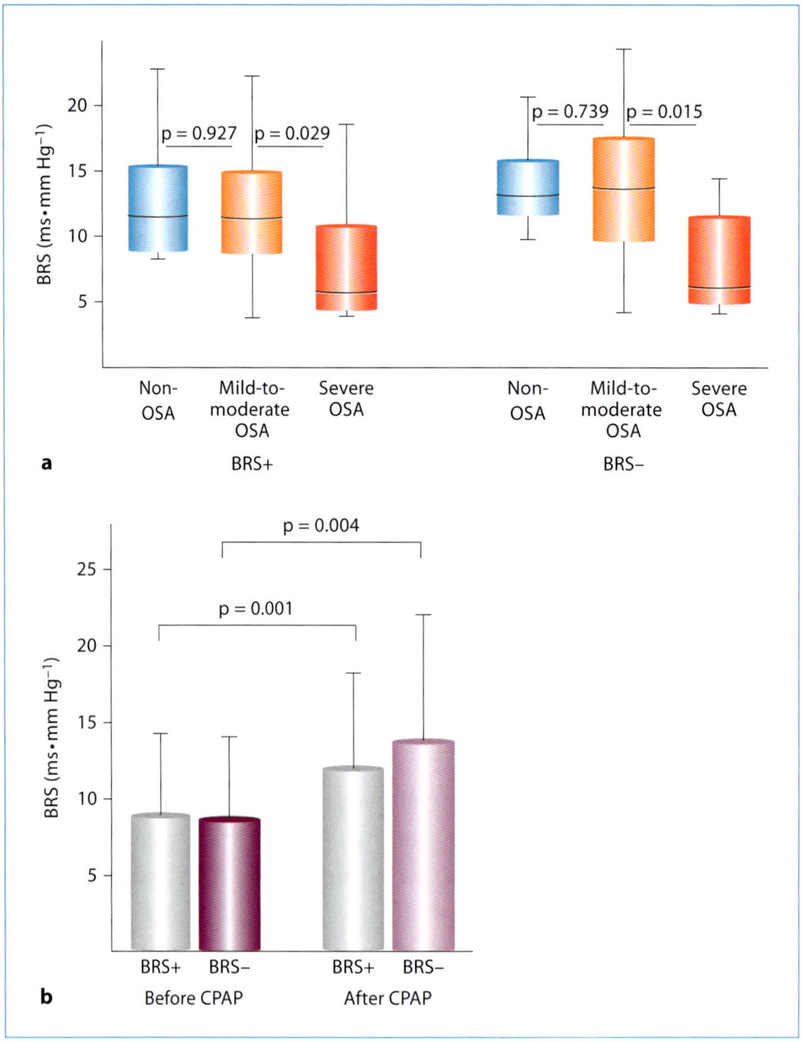

Fig. 15. Depressed baroreflex sensitivity (BRS) in patients with severe OSA during sleep: effect of CPAP treatment. Sequences of 3 or more consecutive beats in which systolic blood pressure (SBP) and pulse intervals (PIs) concurrently increased (+PI/+SBP) or decreased (–PI/–SBP) were identified. Values of +PI/+SBP and –PI/–SBP were averaged to obtain an estimate of BRS+, a measure of baroreceptor activation (a positive ramp), or BRS–, a measure of baroreceptor deactivation (a negative ramp), respectively. **a** Spontaneous BRS during sleep. BRS+ and BRS– were significantly lower in patients with severe OSA (n = 14) than in patients with mild-to-moderate OSA (n = 14) and in non-OSA subjects (n = 10). There was no significant difference between the non-OSA and mild-to-moderate OSA groups. Boxes represent values within the interquartile range, whiskers represent the data range, and lines across the boxes represent the median values. **b** Impact of 6 weeks of CPAP therapy in 8 OSA patients. CPAP therapy significantly improved the BRS measures. Boxes represent mean values, and error bars represent the SD of the mean. After Ryan et al. [89], with permission.

4 Conclusion

Strong evidence has accumulated that indicates the acute and chronic hemodynamic and autonomic changes that occur in OSA. During the apnea-ventilation resumption cycle, these changes are mainly due to reflexes related to chronic intermittent hypoxemia, which is likely to have a major role [32], hypercapnia, lung inflation and blood pressure variations that modulate baroreceptor and chemoreceptor influences on the cardiovascular system. Alterations in the autonomic nervous system observed during sleep in OSA patients are carried over into wakefulness, including a sympathovagal imbalance accompanied with baroreflex and chemoreflex changes that may critically contribute to the development of the cardiovascular disorders associated with OSA. Most importantly, these alterations have been shown to decrease following the treatment of OSA with CPAP.

5 References

1 Rechtschaffen A, Kales AR: Manual of Standardized Terminology: Techniques and Scoring System for Sleep Stages of Human Subjects. Los Angeles, UCLA Brain Information Service, Brain Research Institute, 1968.

2 Iber C, Ancoli-Israel S, Chesson A, Quan SF, American Academy of Sleep Medicine: The AASM Manual for the Scoring of Sleep and Associated Events: Rules, Terminology and Technical Specifications, ed 1. Westchester, American Academy of Sleep Medicine, 2007.

3 Verrier RL, Harper RM, Hobson JA: Cardiovascular physiology: central and autonomic regulation; in Kryger MH, Roth T, Dement WC (eds): Principles and Practice of Sleep Medicine, ed 4. Philadelphia, Saunders, 2005, pp 192–202.

4 Somers VK, Dyken ME, Mark AL, Abboud FM: Sympathetic-nerve activity during sleep in normal subjects. N Engl J Med 1993;328:303–307.

5 Dimsdale JE, Coy T, Ziegler MG, Ancoli-Israel S, Clausen J: The effect of sleep apnea on plasma and urinary catecholamines. Sleep 1995;18:377–381.

6 Heart rate variability: standards of measurement, physiological interpretation and clinical use. Task Force of the European Society of Cardiology and the North American Society of Pacing and Electrophysiology. Circulation 1996;93:1043–1065.

7 Elsenbruch S, Harnish MJ, Orr WC: Heart rate variability during waking and sleep in healthy males and females. Sleep 1999;22:1067–1071.

8 Phillipson EA: Control of breathing during sleep. Am Rev Respir Dis 1978;118:909–939.

9 Bristow JD, Honour AJ, Pickering TG, Sleight P: Cardiovascular and respiratory changes during sleep in normal and hypertensive subjects. Cardiovasc Res 1969;3:476–485.

10 Khatri IM, Freis ED: Hemodynamic changes during sleep. J Appl Physiol 1967;22:867–873.

11 Mancia G: Autonomic modulation of the cardiovascular system during sleep. N Engl J Med 1993;328: 347–349.

12 Baccelli G, Guazzi M, Mancia G, Zanchetti A: Neural and non-neural mechanisms influencing circulation during sleep. Nature 1969;223:184–185.

13 Bonnet MH, Arand DL: Heart rate variability: sleep stage, time of night, and arousal influences. Electroencephalogr Clin Neurophysiol 1997;102: 390–396.

14 Lugaresi E, Coccagna G, Cirignotta F, Farneti P, Gallassi R, Di Donato G, Verucchi P: Breathing during sleep in man in normal and pathological conditions. Adv Exp Med Biol 1978;99:35–45.

15 Raeside DA, Brown A, Patel KR, Welsh D, Peacock AJ: Ambulatory pulmonary artery pressure monitoring during sleep and exercise in normal individuals and patients with COPD. Thorax 2002;57: 1050–1053.

16 Bonsignore MR, Romano S, Marrone O, Chiodi M, Bonsignore G: Different heart rate patterns in obstructive apneas during NREM sleep. Sleep 1997; 20:1167–1174.

17 Tilkian AG, Guilleminault C, Schroeder JS, Lehrman KL, Simmons FB, Dement WC: Hemodynamics in sleep-induced apnea: studies during wakefulness and sleep. Ann Intern Med 1976;85:714–719.

18 Somers VK, Dyken ME, Clary MP, Abboud FM: Sympathetic neural mechanisms in obstructive sleep apnea. J Clin Invest 1995;96:1897–1904.
19 Hoffstein V, Mateika J: Evening-to-morning blood pressure variations in snoring patients with and without obstructive sleep apnea. Chest 1992;101: 379–384.
20 Suzuki M, Guilleminault C, Otsuka K, Shiomi T: Blood pressure 'dipping' and 'non-dipping' in obstructive sleep apnea syndrome patients. Sleep 1996;19:382–387.
21 Portaluppi F, Provini F, Cortelli P, Plazzi G, Bertozzi N, Manfredini R, Fersini C, Lugaresi E: Undiagnosed sleep-disordered breathing among male nondippers with essential hypertension. J Hypertens 1997;15: 1227–1233.
22 Davies CW, Crosby JH, Mullins RL, Barbour C, Davies RJ, Stradling JR: Case-control study of 24 hour ambulatory blood pressure in patients with obstructive sleep apnoea and normal matched control subjects. Thorax 2000;55:736–740.
23 Ancoli-Israel S, Stepnowsky C, Dimsdale J, Marler M, Cohen-Zion M, Johnson S: The effect of race and sleep-disordered breathing on nocturnal BP 'dipping': analysis in an older population. Chest 2002;122:1148–1155.
24 Møller DS, Lind P, Strunge B, Pedersen EB: Abnormal vasoactive hormones and 24-hour blood pressure in obstructive sleep apnea. Am J Hypertens 2003;16:274–280.
25 Routledge FS, McFetridge-Durdle JA, Dean CR: Night-time blood pressure patterns and target organ damage: a review. Can J Cardiol 2007;23:132–138.
26 Garpestad E, Ringler J, Parker JA, Remsburg S, Weiss JW: Sleep stage influences the hemodynamic response to obstructive apneas. Am J Respir Crit Care Med 1995;152:199–203.
27 Leuenberger U, Gleeson K, Wroblewski K, Prophet S, Zelis R, Zwillich C, Sinoway L: Norepinephrine clearance is increased during acute hypoxemia in humans. Am J Physiol 1991;261:H1659–H1664.
28 Anand A, Remsburg-Sailor S, Launois SH, Weiss JW: Peripheral vascular resistance increases after termination of obstructive apneas. J Appl Physiol 2001;91:2359–2365.
29 Imadojemu VA, Gleeson K, Gray KS, Sinoway LI, Leuenberger UA: Obstructive apnea during sleep is associated with peripheral vasoconstriction. Am J Respir Crit Care Med 2002;165:61–66.
30 Garpestad E, Katayama H, Parker JA, Ringler J, Lilly J, Yasuda T, Moore RH, Strauss HW, Weiss JW: Stroke volume and cardiac output decrease at termination of obstructive apneas. J Appl Physiol 1992; 73:1743–1748.
31 Garpestad E, Parker JA, Katayama H, Lilly J, Yasuda T, Ringler J, Strauss HW, Weiss JW: Decrease in ventricular stroke volume at apnea termination is independent of oxygen desaturation. J Appl Physiol 1994;77:1602–1608.
32 Friedman O, Logan AG: Sympathoadrenal mechanisms in the pathogenesis of sleep apnea-related hypertension. Curr Hypertens Rep 2009;11:212–216.
33 Leung RS: Sleep-disordered breathing: autonomic mechanisms and arrhythmias. Prog Cardiovasc Dis 2009;51:324–338.
34 Cutler MJ, Swift NM, Keller DM, Wasmund WL, Smith ML: Hypoxia-mediated prolonged elevation of sympathetic nerve activity after periods of intermittent hypoxic apnea. J Appl Physiol 2004;96:754–761.
35 Leuenberger UA, Brubaker D, Quraishi S, Hogeman CS, Imadojemu VA, Gray KS: Effects of intermittent hypoxia on sympathetic activity and blood pressure in humans. Auton Neurosci 2005;121:87–93.
36 Tamisier R, Anand A, Nieto LM, Cunnington D, Weiss JW: Arterial pressure and muscle sympathetic nerve activity are increased after two hours of sustained but not cyclic hypoxia in healthy humans. J Appl Physiol 2005;98:343–349.
37 Gilmartin GS, Tamisier R, Curley M, Weiss JW: Ventilatory, hemodynamic, sympathetic nervous system, and vascular reactivity changes after recurrent nocturnal sustained hypoxia in humans. Am J Physiol Heart Circ Physiol 2008;295:H778–H785.
38 Somers VK, Mark AL, Zavala DC, Abboud FM: Contrasting effects of hypoxia and hypercapnia on ventilation and sympathetic activity in humans. J Appl Physiol 1989;67:2101–2106.
39 Somers VK, Mark AL, Abboud FM: Interaction of baroreceptor and chemoreceptor reflex control of sympathetic nerve activity in normal humans. J Clin Invest 1991;87:1953–1957.
40 Narkiewicz K, van de Borne PJ, Pesek CA, Dyken ME, Montano N, Somers VK: Selective potentiation of peripheral chemoreflex sensitivity in obstructive sleep apnea. Circulation 1999;99:1183–1189.
41 Leuenberger U, Jacob E, Sweer L, Waravdekar N, Zwillich C, Sinoway L: Surges of muscle sympathetic nerve activity during obstructive apnea are linked to hypoxemia. J Appl Physiol 1995;79:581–588.
42 Richardson DW, Wasserman AJ, Patterson JL Jr: General and regional circulatory responses to change in blood pH and carbon dioxide tension. J Clin Invest 1961;40:31–43.
43 Somers VK, Mark AL, Zavala DC, Abboud FM: Influence of ventilation and hypocapnia on sympathetic nerve responses to hypoxia in normal humans. J Appl Physiol 1989;67:2095–2100.

44 Eckberg DL, Rea RF, Andersson OK, Hedner T, Pernow J, Lundberg JM, Wallin BG: Baroreflex modulation of sympathetic activity and sympathetic neurotransmitters in humans. Acta Physiol Scand 1988;133:221–231.
45 Carlson JT, Hedner JA, Sellgren J, Elam M, Wallin BG: Depressed baroreflex sensitivity in patients with obstructive sleep apnea. Am J Respir Crit Care Med 1996;154:1490–1496.
46 Marrone O, Bellia V, Ferrara G, Milone F, Romano L, Salvaggio A, Stallone A, Bonsignore G: Transmural pressure measurements: importance in the assessment of pulmonary hypertension in obstructive sleep apneas. Chest 1989;95:338–342.
47 Marrone O, Bonsignore MR: Pulmonary haemodynamics in obstructive sleep apnoea. Sleep Med Rev 2002;6:175–193.
48 Marrone O, Bonsignore MR, Romano S, Bonsignore G: Slow and fast changes in transmural pulmonary artery pressure in obstructive sleep apnoea. Eur Respir J 1994;7:2192–2198.
49 Schafer H, Hasper E, Ewig S, Koehler U, Latzelsberger J, Tasci S, Luderitz B: Pulmonary haemodynamics in obstructive sleep apnoea: time course and associated factors. Eur Respir J 1998;12: 679–684.
50 Guilleminault C, Motta J, Mihm F, Melvin K: Obstructive sleep apnea and cardiac index. Chest 1986;89:331–334.
51 Shiomi T, Guilleminault C, Stoohs R, Schnittger I: Leftward shift of the interventricular septum and pulsus paradoxus in obstructive sleep apnea syndrome. Chest 1991;100:894–902.
52 Buda AJ, Schroeder JS, Guilleminault C: Abnormalities of pulmonary artery wedge pressures in sleep-induced apnea. Int J Cardiol 1981;1:67–74.
53 Podszus T, Bauer W, Mayer J, Penzel T, Peter JH, von Wichert P: Sleep apnea and pulmonary hypertension. Klin Wochenschr 1986;64:131–134.
54 Sajkov D, McEvoy RD: Obstructive sleep apnea and pulmonary hypertension. Prog Cardiovasc Dis 2009; 51:363–370.
55 Niijima M, Kimura H, Edo H, Shinozaki T, Kang J, Masuyama S, Tatsumi K, Kuriyama T: Manifestation of pulmonary hypertension during REM sleep in obstructive sleep apnea syndrome. Am J Respir Crit Care Med 1999;159:1766–1772.
56 Podszus T, Mayer J, Penzel T, Peter JH, von Wichert P: Nocturnal hemodynamics in patients with sleep apnea. Eur J Respir Dis Suppl 1986;146:435–442.
57 Sforza E, Laks L, Grunstein RR, Krieger J, Sullivan CE: Time course of pulmonary artery pressure during sleep in sleep apnoea syndrome: role of recurrent apnoeas. Eur Respir J 1998;11:440–446.
58 Laks L, Lehrhaft B, Grunstein RR, Sullivan CE. Pulmonary artery pressure response to hypoxia in sleep apnea. Am J Respir Crit Care Med 1997;155: 193–198.
59 Carlson JT, Hedner J, Elam M, Ejnell H, Sellgren J, Wallin BG: Augmented resting sympathetic activity in awake patients with obstructive sleep apnea. Chest 1993;103:1763–1768.
60 Tamisier R, Pepin JL, Remy J, Baguet JP, Taylor JA, Weiss JW, Levy P: Fourteen nights of intermittent hypoxia elevate daytime blood pressure and sympathetic activity in healthy humans. Eur Respir J 2011;37:119–128.
61 Narkiewicz K, van de Borne PJ, Montano N, Dyken ME, Phillips BG, Somers VK: Contribution of tonic chemoreflex activation to sympathetic activity and blood pressure in patients with obstructive sleep apnea. Circulation 1998;97:943–945.
62 Cutler MJ, Swift NM, Keller DM, Wasmund WL, Burk JR, Smith ML: Periods of intermittent hypoxic apnea can alter chemoreflex control of sympathetic nerve activity in humans. Am J Physiol Heart Circ Physiol 2004;287:H2054–H2060.
63 Weiss JW, Liu MD, Huang J: Physiological basis for a causal relationship of obstructive sleep apnoea to hypertension. Exp Physiol 2007;92:21–26.
64 Grassi G, Facchini A, Trevano FQ, Dell'Oro R, Arenare F, Tana F, Bolla G, Monzani A, Robuschi M, Mancia G: Obstructive sleep apnea-dependent and -independent adrenergic activation in obesity. Hypertension 2005;46:321–325.
65 Grassi G, Seravalle G, Quarti-Trevano F, Mineo C, Lonati L, Facchetti R, Mancia G: Reinforcement of the adrenergic overdrive in the metabolic syndrome complicated by obstructive sleep apnea. J Hypertens 2010;28:1313–1320.
66 Grassi G, Arenare F, Quarti-Trevano F, Seravalle G, Mancia G: Heart rate, sympathetic cardiovascular influences, and the metabolic syndrome. Prog Cardiovasc Dis 2009;52:31–37.
67 Ueno LM, Drager LF, Rodrigues AC, Rondon MU, Mathias W Jr, Krieger EM, Junior RF, Negrao CE, Lorenzi-Filho G: Day-night pattern of autonomic nervous system modulation in patients with heart failure with and without sleep apnea. Int J Cardiol 2011;148:53–58.
68 Chan KH, Wilcox I: Obstructive sleep apnea: novel trigger and potential therapeutic target for cardiac arrhythmias. Expert Rev Cardiovasc Ther 2010;8: 981–994.
69 Grassi G, Seravalle G, Quarti-Trevano F, Mineo C, Lonati L, Facchetti R, Mancia G: Reinforcement of the adrenergic overdrive in the metabolic syndrome complicated by obstructive sleep apnea. J Hypertens 2010;28:1313–1320.

70 Narkiewicz K, Kato M, Phillips BG, Pesek CA, Davison DE, Somers VK: Nocturnal continuous positive airway pressure decreases daytime sympathetic traffic in obstructive sleep apnea. Circulation 1999;100:2332–2335.

71 Waradekar NV, Sinoway LI, Zwillich CW, Leuenberger UA: Influence of treatment on muscle sympathetic nerve activity in sleep apnea. Am J Respir Crit Care Med 1996;153:1333–1338.

72 Grote L, Kraiczi H, Hedner J: Reduced alpha- and beta(2)-adrenergic vascular response in patients with obstructive sleep apnea. Am J Respir Crit Care Med 2000;162:1480–1487.

73 Mills PJ, Dimsdale JE, Coy TV, Ancoli-Israel S, Clausen JL, Nelesen RA: Beta 2-adrenergic receptor characteristics in sleep apnea patients. Sleep 1995; 18:39–42.

74 Nelesen RA, Dimsdale JE, Mills PJ, Clausen JL, Ziegler MG, Ancoli-Israel S: Altered cardiac contractility in sleep apnea. Sleep 1996;19:139–144.

75 Mills PJ, Dimsdale JE, Ancoli-Israel S, Clausen J, Loredo JS: The effects of hypoxia and sleep apnea on isoproterenol sensitivity. Sleep 1998;21:731–735.

76 Bengtsson Bostrom K, Hedner J, Grote L, Melander O, von Wowern F, Rastam L, Groop L, Lindblad U: Polymorphisms in alpha- and beta-adrenergic receptor genes, hypertension, and obstructive sleep apnea: the Skaraborg Sleep Study. Int J Hypertens DOI10.4061/2010/458410.

77 Bartels NK, Borgel J, Wieczorek S, Buchner N, Hanefeld C, Bulut D, Mugge A, Rump LC, Sanner BM, Epplen JT: Risk factors and myocardial infarction in patients with obstructive sleep apnea: impact of beta2-adrenergic receptor polymorphisms. BMC Med 2007;5:1.

78 Pierola J, Barcelo A, de la Pena M, Barbe F, Soriano JB, Sanchez Armengol A, Martinez C, Agusti A: beta3-Adrenergic receptor Trp64Arg polymorphism and increased body mass index in sleep apnoea. Eur Respir J 2007;30:743–747.

79 Hedner JA, Wilcox I, Laks L, Grunstein RR, Sullivan CE: A specific and potent pressor effect of hypoxia in patients with sleep apnea. Am Rev Respir Dis 1992;146:1240–1245.

80 Mahamed S, Duffin J: Repeated hypoxic exposures change respiratory chemoreflex control in humans. J Physiol 2001;534:595–603.

81 Imadojemu VA, Mawji Z, Kunselman A, Gray KS, Hogeman CS, Leuenberger UA: Sympathetic chemoreflex responses in obstructive sleep apnea and effects of continuous positive airway pressure therapy. Chest 2007;131:1406–1413.

82 Laitinen T, Hartikainen J, Vanninen E, Niskanen L, Geelen G, Lansimies E: Age and gender dependency of baroreflex sensitivity in healthy subjects. J Appl Physiol 1998;84:576–583.

83 La Rovere MT, Mortara A, Schwartz PJ: Baroreflex sensitivity. J Cardiovasc Electrophysiol 1995;6:761–774.

84 Narkiewicz K, Montano N, Cogliati C, van de Borne PJ, Dyken ME, Somers VK: Altered cardiovascular variability in obstructive sleep apnea. Circulation 1998;98:1071–1077.

85 Jo JA, Blasi A, Valladares E, Juarez R, Baydur A, Khoo MC: Determinants of heart rate variability in obstructive sleep apnea syndrome during wakefulness and sleep. Am J Physiol Heart Circ Physiol 2005;288:H1103–H1112.

86 Roche F, Court-Fortune I, Pichot V, Duverney D, Costes F, Emonot A, Vergnon JM, Geyssant A, Lacour JR, Barthelemy JC: Reduced cardiac sympathetic autonomic tone after long-term nasal continuous positive airway pressure in obstructive sleep apnoea syndrome. Clin Physiol 1999;19:127–134.

87 Khoo MC, Belozeroff V, Berry RB, Sassoon CS: Cardiac autonomic control in obstructive sleep apnea: effects of long-term CPAP therapy. Am J Respir Crit Care Med 2001;164:807–812.

88 Bonsignore MR, Parati G, Insalaco G, Marrone O, Castiglioni P, Romano S, Di Rienzo M, Mancia G, Bonsignore G: Continuous positive airway pressure treatment improves baroreflex control of heart rate during sleep in severe obstructive sleep apnea syndrome. Am J Respir Crit Care Med 2002;166:279–286.

89 Ryan S, Ward S, Heneghan C, McNicholas WT: Predictors of decreased spontaneous baroreflex sensitivity in obstructive sleep apnea syndrome. Chest 2007;131:1100–1107.

90 Bonsignore MR, Parati G, Insalaco G, Castiglioni P, Marrone O, Romano S, Salvaggio A, Mancia G, Bonsignore G, Di Rienzo M: Baroreflex control of heart rate during sleep in severe obstructive sleep apnoea: effects of acute CPAP. Eur Respir J 2006; 27:128–135.

91 Farrell TG, Odemuyiwa O, Bashir Y, Cripps TR, Malik M, Ward DE, Camm AJ: Prognostic value of baroreflex sensitivity testing after acute myocardial infarction. Br Heart J 1992;67:129–137.

92 La Rovere MT, Bigger JT Jr, Marcus FI, Mortara A, Schwartz PJ: Baroreflex sensitivity and heart-rate variability in prediction of total cardiac mortality after myocardial infarction. ATRAMI (Autonomic Tone and Reflexes after Myocardial Infarction) Investigators. Lancet 1998;351:478–484.

93 Logan AG, Tkacova R, Perlikowski SM, Leung RS, Tisler A, Floras JS, Bradley TD: Refractory hypertension and sleep apnoea: effect of CPAP on blood pressure and baroreflex. Eur Respir J 2003;21:241–247.
94 Kohler M, Pepperell JC, Casadei B, Craig S, Crosthwaite N, Stradling JR, Davies RJ: CPAP and measures of cardiovascular risk in males with OSAS. Eur Respir J 2008;32:1488–1496.
95 Gilmartin GS, Lynch M, Tamisier R, Weiss JW: Chronic intermittent hypoxia in humans during 28 nights results in blood pressure elevation and increased muscle sympathetic nerve activity. Am J Physiol Heart Circ Physiol 2010;299:H925–H931.
96 Escourrou P, Tessier O, Bureau A, Nedelcoux H, Bourgin P: Non-invasive measurement of haemodynamics during sleep apnoea. J Sleep Res 1995;4:78–82.
97 Schneider H, Schaub CD, Andreoni KA, Schwartz AR, Smith PL, Robotham JL, O'Donnell CP: Systemic and pulmonary hemodynamic responses to normal and obstructed breathing during sleep. J Appl Physiol 1997;83:1671–1680.

Cardiovascular Disorders Associated with Obstructive Sleep Apnea

6

Chapter 6

Cardiovascular Disorders Associated with Obstructive Sleep Apnea

Abstract

Epidemiological, longitudinal and therapeutic studies have produced convincing evidence that obstructive sleep apnea (OSA) is associated with an increased risk of cardiovascular morbidity and mortality. The strongest evidence supports an independent causal link between OSA and arterial hypertension. OSA may be independently associated with an increased risk for ischemic heart disease, stroke, arrhythmias and mortality. It remains to be determined whether OSA is an independent cause of congestive heart failure and pulmonary hypertension. Confounders and methodological biases are the main reasons for the lack of definitive conclusions in causality studies. Longitudinal studies, adequately powered randomized controlled studies and therapeutic studies involving well-defined participants are all needed to definitively answer the questions surrounding the relationship between OSA and clinical cardiovascular outcomes, comorbidities and intermediate pathogenic mechanisms. OSA is a modifiable risk factor: continuous positive airway pressure administration, the gold standard treatment of OSA, may reduce the early signs of endothelial dysfunction and atherosclerosis, and improve cardiovascular outcomes, such as the mortality related to cardiovascular events, blood pressure, nonfatal coronary events and cardiac function in heart failure patients. However, cardiac patients may not display the typical signs and symptoms of OSA, such as an excessive body mass index and sleepiness. This fact, and the cardiovascular risk associated with OSA, underlines the need for collaborative guidelines to define a diagnostic strategy specifically oriented toward the evaluation of OSA in cardiovascular patients.

1 Limitations of Studies Found in the Literature

Methodological biases have made the interpretation of studies assessing the relationship between obstructive sleep apnea (OSA) and cardiovascular disorders difficult [1]. These biases include the presence of confounders (i.e. risk factors shared with OSA, such as obesity, insulin resistance, diabetes mellitus and cardiovascular diseases), short study duration, inadequately powered studies and uncontrolled studies. For example, prospective observational or cohort studies comparing patients compliant with continuous positive airway pressure (CPAP) versus non-CPAP-compliant patients are biased by patients who are noncompliant with CPAP possibly engaging in other, less healthy behaviors or being sicker at baseline. Similarly, the large number of epidemiological studies can only prove a correlation and never causation. Almost uniformly, these studies purport to control for the presence of obesity by controlling

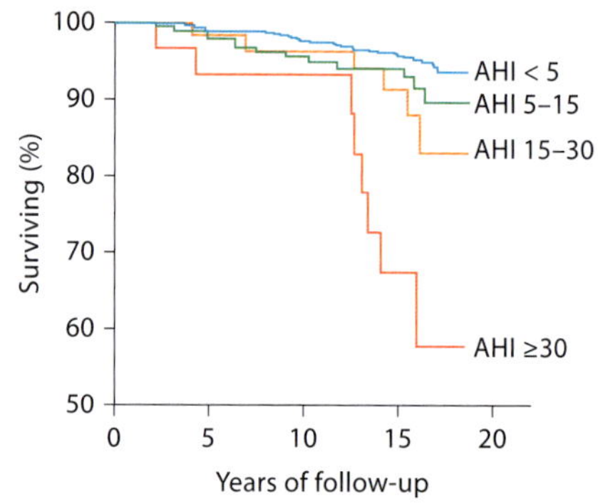

Fig. 1. Kaplan-Meier estimates of survival probability according to the untreated SDB category: none (AHI <5), mild (AHI 5–15), moderate (AHI 15–30) and severe (AHI ≥30). The y-axis is truncated at 50% survival; the log-rank test was used for the differences in survival by SDB category ($p < 0.00001$). Number of participants: 1,396. After Young et al. [13], with permission.

for body mass index (BMI), but BMI is a crude measure of obesity, and other more sophisticated measures, such as visceral fat, may differ markedly in patients with identical BMI. However, in spite of these shortcomings, a causal link between OSA and hypertension is currently accepted. The potential role of OSA in cardiovascular mortality and cardiovascular morbidity, including ischemic heart disease, stroke, congestive heart failure, pulmonary hypertension and arrhythmias, remains to be elucidated. For example, there is a need for randomized trials of treatment for OSA with CPAP or any other treatment to demonstrate a reduction in meaningful cardiovascular endpoints, such as myocardial infarction (MI), stroke or death.

2 Obstructive Sleep Apnea and the Risk of Mortality from Cardiovascular Causes

2.1 Clinical and Epidemiological Studies

Clinically based studies have suggested that OSA may be associated with an increased risk of death [2–11]. This increased risk of death has also been suggested in population-based studies [12–14]. The Australian 13.4-year Busselton Sleep Cohort follow-up study (n = 400) has shown that, after adjustment for confounders, and compared with non-OSA, moderate-to-severe OSA was independently associated with a greater risk of all-cause mortality (adjusted hazard ratio, HR, 6.24, 95% confidence interval, CI, 2.01–19.39) [12]. Mild OSA (apnea-hypopnea index, AHI, from 5 to <15) was not an independent risk factor for higher mortality. However, potential biases in this observational study include the measurement of sleep apnea with MESAM IV rather than polysomnography and the small number of moderate-to-severe OSA cases (n = 18); moreover, the association between sleep apnea and mortality was not controlled for any effects of sleep apnea treatment. An 18-year follow-up study on the population-based Wisconsin Sleep Cohort sample (n = 1,522), with polysomnographically defined sleep-disordered breathing (SDB), revealed that untreated participants with

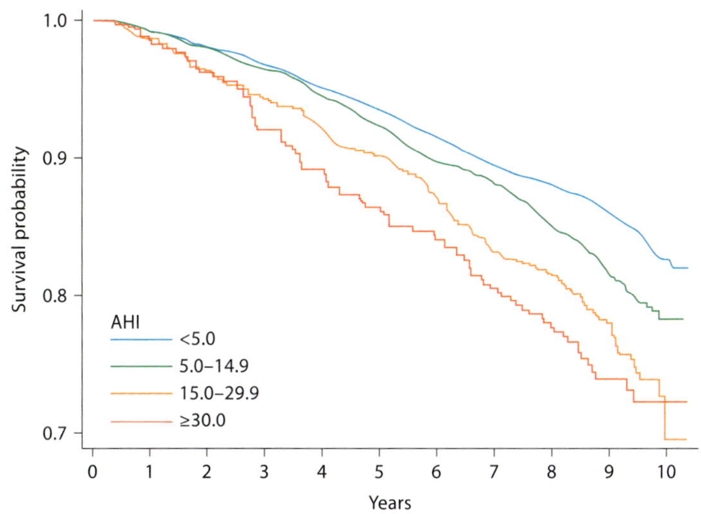

At risk	6,294	6,205	6,110	6,001	5,868	5,732	5,566	5,411	4,756	2,357	300
Deaths	0	59	143	241	359	478	616	757	875	989	1,046

Fig. 2. Kaplan-Meier survival curves across categories of the AHI. After Punjabi et al. [14], with permission.

severe SDB (AHI >30) had a 3.8-fold greater risk for all-cause mortality (95% CI 1.6–9.0; p = 0.004) and a 5.2-fold greater risk for cardiovascular mortality (95% CI 1.4–19.2; p = 0.03) than those without SDB, after adjustment for confounding variables (fig. 1) [13]. The estimates for mortality risk were not significantly greater in patients with mild and moderate SDB compared to those without SDB. These results were unchanged after accounting for daytime sleepiness. The authors drew attention to a potential underestimation of the mortality risk of SDB in ethnic groups other than that in participants (95% white) or in the lowest socioeconomic strata, where there is poor awareness and access to health care (all participants were employed at inclusion). Polysomnographically defined SDB was associated with all-cause and cardiovascular mortality (fig. 2) in the 8.2-year mortality follow-up study of 6,441 men and women from the Sleep Heart Health Study [14]. After adjusting for potential confounders, an AHI ≥30 was associated with a 1.5-fold higher risk for all-cause mortality compared to subjects with an AHI <5 (HR 1.46, 95% CI 1.14–1.86). Stratified analyses by sex and age showed that an AHI ≥30 in men aged 40–70 years was associated with a 2-fold higher risk (HR 2.09, 95% CI 1.31–3.33). Measures of sleep-related intermittent hypoxemia were independently associated with mortality, whereas the arousal frequency and the central sleep apnea (CSA, i.e. the cessation of airflow without respiratory effort) index were not. Patients with mild-to-moderate SDB did not have a significantly increased risk of dying from any cause. Mortality related to coronary artery disease associated with SDB showed a pattern of association similar to all-cause mortality. An association was identified between an AHI ≥15 and deaths related to coronary artery disease in men (adjusted HR 1.69, 95% CI 1.13–2.52), but not in women. It is suggested that SDB is associated with all-cause mortality and specifically that due to coronary artery disease, particularly in men aged 40–70 years with severe SDB. However, a survival bias may have contributed to some of the findings on SDB and mortality, particularly in older participants, as the participants were recruited from ongoing epidemiological studies of cardiovascular and respiratory disease.

Whether the presence of OSA in patients with heart failure accelerates mortality remains unclear. A prospective follow-up trial (mean duration 2.9 years) in heart failure patients with left ventricular ejection fraction (LVEF) ≤45% (n = 164) revealed a higher death rate in heart failure patients with untreated OSA than in mild-to-no sleep apnea subjects, after controlling for confounding factors (8.7 vs. 4.2 deaths per 100 patient-years, respectively; p = 0.029) [15]. The risk of death and the hospitalization rate in heart failure patients with OSA was significantly reduced by CPAP administration, but increased among patients with reduced CPAP compliance (fig. 3) [16]. Potential biases in this clinically based observational study included the relatively small number of patients and the nonrandomization of CPAP therapy. A retrospective cohort study of a large US database (n = 30,719), the 2003–2005 Medicare Standard Analytical Files, which included newly diagnosed heart failure subjects without a prior diagnosis of sleep apnea, revealed that heart failure patients who were treated for sleep apnea had a better 2-year survival rate than subjects with heart failure who were not tested for sleep apnea (HR 0.33, 95% CI 0.21–0.51; p < 0.0001), after adjustment for age, gender and comorbidities [17]. Patients who were treated for sleep apnea had a better 2-year survival rate than those who were tested and diagnosed, but not treated for sleep apnea (HR 0.49, 95% CI 0.29–0.84; p = 0.009). It is suggested that, in Medicare beneficiaries with heart failure, survival is significantly improved in patients with an established diagnosis of sleep apnea and who received treatment. However, this study contained several important biases that limit data interpretation, e.g. the study was retrospective, observational and not controlled for sleep apnea testing and treatment assignment. Conversely, other authors have observed that OSA was not associated with an increased risk for mortality in heart failure patients [18, 19].

Overall, these studies [12–14] suggest that untreated OSA may be a risk factor for all-cause mortality, especially in middle-aged men with more severe OSA. However, the causal link between OSA and an increased risk of death remains to be demonstrated.

2.2 *Day-Night Pattern of Death in Obstructive Sleep Apnea Patients*

The risk of sudden death from cardiac causes in the general population is significantly greater from 6.00 to 12.00 h than during the other 6-hour intervals of the day [20]. In contrast, OSA patients may have a greater risk of death from cardiac causes during the sleeping hours than during the other hours of the nycthemeron [5]. An analysis of polysomnograms and death certificates from OSA patients (n = 78) and patients

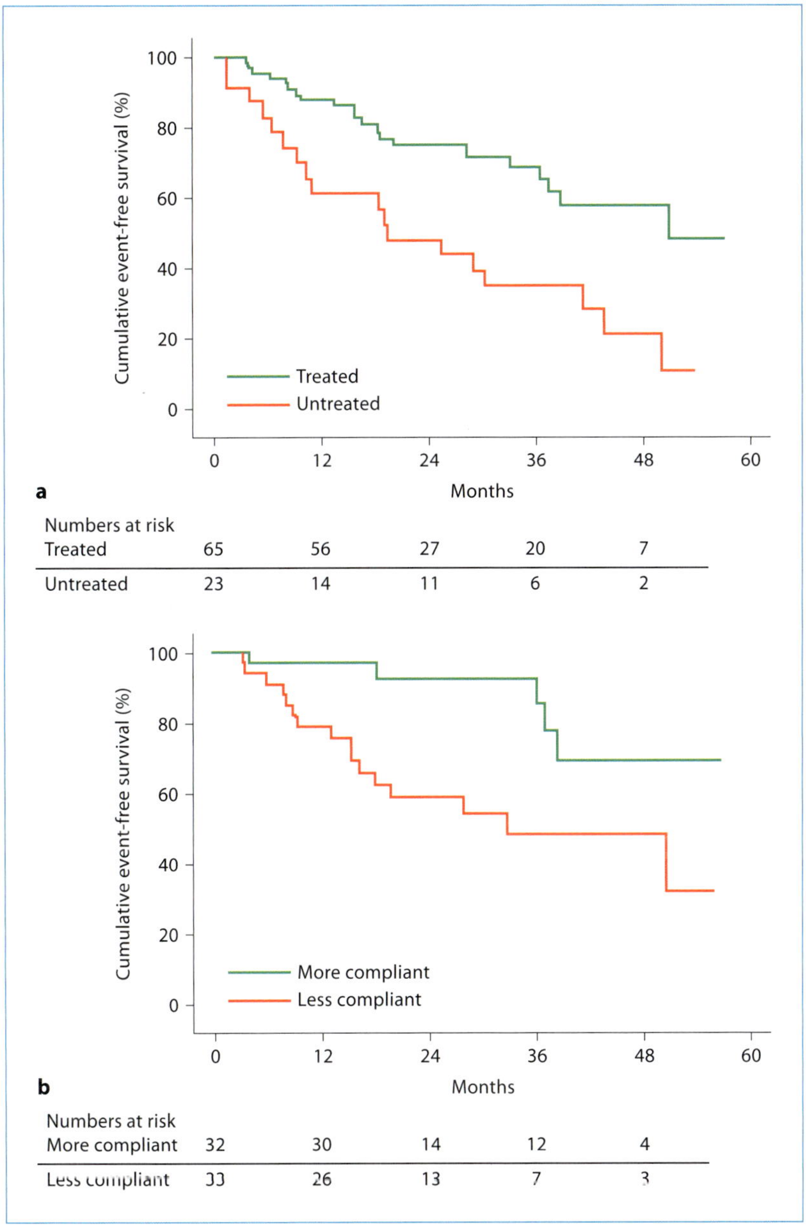

Fig. 3. Cumulative event-free survival in heart failure patients with OSA. **a** Cumulative event-free survival in CPAP-treated and untreated heart failure patients with OSA. The cumulative event-free survival was significantly lower in untreated than in CPAP-treated patients (p = 0.001, log-rank test). **b** Cumulative event-free survival in heart failure patients with OSA determined by the compliance status in CPAP-treated patients. Cumulative event-free survival was significantly lower in patients with poor compliance than in those with good compliance (p = 0.006, log-rank test). After Kasai et al. [16], with permission.

without OSA (n = 34) who had died suddenly from cardiac causes compared the rates of sudden death during 4 intervals of the day among patients without OSA, in the general population, and the expectations of sudden death according to chance [5]. From 0.00 to 6.00 h, sudden death from cardiac causes occurred in 46% of OSA patients, as compared with 21% of subjects without OSA ($p = 0.01$), 16% in the general population ($p < 0.001$) and 25% expected by chance ($p < 0.001$). For OSA patients, the relative risk of sudden death from cardiac causes from 0.00 to 6.00 h was 2.57 (95% CI 1.87–3.52). Pathophysiological pathways that may contribute to increase mortality from cardiac causes during the night in OSA patients remain unknown.

2.3 *Effect of Continuous Positive Airway Pressure Treatment on Mortality from Cardiovascular Causes*

CPAP treatment may reduce the incidence of death in OSA patients. For example, a 7.5-year follow-up study of 168 OSA patients who had begun receiving CPAP therapy at least 5 years previously revealed that deaths from cardiovascular disease were more common in the untreated group than in the CPAP-treated group during follow-up (14.8 vs. 1.9%, respectively; $p = 0.009$), but no significant differences were found in the development of new cases of hypertension, cardiac disorders or stroke [21]. However, only a part of the study population was selected and followed up in a prospective fashion, while the control group was not randomly allocated to conservative therapy and consisted of patients who were noncompliant with CPAP therapy. An observational 10.1-year follow-up study compared the incidence of death from MI or stroke in men with OSA treated with CPAP (n = 372), men with untreated OSA (n = 638), simple snorer men (n = 377) and healthy men recruited from the general population who were matched individually for age and BMI (n = 264) [7]. After adjustment for potential confounders, severe untreated OSA patients had a significantly greater risk of death from cardiovascular events (odds ratio, OR, 2.87, 95% CI 1.17–7.51) than healthy participants. An improvement in mortality rates associated with CPAP therapy was also observed in patients with mild-to-moderate OSA [9]. However, only men were studied (therefore, the findings cannot be readily extrapolated to women) and, as the group treated with CPAP received a more intensive follow-up during the 1st year after diagnosis (2 additional visits), the outcome could have been independently improved in the CPAP treatment group. An observational, nonrandomized 72-month median follow-up study showed a reduction in cardiovascular risk associated with CPAP administration in patients referred for polysomnography (n = 449) [9]. Patients who refused CPAP therapy served as control subjects; however, they could have been different from the treated group (e.g. in terms of healthy behavior), the duration of the observation period was shorter in the untreated patients, and the percentage of women in the treated and untreated patients was 14.1 and 16.5%, respectively, whereas in the general population, the ratio of male-to-female patients with OSA is estimated to be approximately 2:1 to 3:1. Deaths from cardiovascular events (MI or stroke) were more frequent in untreated than in treated patients with

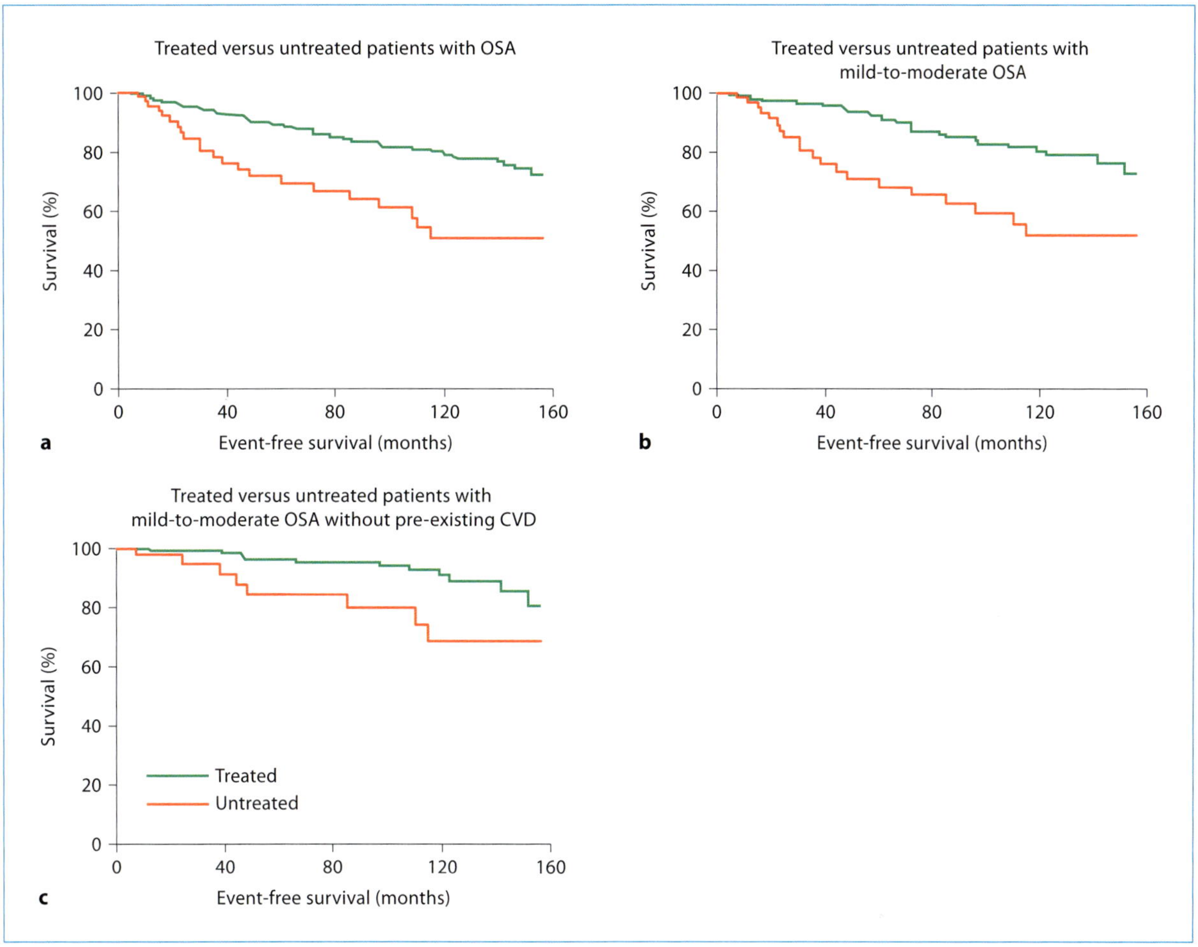

Fig. 4. Kaplan-Meier estimates of the probability of event-free survival in treated versus untreated patients with OSA (**a**), treated versus untreated patients with mild-to-moderate OSA (**b**) and treated versus untreated patients with mild-to-moderate OSA without preexisting cardiovascular disease (**c**). **a** Events were more frequent in untreated than in treated patients (28.3% in untreated vs. 14.3% in treated patients, $p = 0.009$; estimated event-free survival at 10 years 51.8 vs. 79.7%, log-rank test $p < 0.001$; absolute risk reduction 27.9%; treatment of 3.6 patients required to prevent 1 cardiovascular event over 10 years). **b** In patients with mild-to-moderate OSA, more events occurred in untreated (25.3%) than in treated patients (14.4%; $p = 0.021$). The estimated event-free survival after 10 years was 51.8% in untreated and 80.3% in treated patients (log-rank test $p = 0.001$; absolute risk reduction 28.5%; treatment of 3.5 patients required to prevent 1 cardiovascular event over 10 years). **c** In patients with mild-to-moderate OSA without preexisting cardiovascular disease, estimated event-free survival after 10 years was 90.7% in treated versus 68.5% in untreated patients (log-rank test $p = 0.012$). The adjusted HR for OSA treatment in these patients was 0.37 (95% CI 0.17–0.78). After Buchner et al. [9]. Reprinted with permission of the American Thoracic Society. © American Thoracic Society.

mild-to-moderate OSA and for the overall group (fig. 4). After adjustment for confounding factors, the risk reduction from OSA treatment was approximately 60% for patients with mild-to-moderate OSA and for the whole group. This contrasts with the study of Marin et al. [7] described above that only reported a higher incidence of events in untreated patients with severe OSA. This discrepancy may be due to differences between the cohorts studied [9], comorbidities, hypersomnolence and the adherence of the treated groups to CPAP treatment [4].

OSA patients with chronic obstructive pulmonary disease (COPD), i.e. patients with overlap syndrome, receiving long-term oxygen therapy and treated with CPAP, had a greater 5-year survival estimate than untreated patients (treated group: 71%, 95% CI 53–83%; untreated group: 26%, 95% CI 12–43%; $p < 0.01$) [22]. After adjusting for confounders, the patients treated with CPAP showed a significantly lower risk of death (HR of death in treated vs. untreated patients 0.19, 95% CI 0.08–0.48). However, these patients were not randomized to receive or not receive CPAP, the adherence assessment relied on self-reported measurements, and the non-CPAP-treated group included individuals who were withdrawn from CPAP after 3 months due to their nonadherence. Similar findings were reported in a 9.4-year follow-up study that compared mortality rates in CPAP-treated patients, CPAP-untreated patients with overlap syndrome, and in COPD patients without OSA (CPAP therapy was not allocated randomly) [23]. After adjustment for confounders, untreated patients with overlap syndrome had a significantly higher mortality than COPD patients without OSA (relative risk 1.79, 95% CI 1.16–2.77). However, patients with overlap syndrome treated with CPAP did not have a higher risk of mortality than COPD patients without OSA.

Overall, these studies support a potential protective effect of CPAP therapy with regard to death from cardiovascular disease in OSA patients. However, the limitations of these studies contribute to the lack of a definitive conclusion.

2.4 Key Points (table 1)

Table 1.

- OSA, especially more severe OSA, is a risk factor for increased mortality rates from cardiac causes. It remains to be demonstrated whether this association is independent
- This increase in mortality rates may be reduced by CPAP administration in patients who comply with this therapy

3 Systemic Hypertension

3.1 Clinical and Epidemiological Studies

Previous clinical studies have indicated that OSA may be associated with systemic hypertension as approximately 50% of patients with one condition have the other [24–31]. Several cross-sectional studies suggest an independent relationship between

Table 2. Likelihood of arterial hypertension according to the AHI in patients aged ≤50 years and >50 years

AHI	Patients aged ≤50 years (n = 557)		Patients aged >50 years (n = 663)	
	OR	p value	OR	p value
<5	1	–		–
5 to <10	2.9 (1.6–5.5)	0.0006	0.8 (0.4–1.5)	n.s.
10 to <20	3.2 (1.8–5.7)	0.0001	1.4 (0.8–2.5)	n.s.
20 to 40	3.3 (1.9–6.0)	0.0001	1.5 (0.8–2.6)	n.s.
≥40	7.1 (3.8–13.6)	<0.0001	2.7 (1.4–5.1)	0.002

The likelihood was calculated using multiple logistic regression analysis. Figures in parentheses indicate 95% CIs. Hypertension was defined as systolic blood pressure ≥160 mm Hg and diastolic blood pressure ≥95 mm Hg and/or previous diagnosis and/or current treatment of hypertension. After Grote et al. [36]. Reprinted with permission of the American Thoracic Society. © American Thoracic Society.

polysomnographically defined OSA and systemic hypertension [32–38]. The analysis of 1,190 consecutive patients referred for diagnosis of SDB demonstrated that the AHI increased independently of systolic and diastolic blood pressure at rest after controlling for confounders [36]. The relative risk for hypertension (blood pressure ≥160/95 mm Hg) increased with OSA severity, where an AHI ≥40 was associated with a 4-fold risk for hypertension as compared with subjects with an AHI <5. This relative risk was also increased in younger (≤50 years) compared with older (>50 years) patients (table 2). This observation has been confirmed in a cross-sectional analysis of the 6,120 participants of the Sleep Heart Health Study who were stratified by age [39]. After adjustment for confounders, OSA was associated with a 2-fold risk for systolic/diastolic hypertension among patients <60 years, but not among those aged ≥60 years. Isolated systolic hypertension was not associated with OSA in either age category [39]. Overall, these studies suggest that OSA may be an independent risk factor for diastolic hypertension and for systolic/diastolic hypertension, especially in middle-aged patients. Evidence for a causative relationship between OSA and the development of systemic hypertension has been provided by the longitudinal and randomized controlled interventional studies described below and in the following section 3.3.1.

Longitudinal studies have also been used to assess the relationship between polysomnographically defined OSA and systemic hypertension. Analysis of the Wisconsin Sleep Cohort Study, a prospective population-based follow-up study of the natural history of cardiopulmonary sleep disorders, revealed an independent relationship between the severity of OSA and the risk for hypertension over a 4-year period, after adjustment for confounding variables (table 3) [40]. Discrepant findings were observed in the Sleep Heart Health Study, a North American prospective

Table 3. Adjusted ORs for hypertension in a follow-up sleep study, according to the AHI at baseline: data from the Wisconsin Sleep Cohort Study

Baseline AHI	OR for the presence of hypertension in the 4-year follow-up study[a]
0[b]	1.0
0.1–4.9 events • h^{-1}	1.42 (1.13–1.78)
5.0–14.9 events • h^{-1}	2.03 (1.29–3.17)
≥15.0 events • h^{-1}	2.89 (1.46–5.64)
p for trend	0.002

Hypertension was defined as a blood pressure of at least 140/90 mm Hg or the use of antihypertensive medications. Figures in parentheses indicate 95% CIs. p for trend: values are for the linear trend of the logistic regression coefficients (log of the ORs). After Peppard et al. [40], with permission. © 2000 Massachusetts Medical Society.

[a]Adjusted for baseline hypertension status, age, sex, BMI, waist and neck circumference, and alcohol and cigarette use.

[b]This category served as the reference group.

Table 4. Adjusted ORs of the incidence of hypertension at follow-up in relation to the baseline AHI among Sleep Heart Health Study subjects without hypertension at baseline

Baseline AHI	n	Model 1 (adjusted for age, gender, race and time since baseline)	Model 2 (adjusted for factors in model 1 + BMI)
0–4.9	1,511	–	–
5–14.9	629	1.13 (0.90–1.43)	0.92 (0.72–1.17)
15–29.9	234	1.54 (1.12–2.11)	1.12 (0.80–1.56)
>30	97	2.19 (1.39–3.44)	1.51 (0.93–2.47)

Hypertension was defined as blood pressure of at least 140/90 mm Hg or taking antihypertensive medication. Figures in parentheses indicate 95% CIs. Model 2: further adjustment for waist/hip ratio and neck girth did not appreciably change the results (not shown). After O'Connor et al. [41]. Reprinted with permission of the American Thoracic Society. © American Thoracic Society.

cohort follow-up study of the cardiovascular consequences of SDB [41]. The OR for incident hypertension increased with increasing baseline AHI; however, this relationship was attenuated and not statistically significant after adjustment for baseline BMI (table 4). It is suggested that among middle-aged and older persons without hypertension, much of the relationship between AHI and the risk of incident hypertension was accounted for by obesity [41, 42]. The apparently discrepant findings between the Sleep Heart Health Study and the Wisconsin Sleep Cohort Study are likely to be due to differences in the study populations, including differences in age,

Table 5. Discrepancies between the Sleep Heart Health Study (SHHS) and the Wisconsin Sleep Cohort Study (WSCS) that may have contributed to their differing conclusions [40–43]

	SHHS	WSCS	The differences in study findings may reflect
Participants, n	2,470, from 9 ongoing epidemiological studies	709, from a single occupational group in 1 geographical location	the greater heterogeneity and recruitment modalities of the SHHS, in which subjects were, on average, older[1], less heavy and less likely to be male than the WSCS participants
Age at baseline, years	59.6	47	
Mean BMI	27.9	29	
Male sex, %	44.7	56	
Hypertensive patients excluded at baseline, %	51	27	an analysis bias (the so-called 'survivor bias') [43, 340]
Baseline comparison category	AHI <5	AHI = 0	the definition of the non-OSA group in the SHSS may have lowered the size of the estimated associations [43]
OSA assessment technique	unattended in-home polysomnography	attended in-laboratory polysomnography	the use of different OSA severity metrics (differences in OSA measurement methods and scoring) [43][2]

[1] Age >50 years is associated with an increased risk of isolated systolic hypertension [341, 342]. In contrast, OSA may be more related to isolated diastolic hypertension [39] and perhaps systolic/diastolic hypertension; these tend to level off by 65 years of age [219].
[2] The difference in prevalence of moderate-to-severe OSA between the SHHS and WSCS (13.4 and 7.5%, respectively) may reflect the use of different metrics between these studies [43].

sex ratio, BMI, methods of recruitment and methods of OSA assessment (e.g. unattended in-home vs. attended in-laboratory polysomnography; table 5) [41–43].

The effect of gender on the development of hypertension in OSA is controversial. Clinic-based studies have shown that women with OSA were at a higher risk for hypertension than men with OSA [44], whereas the reverse has also been reported [45]. Population-based studies showed no consistent evidence for gender differences in the prevalence of hypertension in adults with SDB [38, 40, 46].

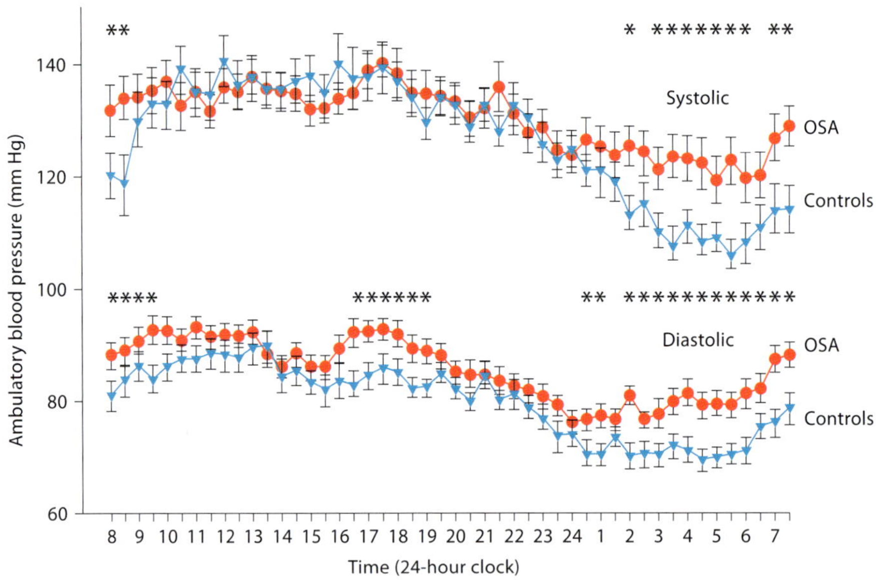

Fig. 5. Mean (±SE) 24-hour systolic and diastolic blood pressure profiles for patients with OSA (n = 45) and matched control subjects (n = 45). Note the clear differences at night, with a reduced nocturnal fall in systolic and diastolic blood pressure in OSA patients, and the increased diastolic blood pressure during the morning and afternoon. OSA patients and control subjects were matched for age, BMI, alcohol and cigarette usage, treated hypertension and ischemic heart disease. * $p < 0.05$: times at which the individual differences reached a statistically significant level (Student's t test). After Davies et al. [53], with permission. © 2000, BMJ Publishing Group Ltd. and the British Thoracic Society.

3.2 *Blood Pressure Profile Abnormalities Associated with an Increased Risk of Obstructive Sleep Apnea*

Masked hypertension (clinically normal, but with a high ambulatory 24-hour blood pressure) is frequently underestimated in OSA patients [47, 48]. For example, in newly diagnosed OSA patients free of recognized cardiovascular disease (n = 130), masked hypertension was reported in 30% of participants, whereas sustained hypertension was observed in 35.4%, white coat hypertension in 3.1% and normotension in 31.5% [47]. Systolic/diastolic hypertension and isolated diastolic hypertension are more likely to be associated with OSA than isolated systolic hypertension (see above) [39, 49].

Patients with isolated nocturnal hypertension, and nonhypertensive or hypertensive patients who do not display the normal physiological reduction of 10–20% in nocturnal blood pressure ('nondippers', fig. 5) have an increased risk for OSA [50–56]. The nondipping profile and nocturnal hypertension have been associated with an increased risk of cardiovascular incidents such as atrial fibrillation, silent cerebral infarction or stroke [56–58]. Nocturnal blood pressure dipping may be masked by variations in blood pressure associated with recurrent apnea-ventilation resumption cycles [59, 60]. Compared with control subjects matched for age, sex and BMI, normotensive patients with sleep apnea (AHI >20) have greater systolic blood pressure variability [61], another variable associated with poor cardiovascular prognosis [62]. However, systolic blood pressure variability may be deceptively increased by repeated blood pressure measurements [63] or arousals from sleep [64].

Resistant hypertension is defined as blood pressure that remains above the therapeutic objective, despite the use of 3 or more antihypertensive drugs (ideally including a diuretic) at effective doses [65, 66]. Patients with resistant hypertension also have an increased risk for OSA [31, 67–72]. For example, in a case-control study, a 5-fold increased risk for OSA (AHI >10) was observed in patients with difficult-to-control hypertension, compared with controlled hypertension; subjects were matched for confounding factors [69]. It is of note that the Hypertension Management Guidelines and the American Heart Association Professional Education Committee of the Council for High Blood Pressure Research highlight OSA as an important identifiable cause of resistant hypertension [65, 73, 74].

3.3 *Effects of Treatment for Obstructive Sleep Apnea on Blood Pressure*

3.3.1 Effect of Continuous Positive Airway Pressure Therapy

3.3.1.1 Clinical Trials. CPAP treatment reduces the increased blood pressure and sympathetic activity associated with OSA during sleep [59]. The interpretation of the results from studies of the blood pressure response to chronic CPAP treatment depends on variables such as study duration (often <6 months), methods and time of measurements of blood pressure, and whether participants have untreated hypertension, treatment-controlled hypertension or are normotensive [60, 75–80]. The type of placebo treatment used may also bias the interpretation of data [76, 81, 82], especially as sham CPAP either increases [77, 83] or decreases daytime blood pressure [75] in OSA patients. Although blood pressure is often assessed manually, 24-hour ambulatory blood pressure monitoring is considered to be more accurate [74]. It should also be borne in mind that the accuracy of blood pressure measurement depends on the sampling interval [84].

Several studies that compared the effects of therapeutic CPAP versus sham or subtherapeutic CPAP on blood pressure levels suggest that CPAP may reduce blood pressure by alleviating OSA:

- Three weeks of CPAP in middle-aged hypertensive patients with and without OSA (patients without OSA received CPAP of 5 cm H_2O) lowered the nocturnal systolic and diastolic blood pressure in the OSA group compared with the non-OSA group (systolic: –7.8 vs. +0.3 mm Hg, p = 0.02; diastolic: –5.3 vs. –0.7 mm Hg, p = 0.03) [85]. A similar but insignificant effect on daytime blood pressure was also observed.
- Analysis of blood pressure changes in 118 men with OSA and a mean Epworth score >9, who were randomly assigned to either therapeutic (n = 59) or

subtherapeutic (n = 59) CPAP (approx. 1 cm H_2O pressure) for 1 month, indicated that therapeutic CPAP reduced mean arterial ambulatory blood pressure by 2.5 mm Hg, whereas subtherapeutic CPAP increased blood pressure by 0.8 mm Hg (p = 0.0013; this may have contributed to overinflating the between-group differences) [77]. The benefit of CPAP treatment was seen for systolic and diastolic blood pressure and during sleep and wakefulness. It was greater in patients with more severe OSA (mean decrease in patients with severe OSA: 5 mm Hg), and in patients taking antihypertensive drugs (mean decrease: 8 mm Hg), but was independent of the baseline blood pressure.

- Sixty patients with moderate-to-severe OSA and excessive daytime somnolence were randomly assigned to either effective or subtherapeutic CPAP for an average of 9 weeks [86]. Two thirds of the patients were hypertensive at inclusion, and 16 patients in each group completed the study. With effective CPAP administration, mean, diastolic and systolic blood pressures all decreased significantly by approximately 10 mm Hg at night and during the day, while no significant changes occurred with subtherapeutic CPAP.
- Four weeks of effective CPAP significantly reduced mean arterial 24-hour ambulatory blood pressure (by a mean ± SD of 2.6 ± 5.4 mm Hg) [87].
- In obese patients with OSA, effective CPAP reduced waking blood pressure within 6 weeks, where mean waking systolic and diastolic blood pressures fell by 6.7 and 4.9 mm Hg, respectively [88]. In CPAP-compliant patients, the fall in blood pressure was greater. In this study, 79% of patients were hypertensive.
- Twelve weeks of effective CPAP reduced the 24-hour mean and diastolic blood pressures by 3.8 and 3.5 mm Hg, respectively, in mildly sleepy patients with OSA [89].
- CPAP administration for 1 year (n = 178) versus conservative treatment (n = 181) in asymptomatic, hypertensive patients with OSA (n = 359, AHI >19, Epworth score <11), decreased systolic blood pressure by 1.89 mm Hg (95% CI –3.90 to 0.11 mm Hg; p = 0.06) and diastolic blood pressure by 2.19 mm Hg (95% CI –3.46 to –0.93 mm Hg; p = 0.0008), after adjusting for confounders [90]. This effect was only evident in patients who used CPAP for >5.6 h • $night^{-1}$.

Conversely, CPAP administration for 1 month was reported to have no significant effect on blood pressure in sleepy OSA patients with well-controlled hypertension (n = 68) [78] and in nonsleepy OSA patients with hypertension at study inclusion (n = 35) [91].

3.3.1.2 *Effect of CPAP Administration in OSA Patients with Resistant Hypertension.* An observational retrospective chart review study of the effects of CPAP therapy on blood pressure in OSA patients with resistant hypertension and subjects with controlled hypertension revealed a decrease of –5.6 and –0.8 mm Hg in mean blood pressure in the resistant and control groups (p = 0.03 and 0.53), respectively [92]. CPAP permitted the reduction of antihypertensive treatment in 71% of subjects with resistant hypertension, but did not significantly alter the antihypertensive regimen in the control group. The beneficial response to CPAP therapy was found mainly in subjects with the most severe hypertensive disease. A single night of CPAP administration in OSA patients with refractory hypertension (n = 11) reduced systolic blood pressure in stage 2 sleep from 138.3 ± 6.8 to 126.0 ± 6.3 mm Hg in a nonrandomized study [93]. CPAP usage for 2 months was accompanied by an 11.0 ± 4.4 mm Hg reduction in the 24-hour systolic blood pressure. In addition, the nocturnal and daytime components of systolic blood pressure fell significantly by 14.4 ± 4.4 and 9.3 ± 3.9 mm Hg, respectively. Diastolic blood pressure was also reduced significantly at night by 7.8 ± 3.0 mm Hg. Overall, these studies suggest that effective CPAP therapy may reduce blood pressure in OSA patients with resistant hypertension, although this should be confirmed with randomized controlled studies.

3.3.1.3 *Meta-Analyses.* Two meta-analyses have shown that CPAP administration is associated with a significant reduction of approximately 2 mm Hg in the mean blood pressure [94, 95]. This reduction was greater among patients with a more severe level of OSA and a more effective nightly use of the CPAP device [95]. A further meta-analysis of 36 trials involving 1,718 subjects from the Cochrane Airways Group Trials Register and reference lists of data from articles indicated that CPAP leads to lower blood pressure than control treatment [96]. In a 4th meta-analysis, CPAP reduced systolic blood pressure by 3.03 mm Hg (95% CI 6.7 to –0.61; p = 0.10) and diastolic blood pressure by 2.03 mm Hg (95% CI 4.1 to –0.002; p = 0.05) in patients with severe OSA (mean AHI >30, n = 313) [97]. However, the effects of CPAP on blood pressure were modest and not statistically significant overall.

In summary, these comparative studies and meta-analyses suggest that CPAP administration may have a modest effect on blood pressure levels. This effect may, however, be greater in:

- patients with more severe OSA [76, 77, 95, 97] and excessive daytime sleepiness [83, 91, 98];
- hypertensive patients [99], nondippers [82], patients with difficult-to-control hypertension [94, 100] or those requiring antihypertensive drugs [77];
- patients who adhere to CPAP therapy [95, 97] for ≥3.5 h • night^{-1} [76].

3.3.2 Effect of a Mandibular Advancement Device

Treatment for 2 months with a mandibular advancement device was associated with a reduction in systolic, diastolic and mean blood pressures (4.5, 3.0 and 3.7 mm Hg, respectively) in OSA patients (mean AHI 17) [101]. Administration of a mandibular advancement device was also associated with a significant reduction of approximately 5 mm Hg in systolic, diastolic and mean blood pressures [102]. In addition, the administration of a mandibular advancement device was associated with significant reductions in systolic and diastolic blood pressures between baseline and at a 3-month evaluation (p < 0.001); the mean reductions were approximately 15 and 10 mm Hg, respectively, and they persisted at the 3-year follow-up [103]. A 4-week randomized, controlled crossover study to compare the effects of mandibular advancement device therapy versus sham oral appliance therapy on 24-hour blood pressure in OSA patients revealed a significant reduction of the mean 24-hour diastolic blood pressure (1.8 mm Hg) with the mandibular advancement device compared with the control at the end of the study ($p = 0.001$); however, 24-hour systolic blood pressure was not affected [104]. Awake blood pressure variables were reduced with the mandibular advancement device by an estimated mean of 3.3 mm Hg for systolic blood pressure ($p = 0.003$) and 3.4 mm Hg for diastolic blood pressure ($p < 0.0001$).

A 3-month randomized, controlled crossover study was used to compare the effects on blood pressure of an advancement device versus CPAP versus a placebo tablet in mild-to-moderate OSA patients (n = 114, AHI ranging from 5 to 30); 16 patients were hypertensive and 44 were nondippers [105]. Treatment with the mandibular advancement device significantly improved the nighttime diastolic blood pressure ($p < 0.05$ compared with placebo and CPAP), but there were no other significant changes with either the mandibular advancement device or CPAP.

Overall, these studies suggest a modest but significant reduction in blood pressure associated with the use of a mandibular advancement device in OSA patients.

3.4 *Effects of Antihypertensive Drugs in Obstructive Sleep Apnea Patients*

Antihypertensive drugs have little effect on nocturnal blood pressure in OSA patients [106–108], and they have not been reported to reduce the severity of OSA [107–109]. Atenolol is more effective than amlodipine, enalapril, hydrochlorothiazide or losartan in lowering daytime blood pressure in OSA patients with hypertension, possibly due to the blocking of sympathetic overreactivity [107]. The respective efficacy of CPAP and valsartan, an angiotensin II receptor blocker (160 $mg \bullet day^{-1}$), in reducing blood pressure in hypertensive patients with OSA never treated for either condition was assessed in an 8-week randomized, controlled crossover trial (n = 23) [110]. Patients whose blood pressure remained uncontrolled by CPAP or valsartan alone continued on to an open-label 8-week study with a combination of CPAP and valsartan. Although the reduction in the 24-hour mean blood pressure was significant under CPAP (-2.1 ± 4.9 mm Hg; $p < 0.01$), valsartan induced a 4-fold greater reduction in the 24-hour mean blood pressure (-9.1 ± 7.2 mm Hg; $p < 0.001$). During the nighttime, the reduction in blood pressure was still significantly greater with valsartan than with CPAP administered alone. When used in combination, the 2 treatments appeared to have significant additive effects on blood pressure. This was true for office blood pressure, while there was only a trend for nighttime blood pressure. The mechanisms leading to such an additive effect are unknown.

3.5 *Mechanisms Potentially Involved in the Development of Sustained Hypertension in Obstructive Sleep Apnea*

The triggers of the intermediate mechanisms that potentially link OSA and the development of systemic hypertension include the chronic intermittent hypoxia and possibly sleep loss and fragmentation associated with the condition. They contribute to alterations in the autonomic nervous system, which appear to play a critical role in the development of hypertension associated with OSA [111]. They may increase inflammatory and oxidative stress and coagulation and thrombotic activity, which may in turn lead to vascular inflammation, vascular endothelial dysfunction, atherosclerosis and hypertension.

3.6 *Key Points (table 6)*

Table 6.

- It is recognized that OSA is a cause of systemic hypertension
- Patients with nondipping blood pressure or hypertension during sleep, and patients with resistant hypertension should be assessed for OSA
- Some studies have shown that CPAP administration may modestly, but significantly, decrease blood pressure
- The effects of CPAP administration on blood pressure may be greater in patients with better CPAP adherence, in patients with more severe OSA and in those with refractory hypertension

4 Heart Failure

4.1 *Obstructive Sleep Apnea Prevalence in Patients with Heart Failure*

OSA and CSA are common among patients with heart failure secondary to systolic dysfunction and may coexist in the same individual [112–115]. A high proportion of patients with heart failure may demonstrate a shift in the type of their SDB throughout the night (from CSA to OSA or vice versa), whereas the AHI remains fairly stable between nights [112, 114–116]. It is of note that current evidence does not support grouping OSA with CSA with regard to risk factors, outcomes and response to therapy [117].

Clinical and epidemiological cross-sectional studies have shown that up to 70% of patients with heart failure may have OSA [15, 113, 118–125]. In a retrospective study of 450 patients with cardiac heart failure who were referred to a sleep clinic, OSA was significantly more prevalent in men (38%) than in women (31%; $p < 0.005$) [120]. The risk factors for OSA differed by gender: in men, only the BMI was significantly associated with OSA, whereas in women, age was the only important risk factor [120]. In a prospective study of 81 patients with cardiac failure and an LVEF <45%, OSA had a prevalence of 11% and CSA had a prevalence of 40% [119]. Heart failure patients with OSA had a significantly greater mean body weight (112 vs. 75 kg) and prevalence of habitual snoring (78 vs. 28%) than those with CSA [119]. In patients with heart failure (n = 218), 26% presented with moderate-to-severe OSA in a prospective study performed in a hospital heart failure clinic [125]. The predictors for OSA in these patients were older age, male sex and greater BMI [125]. In the Sleep Heart Health Study, cross-sectional analysis (n = 6,424) revealed a 2.38-fold increased risk for heart failure associated with OSA (fig. 6) [126].

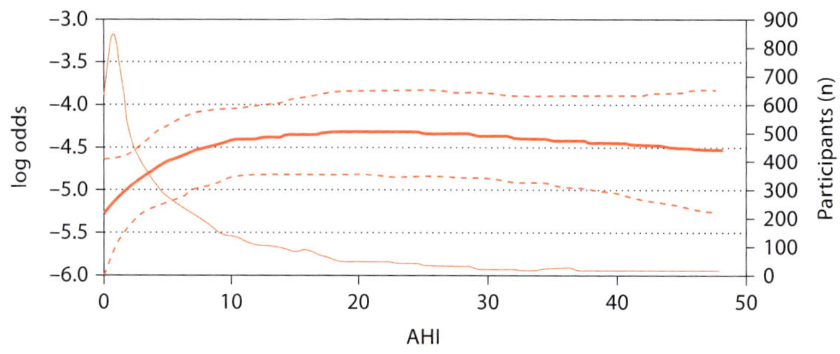

Fig. 6. Restricted cubic spline regression of the log odds of heart failure on the AHI. The left y-axis is a measure of the risk for heart failure (quantified as the log of the prevalence odds), with larger values (smaller absolute values) indicating greater risk. The prevalence odds of heart failure appear to increase within the range of mild-to-moderate SDB (AHI <10) and to plateau thereafter. Note that inference on the dose-response pattern at the right tail (for example, AHI >20) is based on a limited amount of data. The solid thick line indicates the predicted log odds, dashed lines are the 95% CIs, and the solid thin line indicates the number of participants at various AHI values (frequency distribution; right y-axis). After Shahar et al. [126]. Reprinted with permission of the American Thoracic Society. © American Thoracic Society.

Several studies have reported an independent association between OSA and diastolic dysfunction [127–130]. In OSA patients, the pattern of early and late mitral inflow velocities (E/A ratio) and the duration of early mitral inflow (deceleration time) correlate with the level and duration of oxygen desaturation during sleep [127–129].

4.2 Characteristic Clinical Features of Obstructive Sleep Apnea in Patients with Chronic Heart Failure

OSA patients with chronic heart failure may be less sleepy and obese than OSA patients without chronic heart failure [131–133]. Sleepiness (evaluated using the Epworth Sleepiness Scale), BMI and sleep structure were assessed according to OSA severity (assessed using polysomnography) in patients with chronic heart failure (n = 155) and in a random community sample (n = 1,139) [131]. Compared with the community sample, for any given severity of OSA, patients with chronic heart failure had lower BMIs and lower Epworth Sleepiness Scale scores (fig. 7). However, chronic heart failure patients with SDB were sleepier during the day than those without SDB when sleepiness was assessed objectively (using the OSLER test or actigraphy) [134], but not when assessed subjectively (using the Epworth Sleepiness Scale). OSA symptoms may be difficult to distinguish from fatigue and dyspnea related to chronic heart failure [135]. A cross-sectional study that evaluated the clinical and demographic characteristics of stable chronic heart failure patients (n = 170; mean LVEF ± SD 32 ± 14.6%) revealed that 51% of patients had significant SDB and 9% had CSA [136]. SDB was associated with clinical

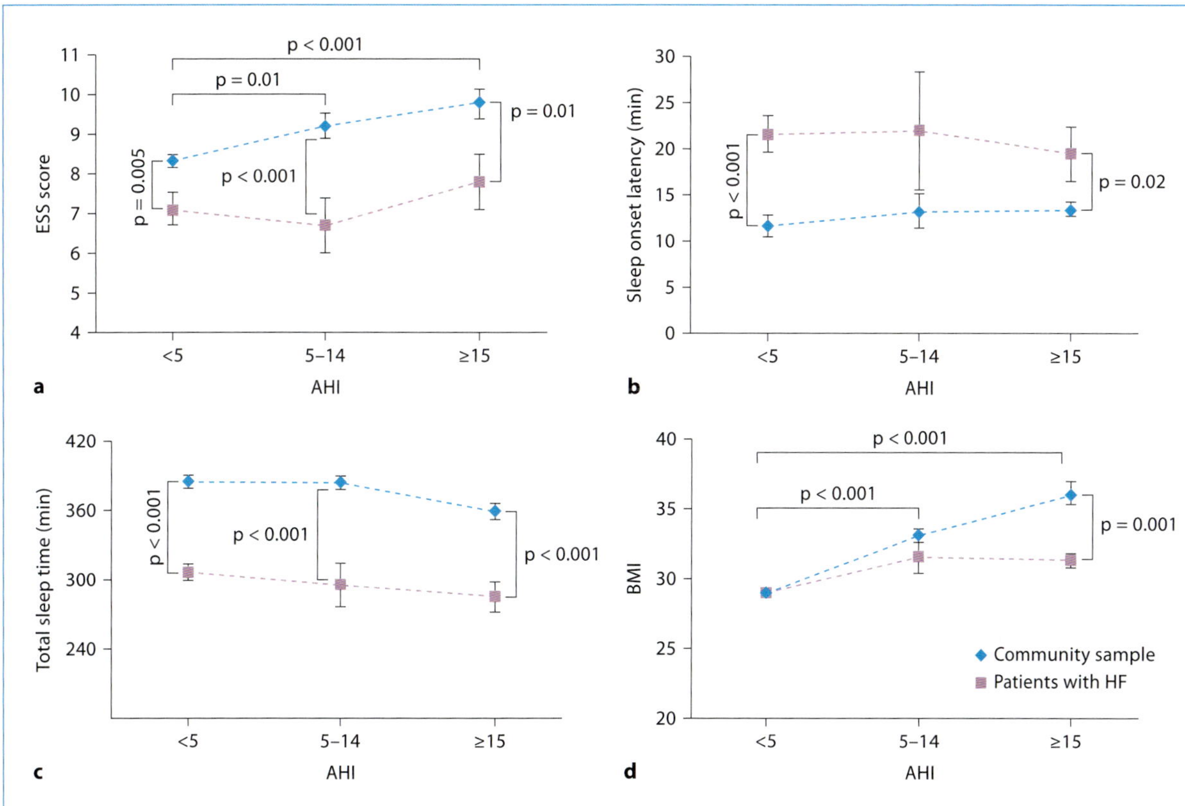

Fig. 7. Epworth Sleepiness Scale (ESS) score, sleep structure and BMI by AHI categories in patients with OSA and heart failure (HF), compared to a community sample with no history of HF. Patients with OSA and HF have lower Epworth scores (**a**) and longer sleep onset latencies (**b**) compared with those without a history of HF in all AHI categories. In addition, they have a shorter total sleep time (**c**), indicating that they are less sleepy despite sleeping less. In patients with OSA and HF, there were no significant differences in the mean Epworth scores with increasing AHI category. In contrast, in the community sample, these scores increased significantly with increasing AHI category. In patients with OSA and HF, there was no significant increase in the AHI category with increasing BMI (**d**). In contrast, in the community sample, this category increased significantly in association with an increasing BMI. In those with an AHI ≥15, the BMI was significantly greater in the community sample compared with the patients with HF. Values are means ± SE. After Arzt et al. [131], with permission. © 2006 American Medical Association.

and demographic characteristics similar to those of the general adult population, including male gender, age, obesity and hypertension. In contrast, there were no significant differences in the self-reported sleep quality, depressive symptoms, fatigue or self-reported excessive sleepiness between groups characterized by the severity of SDB or categorized as CSA, OSA or no SDB, when adjusted for age and gender. Therefore, it is suggested that clinical and demographic characteristics rather than self-reported symptoms may be the best indicators of the need to evaluate and treat SDB in chronic heart failure patients.

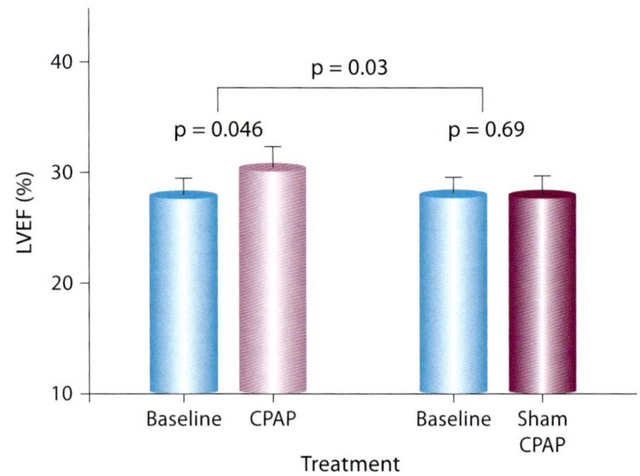

Fig. 8. LVEF at baseline and after 3 months of CPAP or sham CPAP treatment in OSA patients with heart failure. An improvement in the LVEF is observed in the CPAP group, but not in the sham group. After Egea et al. [140], with permission.

Overall, these findings suggest that daytime symptoms do not accurately predict OSA in chronic heart failure patients, and that the absence of subjective sleepiness or obesity is not a reliable measure to rule out OSA.

4.3 *Effects of Continuous Positive Airway Pressure Therapy*

Several controlled studies have assessed the effects of CPAP treatment on left ventricular function in patients with systolic heart failure. One month of CPAP administration plus optimal heart failure medical treatment (n = 12) improved the mean LVEF from 25.0 to 33.8% ($p < 0.001$) [137]. In the control group (n = 12), which consisted of patients with OSA (mean AHI ≥20) and systolic heart failure (mean LVEF ≤45%) who were treated with medical treatment alone, there were no significant changes in the LVEF during the study. When the effects of acute or a mean CPAP administration of 6.9 weeks on left ventricular systolic function were assessed in congestive heart failure patients with (n = 7) and without (n = 5) OSA, acute CPAP administration resulted in a significant decrease in the mean stroke volume (44 vs. 50 ml; $p = 0.002$) and mean LVEF (34.8 vs. 38.4%; $p = 0.006$) compared with baseline [138]. Conversely, 6.9 weeks of CPAP therapy resulted in a trend towards an increase in the mean stroke volume (59 vs. 50 ml; $p = 0.07$) and a significant increase in the mean LVEF (43.4 vs. 38.4%; $p = 0.01$) compared with baseline. A parallel, randomized controlled study of CPAP versus no CPAP revealed a mean 5% increase in the LVEF in the treated group versus a 1.5% increase in the untreated group ($p = 0.04$) [139]. Similar results were observed in a randomized, multicenter placebo (sham-CPAP)-controlled study (fig. 8) [140]. Bilevel positive airway pressure administration was suggested to be superior to CPAP in improving the LVEF (8.5 vs. 0.5%, respectively; 95% CI 2.3–13.4; $p = 0.01$) in a pilot randomized controlled trial in OSA patients with stable systolic dysfunction (n = 24) [141]. In contrast, no significant effect of CPAP administration on the

LVEF was observed in a randomized controlled study (autotitrating CPAP compared with sham CPAP for 6 weeks each in a crossover design) [142]. It was suggested that the potential therapeutic benefits of CPAP in heart failure are achieved by alleviating OSA rather than by improving cardiac function.

Although it was targeted at CSA rather than OSA, the Canadian Continuous Positive Airway Pressure Patients with Central Sleep Apnea and Heart Failure trial (CANPAP study) should be considered, which remains by far the largest randomized controlled trial of CPAP for the treatment of SDB in heart failure patients (n = 258) [143]. At baseline, the AHI (mean ± SD) was 40 ± 17 (87 ± 14% of CSA) and 40 ± 15 (91 ± 12% of CSA) in the control and CPAP-treated groups, respectively. Treatment with CPAP attenuated CSA, improved nocturnal oxygenation, increased the ejection fraction (similar to the reported findings for treating OSA), lowered norepinephrine levels and increased the distance walked in 6 min, but did not affect survival. Adaptive servoventilation may be more effective than CPAP and bilevel pressure support ventilation in alleviating OSA and CSA in heart failure patients (adaptive servoventilation provides a small but varying amount of ventilatory support, against a background of low-level positive airway pressure) [144–147]. This observation should be confirmed in randomized, controlled long-term studies in large populations.

Only a few studies have assessed the effect of CPAP therapy in OSA patients with diastolic heart failure. The study by Johnson et al. [138], cited above, did not reveal any effect of CPAP on diastolic function. A prospective, randomized, placebo-controlled, double-blind crossover study assessed men with OSA (n = 27), who were randomized to 12 weeks of sham CPAP and 12 weeks of effective CPAP application, and 15 healthy control subjects [148]. At baseline, an abnormal left ventricular filling pattern was observed in 15 OSA patients and in 3 control subjects (p = 0.02). Compared with sham CPAP, 3 months of CPAP administration improved diastolic function, which was evaluated echocardiographically by the E/A ratio, deceleration and the isovolumic relaxation time (fig. 9). It was suggested that OSA may independently affect left ventricular diastolic function, and that chronic CPAP application could prevent the progression of diastolic abnormalities. In addition, chronic CPAP may reverse these abnormalities, at least in the initial stages before severe structural changes have occurred. Adaptive servoventilation effectively attenuated Cheyne Stokes respiration by improving heart failure symptoms and cardiac function in patients with diastolic heart failure and Cheyne-Stokes respiration [149]. Whether this is accompanied by an improved prognosis remains to be determined in randomized controlled studies of well-defined diastolic heart failure patients.

4.4 Mechanisms Potentially Involved in the Development of Heart Failure in Obstructive Sleep Apnea Patients

4.4.1 Increased Blood Pressure and Other Cardiac Disorders

The surges in blood pressure associated with ventilation resumption following obstructive respiratory events during sleep, sustained daytime and nighttime

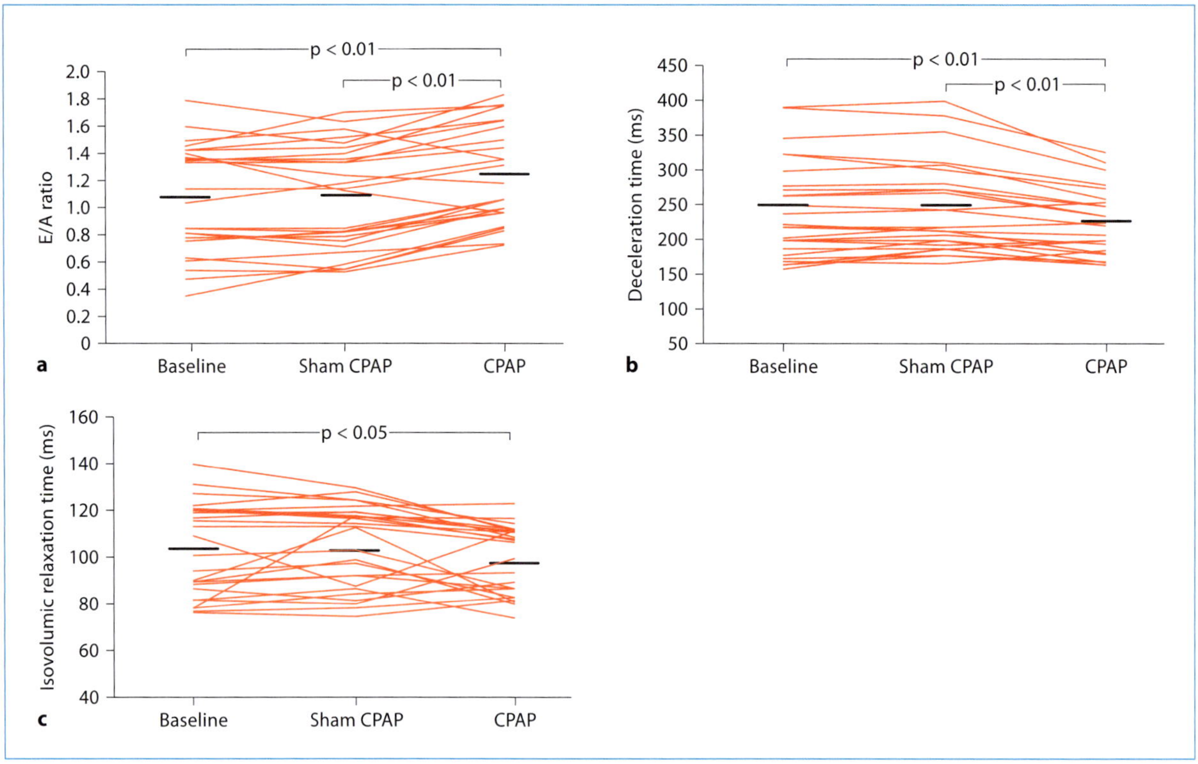

Fig. 9. Echocardiographic features of diastolic dysfunction in OSA patients at baseline and after 3 months of sham and therapeutic CPAP treatment. **a** Individual values of the E/A ratio (the ratio between peak early and late left ventricular filling velocities). **b** Deceleration time. **c** Isovolumic relaxation time at baseline, after sham CPAP and after CPAP therapy in OSA patients. After Arias et al. [148], with permission

hypertension, coronary artery disease and arrhythmias associated with OSA may contribute to the development of heart remodeling and heart failure observed in OSA patients [150].

4.4.2 Chronic Intermittent Hypoxia

During the apnea-ventilation resumption cycle, myocardial oxygen demand increases at times of recurrent hypoxia. This may contribute to reduce myocardial contractility [151, 152] and the ventricular ejection fraction. It may also increase the risk of myocardial ischemia and infarction, and consequently worsen ventricular function in OSA patients with chronic heart failure [7, 60, 153]. Chronic intermittent hypoxia also triggers the production of reactive oxygen species, cytokines and growth factors, and increases nighttime and daytime sympathetic nervous system activity [see chapters 2 and 5, this vol., pp. 43–66 and pp. 171–195]. These factors may all contribute to the development and aggravation of heart failure.

4.4.3 Sympathetic Overactivation

Sympathetic activity is increased in all patients with heart failure, and its magnitude in this context is an independent predictor of increased mortality [154, 155]. The additional presence of OSA may further increase its level [156]. When daytime muscle sympathetic nerve activity (SNA) was assessed during wakefulness in heart failure patients (LVEF <45%) with OSA (n = 29, mean AHI 39) and without OSA (n = 17, mean AHI <15), muscle SNA was significantly higher in patients with OSA than in those without OSA (p = 0.032), and CPAP administration significantly lowered muscle SNA in the OSA patients (n = 8) [156]. It is suggested that OSA: (1) may be an additional stimulus to central sympathetic outflow; (2) may accelerate the progression of heart failure, and (3) may be a risk factor for chronic heart failure that is potentially treatable with CPAP. When the effects of 4 months of exercise training on sleep apnea severity, muscle SNA and LVEF were prospectively evaluated in patients with systolic heart failure with OSA (n = 8), CSA (n = 9), no sleep apnea (n = 7) and healthy subjects (n = 9), exercise training improved the AHI and the minimum O_2 (oxyhemoglobin) saturation (Sao_2; $p < 0.05$) in OSA patients, and produced an increase in LVEF that approached statistical significance (p = 0.056) [157]. No significant changes were observed in CSA patients. Exercise training was associated with a significant reduction in muscle SNA in all groups ($p < 0.001$), independently of the presence of sleep apnea. The mechanisms by which exercise training may contribute to reduce OSA severity in patients with heart failure and OSA have been reviewed by Morgan [158]. They may include the reduction in SNA and the improvement in cardiac function resulting from the exercise. Overall, these findings suggest that sympathetic overactivity may contribute to the development of heart failure in OSA.

4.4.4 Fluid Retention and Obstructive Sleep Apnea Severity

Some evidence suggests that, in recumbent patients with heart failure, the development of edema in the upper airway tract can cause its narrowing and be a predisposing factor for pharyngeal collapsibility. In awake healthy subjects, fluid displacement from the legs into the neck induced by lower-body positive pressure increased the neck circumference, reduced the size of the upper airway and increased its collapsibility [159–162]. These findings were confirmed in nonobese men with OSA without other chronic disorders [163]. The overnight rostral volume of fluid displacement from the legs strongly correlated with the AHI ($r = -0.773$; $p < 0.001$) and the change in the neck circumference ($r = -0.792$; $p < 0.001$), which together explained 68% of the variability in the AHI among subjects (fig. 10). In another study, the same group confirmed that OSA severity was related to overnight rostral leg fluid displacement and the increase in neck circumference, and that CPAP alleviated OSA in association with the prevention of fluid accumulation in the neck [164]. The effects of a short course of diuretic treatment (intravenous furosemide, 20 mg, and spironolactone, 100 mg, b.i.d. for 3 days) on OSA severity and upper airway patency were assessed in patients with severe OSA, hypertension and diastolic heart failure [165]. Upper airway patency was assessed by measuring the oropharyngeal junction area using acoustic

Fig. 10. Relationship between the overnight change in leg fluid volume and the AHI. The more fluid was displaced from the leg at night, the greater the AHI. This relationship was best described by an exponential curve ($r = -0.802$; $p < 0.001$), although the linear relationship was also significant ($r = -0.773$; $p < 0.001$). After Redolfi et al. [163]. Reprinted with permission of the American Thoracic Society. © American Thoracic Society.

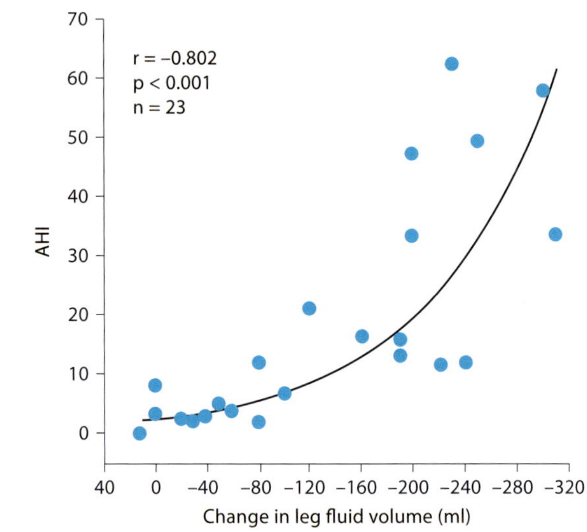

pharyngometry and the forced mid-inspiratory flow percentage. Diuretic treatment significantly decreased the mean AHI (from 75 to 57; $p < 0.001$), improved the mean oropharyngeal junction area (from 1.3 to 1.8 cm^2; $p = 0.007$) and decreased the mean forced mid-inspiratory flow percentage (from 118 to 93%, $p = 0.002$). Overall, these studies suggest that fluid overload in heart failure patients may alter the properties of the soft tissues in the upper airway and increase their tendency to collapse during sleep. This may account for the high prevalence of OSA in these patients.

4.4.5 Ventricular Hypertrophy

An independent association between OSA and left ventricular hypertrophy was observed in adults with nonischemic dilated cardiomyopathy [166]. An increased left ventricular thickness or mass associated with OSA has also been observed, although they were not significant after adjustment for body weight [148, 167].

4.4.6 Recurrent Exaggerated Negative Intrathoracic Pressure during Apnea-Ventilation Resumption Cycles

Over the course of an apnea, the negative intrathoracic pressure swings caused by repetitive inspiratory efforts elicit 3 main effects. Firstly, there is an increase in transmural pressure on the intrathoracic cardiovascular structures [168–170]. Secondly, there is an increase in inspiratory afterload to the left ventricle that impairs its emptying. Thirdly, there is an increase in venous return and filling of the right ventricle that result in its distension and a left-forward shift in the interventricular septum [171]. Altogether, the recurrence of these effects throughout sleep may contribute to the development of left ventricular dysfunction.

4.5 *Diagnosis of Obstructive Sleep Apnea in Patients with Heart Failure*

Patients with classical signs or symptoms associated or correlated with OSA, e.g. snoring, excessive daytime sleepiness, increased BMI, neck size or hypertension, may need to be evaluated for OSA. However, self-reported symptoms of sleepiness, poor sleep, fatigue or depression are not reliable indicators of OSA, and the absence of these symptoms should not rule out the evaluation of OSA in patients with heart failure [131–133, 136]. Whether simplified tests such as type 3 or 4 monitoring are useful in diagnosing OSA in heart failure patients is not known. For example, the agreement in diagnostic outcome between home-limited sleep studies and in-laboratory polysomnography in the identification of SDB in patients with heart failure was prospectively assessed using synchronous in-laboratory Embletta and polysomnography and home Embletta studies in 20 consecutive patients with stable heart failure [172]. Unlike synchronous in-laboratory Embletta (kappa coefficient 0.63; $p < 0.01$), home Embletta did not correlate with polysomnography (kappa coefficient 0.27; $p = 0.06$). The positive and negative predictive values for home Embletta in detecting SDB were 83 and 57%, respectively. However, patients with heart failure may have other sleep disorders, such as insomnia, leg movements [173, 174], sleep disturbances brought on by drug side effects, nocturia etc. Overall, routine polysomnography may be indicated in congestive heart failure [175], but this is still a controversial issue [176].

4.6 *Key Points (table 7)*

Table 7.

- OSA is associated with heart failure, but it remains to be demonstrated whether this association is independent
- OSA patients with heart failure may be less sleepy and obese than OSA patients without heart failure. Whether OSA should be routinely assessed in heart failure patients is not clear, and the strategy for this possible assessment has not yet been defined [175, 176]
- Short-term CPAP administration in heart failure patients with OSA may decrease left ventricular afterload, heart rate and blood pressure during sleep [343, 344]
- The effects of long-term positive airway pressure therapy on cardiac function, quality of life and risks associated with heart failure in heart failure patients with OSA remain to be demonstrated

5 Stroke

5.1 *Prevalence of Obstructive Sleep Apnea in Patients with Stroke*

5.1.1 Clinical Studies

Clinical studies have shown that OSA is common among stroke patients, with a prevalence exceeding 50% [177–184]. The presence and severity of OSA has not been associated with stroke severity or lesion site [180, 182]. The prevalence of central apneas progressively decreased during the 3 months following an acute stroke, while that

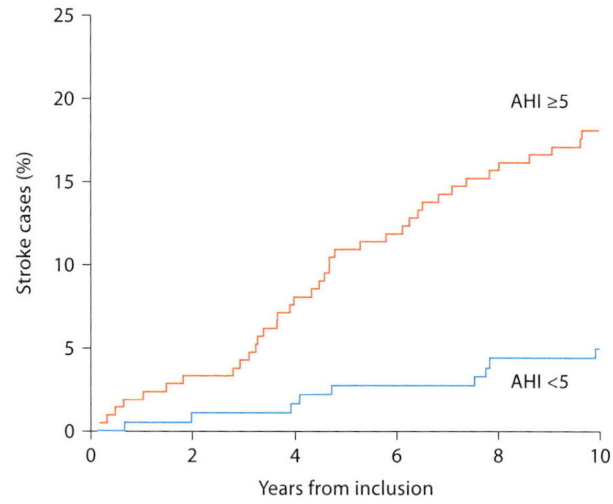

Fig. 11. Cumulative risk of stroke during 10 years of follow-up. Patients with sleep apnea and an AHI ≥5 had an increased risk of stroke compared to those with an AHI <5 ($p < 0.001$). After Valham et al. [188], with permission.

of obstructive apneas remained unchanged [182, 185]. It was suggested that patients may have had a tendency for obstructive events prior to the stroke, whereas central events could occur as its consequence [80, 182].

5.1.2 Population Studies

• Cross-sectional and longitudinal analyses were performed on 1,475 and 1,189 subjects, respectively, from the general population [186]. In the cross-sectional analysis, subjects with an AHI ≥20 had a 4.3-fold increase in risk for stroke ($p = 0.02$) compared with those with an AHI <5, after adjustment for confounding factors. In the longitudinal analysis, patients with an AHI ≥20 had an increased risk of suffering a first-ever stroke over the next 4 years (unadjusted OR 4.31, 95% CI 1.31–14.15; $p = 0.02$). However, after adjustment for confounders, the OR was still raised, but it was no longer statistically significant (OR 3.08, 95% CI 0.74–12.81; $p = 0.12$) [186].

• An observational study assessed whether OSA was an independent risk for a composite endpoint of 'stroke or death from any cause' in OSA patients (n = 697, mean AHI 35) and control subjects without OSA (n = 325, mean AHI 2) [8]. OSA was significantly associated with the composite endpoint (HR 1.97, 95% CI 1.12–3.48; $p = 0.01$) after adjustment for confounders. The increased severity of OSA at baseline was associated with an increased risk for the development of the composite endpoint. There was no significant association between OSA and stroke, transient ischemic attacks or death alone. However, patients with treated OSA were also included in the analysis, thus making it more difficult to determine the role of OSA in the risk of stroke or death.

• A prospective cohort study of patients aged ≤70 years with verified coronary disease (n = 408) revealed that OSA independently increased the risk of cerebrovascular events (HR 2.98, 95% CI 1.43–6.20; $p = 0.004$) [187].

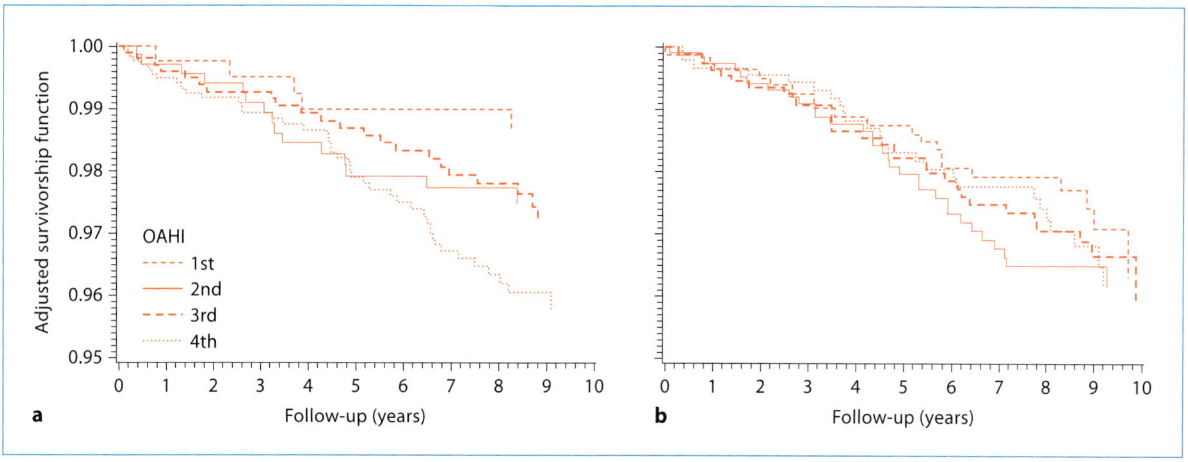

Fig. 12. Adjusted Kaplan-Meier stroke-free survival estimates as a function of the obstructive AHI (OAHI) quartiles. Values are modeled in this graph for Caucasian current smoker men (**a**) and women (**b**) who did not use antihypertensive medications, and with mean values of other covariates. The 1st (OAHI <4.5), 2nd (4.5–9.5), 3rd (9.5–19.1) and 4th quartiles (>19.1) of the OAHI are shown. After Redline et al. [189]. Reprinted with permission of the American Thoracic Society. © American Thoracic Society.

- When the effects of OSA on the incidence of stroke, acute MI and death were assessed in a 10-year follow-up study of patients with angina pectoris who were referred for coronary angiography (n = 392), the frequency of CSA was thought to be low as none of the patients had symptoms of congestive heart failure [188]. Compared to patients with coronary artery disease without sleep apnea, patients with an AHI ≥5 had an approximately 3-fold increase in the risk of stroke during the 10-year follow-up (fig. 11), independently of confounding variables. There was a dose-response relationship between the severity of sleep apnea and the risk of stroke, where patients with an AHI of 5–15 and patients with an AHI ≥15 had a 2.44- and 3.56-fold increased risk of stroke, respectively, compared to patients without sleep apnea, independently of confounders (p for trend = 0.011). Death and MI were not related to sleep apnea.
- Cross-sectional analysis on the Sleep Heart Health Study (n = 6,424) has shown a 1.58-fold increased risk for stroke in OSA patients with an AHI ≥11 (upper AHI quartile) versus those with an AHI ≤1.3 (lower AHI quartile) [126]. Longitudinal analysis of the data set, using 5,422 participants without a history of stroke at baseline, who were untreated for sleep apnea and were followed for a median of 8.7 years, demonstrated that men with moderately severe sleep apnea had a 2.86-fold increased risk of ischemic stroke after adjusting for confounders (95% CI 1.1–7.4) compared with men in the lowest sleep apnea quartile (fig. 12) [189]. The risk of stroke increased by 6% (95% CI 2–10%) with every unit increase in the baseline obstructive AHI (OAHI) from 5 to 25. In women, stroke was not significantly associated with OAHI quartiles,

but an increased risk was observed at an OAHI >25. It is suggested that ischemic stroke is strongly associated with OAHI in community-dwelling men with mild-to-moderate sleep apnea.

5.1.3 Meta-Analysis of the Frequency of Sleep Apnea in Stroke and Transient Ischemic Attack

A meta-analysis confirmed that OSA is very common in ischemic and hemorrhagic stroke and transient ischemic attack patients [185]. In 2,343 patients with these conditions (29 studies), the frequency of SDB with an AHI >5 was 72 and 38% for an AHI >20. Only 7% of the SDB was primarily central apnea. There was no significant difference in the prevalence of SDB by event type, timing after stroke or type of monitoring. An unknown cause for stroke was associated with higher frequencies of SDB; a cardioembolic cause was associated with a lower frequency of SDB. Men had a higher percentage of SDB (AHI >10) than women (65% compared to 48%, respectively; p = 0.001). Patients with recurrent strokes had a higher percentage of SDB (AHI >10) than initial strokes (74% compared to 57%, respectively; p = 0.013).

5.2 *Effects of Obstructive Sleep Apnea on Stroke Outcome*

5.2.1 Effects of Untreated Obstructive Sleep Apnea on Stroke Outcome

OSA is an independent predictor of worse functional outcome, increased duration of poststroke hospitalization and rehabilitation, and an increased risk of death or new vascular events [177, 178, 184, 190–195]. An increased severity of OSA in the supine position (positional OSA) may be a predominant feature of acute stroke [183, 196], and its incidence may decrease significantly during the months following the stroke [196]. OSA may reduce the long-term survival of patients with stroke or transient ischemic attack [179, 182–184]. OSA (OAHI ≥15) and CSA (central AHI ≥15) were assessed to determine whether they reduced long-term survival in patients with stroke over a mean period of 10 years [184]. The risk of death was higher among OSA patients than controls (adjusted HR 1.76, 95% CI 1.05–2.95; p = 0.03), independently of age, sex, BMI, smoking, hypertension, diabetes mellitus, atrial fibrillation, Mini Mental State Examination score and the Barthel Index of activities of daily living (fig. 13). Conversely, there was no difference in mortality between the CSA patients and controls.

5.2.2 Effects of Treated Obstructive Sleep Apnea on Stroke Outcome

CPAP administration in stroke patients with OSA has been associated with an improvement in well-being and decreased nocturnal blood pressure in those who accepted the treatment, but not in those who did not [197]. CPAP administration for 28 days in stroke patients with sleep apnea also improved depressive symptoms, but not delirium or functional and cognitive functioning, compared with those with

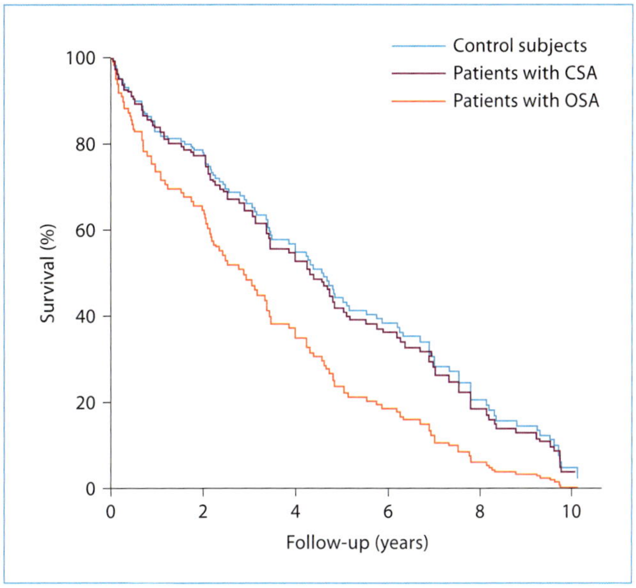

Fig. 13. Survival curves calculated from a Cox proportional hazards regression model after adjustment for confounders. Stroke patients with obstructive and central AHI <15 served as control subjects. Mortality was higher among stroke patients with OSA versus control subjects (p = 0.03). There was no difference in mortality between stroke patients with CSA and controls (p = 0.80). After Sahlin et al. [184], with permission. © 2008 American Medical Association.

untreated OSA [198]. Conversely, no improvement of mood, sleepiness or physical functioning was observed in stroke patients; however, the use of CPAP in this study was poor, averaging only 1.4 h • night^{-1} [199]. In fact, compliance with CPAP is poor in OSA patients with stroke compared with OSA patients without stroke [199–202]. However, 70.5% of stroke patients continued CPAP treatment at home whereas 29.5% rejected it; nonacceptance was associated with a lower functional status, as measured by the Barthel Index, and the presence of aphasia [197]. The feasibility to provide auto-CPAP in the acute transient ischemic attack period has been reported by other authors [203].

Stroke patients with OSA (AHI ≥20) who could not tolerate CPAP had a higher risk of new vascular events (especially another stroke) than those who tolerated the treatment (36.1 vs. 6.7%, respectively; p = 0.03) in an 18-month follow-up study [194]. However, the mortality rate was not significantly different between these 2 groups. When this study was expanded and extended to 5 years of prospective observations, it was suggested that CPAP may reduce mortality in patients with moderate-to-severe OSA and ischemic stroke (fig. 14) [204]. Patients with an AHI ≥20 who did not tolerate CPAP (n = 68) showed an increased adjusted mortality risk compared with patients with an AHI <20 (n = 70; HR 2.69, 95% CI 1.32–5.61). They also showed an increased adjusted mortality risk compared with patients with moderate-to-severe OSA who tolerated CPAP (n = 28; HR 1.58, 95% CI 1.01–2.49; p = 0.04). There were no differences in mortality among patients without OSA, patients with mild disease and patients who tolerated CPAP. It is of note that the low percentage of adherence to CPAP treatment among these patients (nearly 30%) and the comparison of a group of

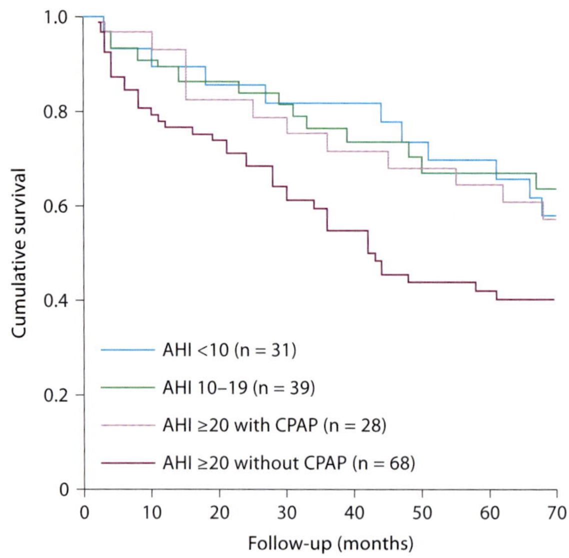

Fig. 14. Accumulated survival curve for study groups of patients with stroke, according to the AHI cutoff point and CPAP tolerance. The group of patients with an AHI ≥20 and poor tolerance of CPAP showed increased mortality compared with the other patients after 5 years of follow-up. After Martinez-Garcia et al. [204]. Reprinted with permission of the American Thoracic Society. © American Thoracic Society.

patients who tolerated CPAP with one that did not tolerate CPAP introduced a selection bias as the 2 groups may be different in terms of health risks and behavior. It is suggested that CPAP therapy may provide protection from increased mortality and new vascular events in this population.

In summary, these studies suggest that the diagnosis and treatment of OSA are possibly important in stroke patients; however, prospective studies are needed to draw definitive conclusions [205–207].

5.3 Characteristic Clinical Features of Obstructive Sleep Apnea in Patients with Stroke: Diagnosis of Obstructive Sleep Apnea in the Poststroke Period

The presence of symptoms such as snoring, sleepiness and witnessed apneas in stroke patients may increase their risk of having OSA and could indicate the need for the evaluation of this condition. However, a significant number of patients may be missed if history alone is used to implement an OSA diagnostic and treatment strategy. For example, a meta-analysis revealed that the frequency of SDB was high in stroke patients despite a relatively low average BMI (26.4), and over 25% of patients with SDB did not snore, while over 50% of patients without SDB did snore [185]. These findings are consistent with those of other authors [208]. Similarly [209], according to OSA severity levels, OSA patients with stroke had lower levels of sleepiness and BMI than a community sample of subjects with OSA, but without a history of stroke: for mild OSA, the Epworth Sleepiness Scale score was 5.6 ± 0.5 vs. 9.3 ± 0.3 ($p < 0.001$) and the BMI was 28.5 ± 1.1 vs. 33.1 ± 0.5 ($p < 0.048$), respectively; for moderate-to-severe OSA, the Epworth Sleepiness Scale score was 7.1 ± 0.9 vs. 9.7 ± 0.4 ($p = 0.043$) and the BMI was 27.2 ± 0.8 vs. 36.4 ± 0.8 ($p < 0.025$), respectively.

Overall, these findings suggest that clinical assessment alone cannot rule out the diagnosis of OSA in stroke patients. In 2006, a guideline for the primary prevention of ischemic stroke from several major organizations considers that 'SDB may independently contribute to stroke risk' [210]. In order to identify this potential risk factor for stroke, it has been recommended that physicians should question 'bed partners and patients, particularly those with abdominal obesity and hypertension, about symptoms of SDB, and referral to a sleep specialist for further evaluation as appropriate may be reasonable, especially in the setting of drug-resistant hypertension' [210]. In 2010, a new version of the guideline suggests: 'Because of its association with other vascular risk factors and cardiovascular morbidity, evaluation for SDB through a detailed history and, if indicated, specific testing is recommended, particularly in those with abdominal obesity, hypertension, heart disease or drug-resistant hypertension' and 'Treatment of sleep apnea to reduce risk of stroke might be reasonable, although its effectiveness is unknown' [211]. Some authors consider that evaluating SDB may be warranted in all stroke patients [185]; however, others believe it should only be carried out in those who may potentially accept CPAP treatment [207]. Studies and collaborative guidelines are needed to define a diagnostic strategy for OSA evaluation in the poststroke period, during which time OSA is frequent and may increase morbidity and mortality. The potential beneficial effects of CPAP administration should also be investigated in further studies.

5.4 Key Points (table 8)

Data from the literature tend to show that OSA is associated with an increased risk for stroke, but the causal link remains to be demonstrated. The use of composite endpoints and selected population studies (e.g. in sleep clinics) have made the overall risk of stroke in relationship to OSA unclear. Studies and collaborative guidelines are needed to identify those clinical profiles of OSA with a higher risk for stroke in which OSA evaluation may be routinely recommended.

Table 8.

- OSA is associated with an increased risk of stroke, but whether this association is independent remains to be determined
- In patients with stroke, OSA may aggravate poststroke physical and cognitive functioning, increase the duration of poststroke hospitalization and rehabilitation, and increase the risk of death and the occurrence of a new vascular event. These factors may be reduced by CPAP administration, but this remains to be confirmed
- Stroke patients with symptoms suggesting that the OSA preceded the stroke may benefit from a sleep study [200, 345], but sleepiness may not be related to OSA in stroke patients
- Clinical assessment cannot rule out the diagnosis of OSA in stroke patients. Routine evaluation of OSA may be warranted in all stroke patients who could accept CPAP treatment [185, 207]

6 Coronary Artery Disease

6.1 Clinical and Epidemiological Studies

Clinical studies have shown that OSA is common in patients with coronary artery disease, with a prevalence that may exceed 60% [153, 212–221]. For example, a comparison of unselected male survivors of acute MI (n = 101, aged <66 years) and age-matched male patients without evidence of ischemic heart disease (n = 53) indicated that, after adjustment for confounders, an apnea index >5.3 was associated with a 23.3-fold increased risk for MI (upper vs. lower apnea index quartile, 95% CI 3.9–139.9) [213].

Epidemiological studies have also suggested an independent link between OSA and coronary artery disease. The cross-sectional analysis of data from the Sleep Heart Health Study (n = 6,424) demonstrated that SDB (AHI >11) gave a modest, but significant, 1.27-fold increase in risk for coronary artery disease (upper vs. lower AHI quartile, 95% CI 0.99–1.62) [126]. Longitudinal analysis of the 8.2-year follow-up of this study has shown, after adjustment for confounders, an association between SDB and coronary artery disease-related deaths in men with an AHI ≥15 (HR 1.69, 95% CI 1.13–2.52) [14]. However, this association was not identified in women.

In a 5-year longitudinal study that assessed a composite primary endpoint of risk for MI, stroke and death in patients with verified coronary artery disease (n = 408), OSA was not associated with an increased risk of MI when evaluated as an individual endpoint [187]. Similar findings were also observed in a comparable 10-year longitudinal study of 392 men and women with coronary artery disease referred for coronary angiography [188].

OSA was associated with an increased incidence of restenosis after elective percutaneous intervention [221, 222]. OSA was found in 51 patients (57%) during a 7.5-month follow-up study in patients with acute coronary syndrome treated with percutaneous coronary intervention (n = 89) [221]. The incidence of major adverse cardiac events, e.g. cardiac death, reinfarction and target vessel revascularization, was significantly higher in the OSA patients (23.5 vs. 5.3%, respectively; p = 0.022). The presence of OSA was an independent predictor for major adverse cardiac events (HR 11.61, 95% CI 2.17–62.24; p = 0.004). The incidence of restenosis was greater in patients with OSA than in those without OSA (36.5 vs. 15.4%, respectively; p = 0.026). Similar findings have also been observed by other authors [222].

6.2 Day-Night Pattern of Myocardial Ischemia and Infarction in Obstructive Sleep Apnea Patients

6.2.1 Myocardial Ischemia

Nocturnal myocardial ischemia may be more common in coronary artery disease patients with OSA than in those without OSA [153, 223–226]. Analysis of nocturnal ischemic events in OSA patients with ischemic heart disease (n = 51) and control OSA patients free from ischemic heart disease (n = 17), after the withdrawal of β-adrenergic blocking agents and antianginal treatment, revealed that nocturnal ST segment depression occurred in 10 patients (a total of 15 events, 182 min), of whom 6 also had morning ischemia (6.00–8.00 h) [227]. These were observed predominantly during the rebreathing phase of the obstructive apneas, during which time there is an increase in the heart rate, blood pressure and myocardial oxygen consumption, and a decrease in oxygen supply. No ischemic events occurred in the control group. Such a temporal relationship between myocardial ischemia and the apnea-ventilation resumption cycle was also observed in a minority of patients, but occurred more frequently in men and in patients with more severe OSA [225].

The increasing respiratory efforts, increased cardiac oxygen demand and hypoxemia associated with recurrent apnea-ventilation resumption cycles may trigger myocardial ischemia during sleep in OSA patients. When OSA patients (n = 10) undergoing elective percutaneous coronary intervention were assessed to determine whether abnormalities of coronary blood flow associated with obstructive apneas may predispose them to ischemia, myocardial work was observed to increase at the termination of each obstructive apnea [228]. Following the rise in myocardial work, there was an 8-second delay before coronary blood flow began to increase ($p < 0.001$). This delay was associated with an increase in coronary vascular resistance of 16 ± 4% ($p < 0.05$; fig. 15). The increase in coronary blood flow was independently predicted by the rise in myocardial work ($r = 0.52$; $p < 0.001$) and the presence of arousal from sleep ($r = 0.30$; $p < 0.05$), but not by the degree of oxygen desaturation. Therefore, it is suggested that the disturbed flow-metabolic coupling may lead to nocturnal myocardial ischemia in patients with OSA and coronary artery disease [228, 229].

6.2.2 Myocardial Infarction

OSA may affect the timing of MI. In the general population, the risk of acute MI is significantly greater during the morning hours after waking (i.e. from 6.00 to 12.00 h) than during the rest of the day [20]. There is also a marked nadir in this risk during sleep (i.e. from 0.00 to 6.00 h). However, in OSA patients, MI had a 6-fold higher risk of occurring between 0.00 and 6.00 h than during the rest of the day (95% CI 1.3–27.3; $p = 0.01$; fig. 16) [230]. Similar findings have been reported by other authors [231], and this is probably related to the greater risk of sudden death from cardiovascular causes from 0.00 to 6.00 h in OSA patients, whereas it ranges mainly between 6.00 and 12.00 h in the general population (see above) [5].

6.3 *Coronary Artery Calcification in Obstructive Sleep Apnea Patients*

Coronary artery calcification is a subclinical predictor of coronary heart disease. Several authors have reported that OSA patients may have a greater coronary atherosclerotic plaque volume than non-OSA controls [232, 233], although this is controversial [234]. Coronary artery calcification was present in 67% of OSA patients and

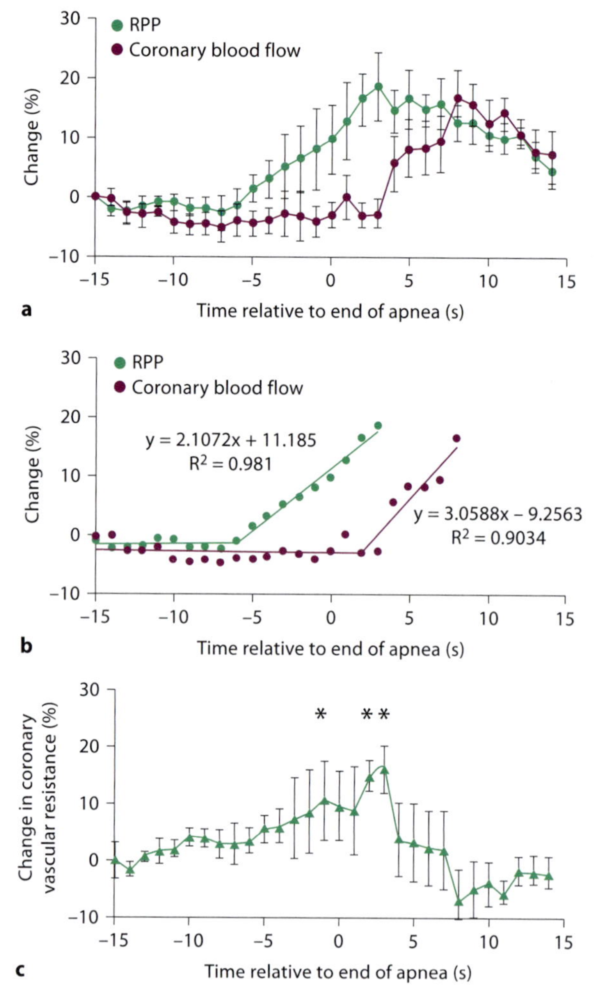

Fig. 15. Change in coronary blood flow, myocardial work and coronary vascular resistance from 15 s before to 15 s after the end of obstructive apnea. **a** Change in coronary blood flow and myocardial work (assessed by measuring the rate-pressure product, RPP). Note the dissociation between coronary blood flow and RPP. **b** Bilinear regression curves demonstrating the relationship between coronary blood flow and RPP. The increase in coronary blood flow follows the increase in RPP after a delay of 8 s, and with a steeper slope of rise ($p < 0.001$ for difference of intercept, slope and coincidence). **c** Change in coronary vascular resistance. Coronary vascular resistance increases after apnea, peaking at 16 ± 4% above baseline, 3 s after the apnea has finished (* $p < 0.05$). Data represent means ± SEM for pooled results of 5 patients with obstructive apneas. After Hamilton et al. [228], with permission.

31% of non-OSA patients ($p < 0.001$) with no history of coronary disease (n = 202) who underwent electron beam computed tomography within 3 years of polysomnography. After adjustment for confounders, the median coronary artery calcification score (Agatston units) became higher as OSA severity increased (p for trend by AHI quartile <0.001; fig. 17) [232]. When patients with stable coronary artery disease were assessed using a 3-dimensional intravascular ultrasound technique, patients with an AHI ≥15 had a larger mean coronary atherosclerotic plaque volume than those with an AHI <15 (238 vs. 169 mm^3, respectively; p = 0.047); this difference was larger in OSA patients than in patients without OSA (243 vs. 170 mm^3, respectively; p = 0.03) [233]. There was a significant positive correlation between coronary atherosclerotic plaque volume and OAHI (r = 0.6; p = 0.01). There was also a significant correlation

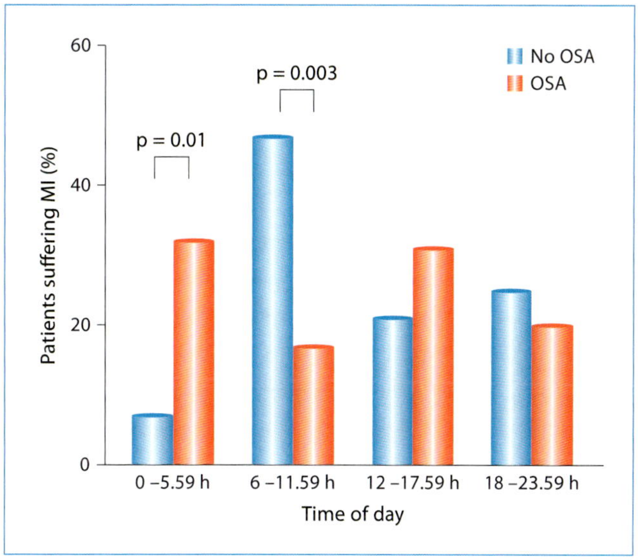

Fig. 16. Day-night pattern of MI based on four 6-hour time intervals in OSA (n = 64) and non-OSA (n = 28) patients. From 0.00 to 6.00 h, the frequency of MI was significantly higher in OSA patients than in non-OSA patients (32 vs. 7%; p = 0.01). From 6.00 to 12.00 h, the frequency of MI was higher in non-OSA patients than in OSA patients (47 vs. 17%; p = 0.003). After Kuniyoshi et al. [230], with permission.

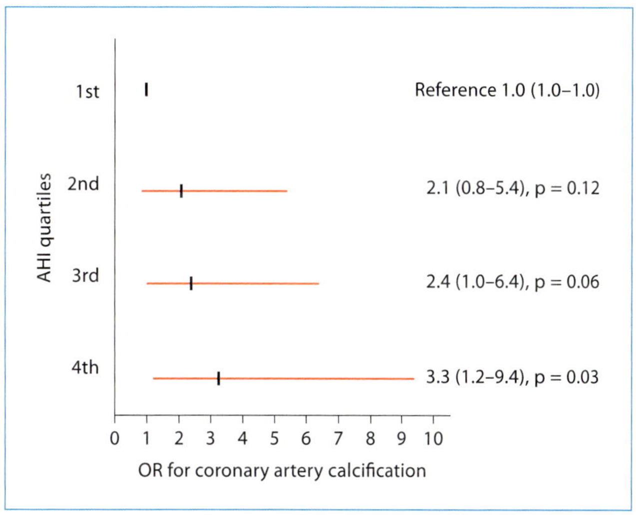

Fig. 17. Association between the severity of OSA measured by the AHI quartiles and coronary artery calcification. Using the 1st AHI quartile as a reference, the adjusted ORs for the 2nd, 3rd and 4th quartiles were 2.1 (p = 0.12), 2.4 (p = 0.06) and 3.3 (p = 0.03), respectively. AHI quartiles (in the figure, ranges are given in parentheses): 1st = 0–5; 2nd = 6–13; 3rd = 14–32; 4th >33. After Sorajja et al. [232], with permission.

between coronary atherosclerotic plaque volume and indices of sleep fragmentation, including the respiratory arousal index (r = 0.6; p = 0.02) and the total arousal index (r = 0.5; p = 0.03), suggesting that coronary atherosclerotic plaque volume may be associated with the severity of OSA and OSA-induced sleep fragmentation. Conversely, cross-sectional analysis of the relationship between coronary artery calcification with polysomnographically defined OSA and obesity in middle-aged men (n = 258, aged 40–49 years) randomly selected from a population-based cohort, demonstrated that the presence of coronary artery calcification was significantly greater in the 4th quartile versus the 1st quartile of AHI severity (OR 2.21, 95% CI 1.01–4.86) after adjustment for confounders, excluding BMI [234]. However, this association was no longer significant after adjusting for BMI. This could indicate that obesity was the significant independent contributor for coronary artery calcification after adjustment for potential cardiovascular risk factors, irrespective of OSA.

6.4 *Effect of Obstructive Sleep Apnea Treatment on Nonfatal Coronary Events*

CPAP treatment reduces nocturnal ST depression in OSA patients [153, 227, 235]. In a prospective study of coronary artery disease patients with moderate-to-severe OSA (n = 54, median follow-up 86.5 months), 25 patients were treated with CPAP (n = 21) or upper airway surgery (n = 4), while the remaining 29 patients declined treatment [236]. Compared with untreated patients, treated patients had a significantly reduced risk of the composite endpoint of cardiovascular death, acute coronary syndrome, hospitalization for heart failure or need for coronary revascularization (adjusted HR 0.24, 95% CI 0.09–0.62; $p < 0.01$). The effects of OSA treatment (n = 175) were retrospectively assessed in 371 OSA patients (AHI ≥15) who underwent a percutaneous coronary intervention on: (1) cardiac death; (2) general mortality; (3) major adverse cardiac events (severe angina, myocardial infarction, percutaneous coronary intervention, coronary artery bypass grafting or death), and (4) major adverse cardiac or cerebrovascular events [237]. Compared with untreated OSA patients, treatment of OSA did not significantly reduce the number of major adverse cardiac events or major adverse cardiac or cerebrovascular events on follow-up ($p = 0.91$), but reduced the number of deaths from cardiac causes at a 5-year follow-up (treated patients: 3%, 95% CI 0–6; untreated patients: 10%, 95% CI 5–14; $p = 0.027$). An observational 10.1-year follow-up study compared the incidence of nonfatal cardiovascular events (MI, stroke, coronary artery bypass surgery and percutaneous transluminal coronary angiography) in simple snorers (n = 377), patients with untreated OSA (n = 638), patients treated with CPAP (n = 372) and healthy men recruited from the general population individually matched for age and BMI (n = 264) [7]. Patients with untreated severe disease had a higher incidence of nonfatal cardiovascular events (2.13 per 100 person-years) than did untreated patients with mild-to-moderate disease (0.89 per 100 person-years; $p < 0.0001$), simple snorers (0.58 per 100 person-years; $p < 0.0001$), patients treated with CPAP (0.64 per 100 person-years; $p < 0.0001$) and healthy participants (0.45 per 100 person-years; $p < 0.0001$). After adjustment for confounders, untreated severe OSA patients had a significantly greater risk of nonfatal cardiovascular events than healthy participants (OR 3.17, 95% CI 1.12–7.51). This suggests that, in men, severe OSA may significantly increase the risk of nonfatal cardiovascular events that may be reduced by CPAP administration.

Overall, CPAP administration may have a beneficial effect on composite cardiovascular endpoints. Randomized controlled studies are required to determine whether CPAP treatment specifically reduces the risk of coronary artery disease.

6.5 *Mechanisms Potentially Linking Obstructive Sleep Apnea and Coronary Artery Disease*

Chronic intermittent hypoxia may increase the levels of various markers of inflammation, oxidative stress, and procoagulant and thrombotic activity. These alterations may contribute to the development of endothelial and metabolic dysfunction, and the development or aggravation of atherosclerosis and other cardiovascular diseases (including coronary artery disease and coronary artery calcification) associated with OSA.

Sleep loss and fragmentation may also contribute to the development of endothelial dysfunction, atherosclerosis and coronary disease in OSA. However, this still remains to be demonstrated, and it is important to distinguish sleep deprivation per se from sleep fragmentation secondary to sleep apnea because the former can occur without the coexistence of sleep apnea. Sleep loss may be a potential mechanism that increases the risk for coronary calcification. Sleep duration has been associated with a 5-year increased incidence of coronary artery calcification; in an observational study of 495 healthy subjects (the Coronary Artery Risk Development in Young Adults cohort) [238], longer sleep duration was significantly associated with the reduced incidence of coronary calcification (adjusted OR $0.67 \bullet h^{-1}$, 95% CI $0.49–0.91 \bullet h^{-1}$; $p = 0.01$). Sleep loss and fragmentation have also been shown to increase cardiovascular mortality and morbidity, including hypertension and coronary artery disease [14, 238–243]. The mechanisms by which sleep loss and fragmentation may increase the risk for atherosclerosis may include insulin resistance and diabetes [244–248], and increased levels of inflammatory and prothrombotic factors [249–251].

6.6 *Assessment of Obstructive Sleep Apnea in Coronary Artery Disease Patients*

OSA is prevalent in patients with coronary artery disease and may be a risk factor for poor prognosis; however, it is not routinely assessed in this population [252, 253], perhaps due to the fact that these patients often display little or no sleepiness [233]. This may be a characteristic feature of OSA in this situation, and clinicians should therefore be alert to the possibility of this condition, even if the patient does not suffer from sleepiness [254]. Compliance with CPAP treatment has been reported to be similar in coronary artery disease patients with or without excessive sleepiness [254].

6.7 *Key Points (table 9)*

Table 9.

- OSA may be associated with an increased risk of coronary artery disease, but whether this association is independent remains to be determined. It may also be a risk for recurrent cardiovascular events in untreated OSA patients with coronary artery disease
- OSA patients with coronary artery disease may have little or no sleepiness. This should not rule out these patients for the diagnosis and treatment of OSA
- Whether CPAP administration specifically reduces the incidence of coronary events in OSA patients remains to be fully elucidated
- There is a need for guidelines for the diagnosis of OSA in patients with coronary artery disease

7 Pulmonary Hypertension and Right Ventricular Dysfunction

7.1 *Pulmonary Hypertension*

7.1.1 Definition of Pulmonary Hypertension

Pulmonary hypertension is currently defined by a mean pulmonary arterial pressure ≥25 mm Hg at rest, as assessed by right heart catheterization [255]. The normal mean pulmonary arterial pressure at rest is considered to be 14.0 ± 3.3 mm Hg, with an upper normal limit of approximately 20 mm Hg [255, 256]. However, the significance of a mean pulmonary arterial pressure between 21 and 24 mm Hg remains to be clarified [255, 256]. The definition of pulmonary hypertension during exercise as a mean pulmonary arterial pressure >30 mm Hg (as assessed by right heart catheterization) is not currently considered supported by the medical literature, as healthy subjects can reach much higher values [255, 256].

7.1.2 Clinical Studies

Methodological biases make it difficult to draw definitive conclusions concerning the link between OSA and pulmonary hypertension. In addition, there are frequently differences in measurement techniques and definitions of variables between studies. Pulmonary hemodynamics are most often measured using Doppler echocardiography, providing several variables correlating with right heart hemodynamics, including pulmonary arterial pressure [255]. In previous studies, right heart hemodynamic measurements have been mostly performed in patients with OSA and comorbidities at risk for hypoxemia and, consequently, for pulmonary hypertension and right ventricular dysfunction (such as obesity, chronic lung or cardiac disorders). For example, patients with overlap syndrome develop more pronounced nocturnal oxygen desaturation than patients with COPD or OSA alone, which predisposes to pulmonary hypertension [257]. It was suggested that only OSA patients with such confounders may develop pulmonary artery hypertension [258–264].

Recent studies have provided some evidence for a causal link between OSA and pulmonary hypertension, independently of confounding variables. In clinical studies of OSA patients free from comorbidities involving a risk for pulmonary hypertension, the prevalence of pulmonary hypertension ranged between 20 and 40% [264]. In these populations, OSA is independently associated with pulmonary hypertension [60, 263–271], but it is unclear whether the pulmonary hypertension was related to the severity of OSA [265, 266]. The increase in pulmonary pressure associated with OSA has been shown to be mild, with a mean pulmonary artery pressure of approximately 20–30 mm Hg [264]. For example, from 27 patients (mean age 49 years) with OSA in whom clinically significant lung or cardiac diseases were excluded, 11 OSA patients (41%) were found to have mild pulmonary hypertension (≤26 mm Hg). There were no differences between patients with and without pulmonary hypertension in terms of BMI, smoking history or lung function. Patients with pulmonary hypertension were

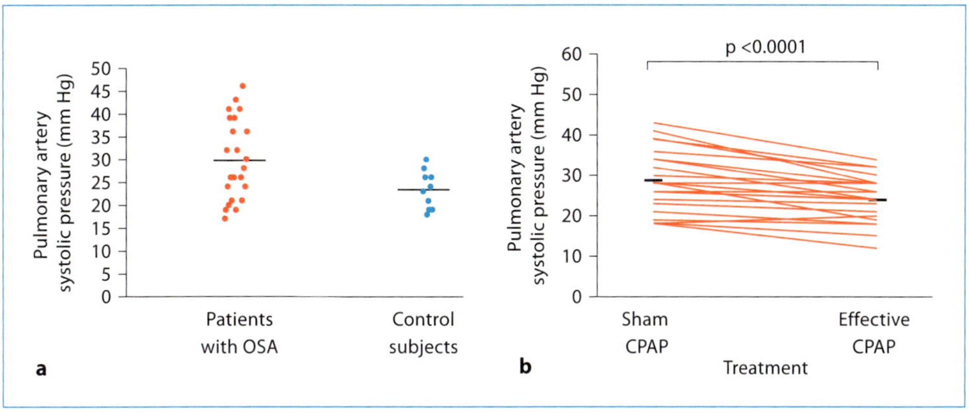

Fig. 18. Pulmonary artery systolic pressure at baseline in OSA patients and control subjects and after sham and effective CPAP treatment in OSA patients. **a** Individual values for the pulmonary artery systolic pressure in OSA patients and control subjects at baseline. **b** Individual values for the pulmonary artery systolic pressure after sham and effective CPAP treatment in OSA patients. After Arias et al. [271], with permission.

more hypoxemic when awake than those without pulmonary hypertension, but did not differ in the severity of OSA or indices of sleep desaturation. The hypoxemia in patients with pulmonary hypertension could not be explained by the impairment of lung function, greater body mass or a higher prevalence of smoking. Pao_2 in the study population was significantly correlated with pulmonary artery pressure (r = –0.46; p < 0.02), but not with forced expiratory volume in 1 second or BMI. Similarly, daytime hypoxemia has also been observed in OSA patients without significant comorbidity [268, 269].

7.1.3 Therapeutic Studies

There are a limited number of studies assessing the effect of CPAP application on pulmonary artery pressure; however, CPAP administration for up to 6 months significantly reduced pulmonary artery pressure in OSA patients [269, 271, 272]. The first randomized controlled study to assess the effect of CPAP administration on pulmonary artery pressure was conducted on 23 middle-aged OSA and otherwise healthy patients (mean AHI 44.1) and in 10 control subjects [271]. OSA patients randomly received either sham or effective CPAP for 12 weeks, and pulmonary pressure was assessed using echography. At baseline, OSA patients had higher pulmonary artery systolic pressure than control subjects (mean ± SD 29.8 ± 8.8 vs. 23.4 ± 4.1 mm Hg, respectively; p = 0.036; fig. 18). Effective CPAP induced a significant reduction in pulmonary systolic pressure (from 28.9 ± 8.6 to 24.0 ± 5.8 mm Hg; p < 0.0001). A greater reduction in pulmonary artery systolic pressure after effective CPAP therapy was observed in OSA patients with either left ventricular diastolic dysfunction (7.3 ± 3.3 vs. 1.6 ± 1.8 mm Hg; $p < 0.001$) or pulmonary hypertension at baseline (8.5 ± 2.8 vs. 2.6 ± 2.8 mm Hg; $p < 0.001$). However, these findings need to be confirmed.

In summary, clinical and therapeutic studies suggest that OSA may cause mild pulmonary artery hypertension in some patients who have no clinically identifiable comorbidity that can cause pulmonary hypertension. However, the clinical significance of such mild pulmonary hypertension is not known [60, 264, 266–269, 271].

7.2 *Right Ventricular Dysfunction*

7.2.1 Clinical Studies

The relationship between OSA and alterations in right ventricular structure and function has been assessed in OSA patients who did not have any comorbidity associated with the risk for pulmonary hypertension [273–276]. For example, the right ventricular ejection fraction, as assessed by radionuclide ventriculography, was impaired in 19 OSA patients (18%) without coexisting lung disease or left ventricular failure [273], and this was significantly associated with the AHI (r = –0.68; p = 0.0009) and the extent of nocturnal Sao_2 (r = 0.42; p = 0.035), but not with age, BMI, blood gas analysis, gender, lung function, pulmonary artery pressure or LVEF. In another study, the echocardiographic features were examined in subjects with SDB from the Framingham Heart Study site of the Sleep Heart Health Study [277]. Patients with severe OSA (n = 90, mean AHI 42) were compared with low-AHI subjects (n = 90, mean AHI 5) matched for age, sex and BMI. Right ventricular wall thickness was significantly greater (p = 0.005) in the OSA patients (mean ± SD 0.78 ± 0.02 cm) than in the low-AHI subjects (0.68 ± 0.02 cm); however, right atrial and ventricular dimensions and right ventricular systolic function were not significantly different between the groups.

7.2.2 Therapeutic Studies

CPAP administration improved right ventricular function in OSA patients [278–280]. For instance, right ventricular function was assessed using cardiac magnetic resonance imaging at baseline and after 3 months of CPAP therapy in obese patients with severe OSA, who were free of other significant comorbid conditions (n = 13, mean BMI 35.3, mean AHI 60.2) [280]. CPAP treatment significantly reduced the right ventricular end-systolic and end-diastolic volumes ($p < 0.05$). There was a trend toward an improvement in right ventricular ejection fraction, but the improvement did not reach significance.

In summary, these studies suggest that OSA (especially its severe form) appears to be a risk factor for mild alterations in right ventricular structure and function. Whether this association is independent of confounding variables remains to be demonstrated [60, 264]. In addition, the clinical significance of such mild alterations is unknown [264].

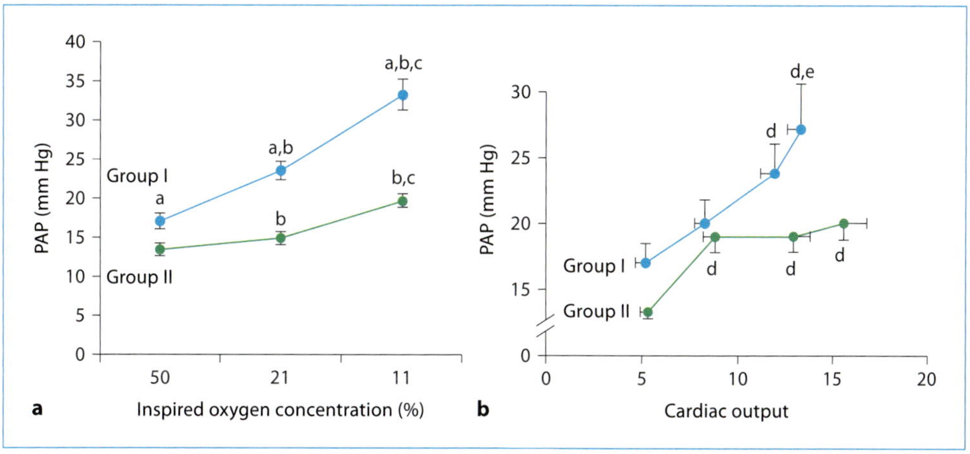

Fig. 19. Mean pulmonary artery pressure (PAP) in response to differences in inspired O_2 concentration (**a**) and increasing dobutamine infusion concentrations (**b**) in OSA patients with a mean PAP ≥20 mm Hg (group I) or a mean PAP <20 mm Hg (group II) at baseline. **a** Both groups of patients demonstrated a reduction in mean PAP during 50% O_2 breathing compared with room air breathing. Compared with group II, group I patients had (1) a greater mean PAP at all levels of inspired O_2 and (2) a greater hypoxic pressor response measured as the difference in PAP between 50% and 11% O_2 breathing. [a] $p < 0.05$ compared with group II; [b] $p < 0.05$ compared with PAP at 50% O_2 breathing; [c] $p < 0.05$ compared with PAP at 21% O_2 breathing. **b** The points on each curve correspond to different dobutamine infusion rates (from left to right): 0, 10, 20 and 30 $\mu g \cdot kg^{-1} \cdot min^{-1}$. Patients breathed 50% O_2 to abolish hypoxic pulmonary vasoconstriction. In group I patients, note the progressive rise in mean PAP with increasing dobutamine infusion rates. In contrast, group II patients showed an increase in PAP with the first increment in cardiac output, but it thereafter stabilized despite marked increases in cardiac output. [d] $p < 0.05$ compared with PAP at 0 $\mu g \cdot kg^{-1} \cdot min^{-1}$ dobutamine; [e] $p < 0.05$ compared with PAP at 10 $\mu g \cdot kg^{-1} \cdot min^{-1}$ dobutamine. After Sajkov et al. [267]. Reprinted with permission of the American Thoracic Society. © American Thoracic Society.

7.3 Potential Mechanisms That May Lead to Pulmonary Hypertension and Right Ventricular Dysfunction in Obstructive Sleep Apnea

Hypoxemia is likely to be a critical factor contributing to the development of pulmonary hypertension and alterations in right ventricular structure and function in OSA patients [258, 265, 266, 268, 269], especially in patients with comorbidities linked to hypoxemia, such as chronic cardiac or lung disorders and severe obesity [257, 264, 267, 268].

Remodeling of the pulmonary circulation, i.e. structural changes in the pulmonary vasculature, may contribute to the development of sustained pulmonary hypertension in OSA patients [264, 265, 267, 281, 282]. In OSA patients with and without (control group) pulmonary hypertension (and no coexisting lung disorder), there was increased closure of small airways during tidal breathing, more ventilation-perfusion inequality, a greater pulmonary artery pressor response to hypoxia and a marked rise in pulmonary artery pressure during increased pulmonary blood flow (fig. 19)

[267]. These findings may be consistent with remodeling of the pulmonary vascular bed. In another study, the same authors reported that CPAP treatment may reduce pulmonary artery pressure and hypoxic pulmonary vascular reactivity in OSA [272]. It is speculated that this may be due to an improvement in pulmonary endothelial function.

Pulmonary vascular reactivity was assessed in patients with moderate-to-severe OSA, before and after 3 months of CPAP treatment, at baseline and in response to acetylcholine (an endothelium-dependent dilator), sodium nitroprusside (an endothelium-independent dilator), L-NMMA (N^G-monomethyl-L-arginine, a competitive antagonist of nitric oxide synthesis), and L-arginine (the substrate of nitric oxide) [283]. At baseline, pulmonary flow fell in response to L-NMMA and increased in response to acetylcholine and sodium nitroprusside. Following CPAP treatment, the decrease in flow following L-NMMA administration was significantly greater, consistent with the enhanced basal release of nitric oxide.

Overall, these findings suggest that chronic intermittent hypoxia, endothelial dysfunction and pulmonary vascular remodeling may all contribute to the development of pulmonary hypertension in OSA.

7.4 Key Points (table 10)

Table 10.

- OSA may be an independent risk factor for mild pulmonary hypertension. It may also be a risk factor for alterations in the structure and function of the right ventricle, probably in association with comorbidities such as chronic obstructive lung disease [60, 264]
- The clinical classification of pulmonary hypertension and European guidelines consider OSA as a condition associated with pulmonary hypertension [255, 346]. As a consequence, patients with pulmonary artery hypertension may benefit from sleep studies to diagnose OSA [255, 346]. The Task Force for the Diagnosis and Treatment of Pulmonary Hypertension of the European Society of Cardiology and the European Respiratory Society, endorsed by the International Society of Heart and Lung Transplantation, has stated that 'if clinically suspected, screening overnight by oximetry or polysomnography will exclude significant OSA' [255]

8 Arrhythmias

8.1 Atrial Fibrillation

8.1.1 Clinical, Epidemiological and Therapeutic Studies

8.1.1.1 Prevalence of Sleep Apnea in Patients with Atrial Fibrillation. In a prospective study, consecutive patients undergoing electrocardioversion for atrial fibrillation (n = 151) and patients without past or current atrial fibrillation referred to a general cardiology practice (n = 312) were assessed. The Berlin questionnaire was used to diagnose OSA, and its accuracy was compared with polysomnographic results.

The proportion of patients with OSA was significantly higher in the atrial fibrillation group than in the general cardiology group (49 vs. 32%, respectively; $p = 0.0004$). The adjusted OR for the association between atrial fibrillation and OSA was 2.19 (95% CI 1.40–3.42; $p = 0.0006$). In patients with normal left ventricular function, those with paroxysmal and persistent atrial fibrillation (n = 90, mean age 56 years) had a significantly greater proportion of OSA (AHI >15) than those without atrial fibrillation, matched for age and gender (n = 45, mean age 54 years; 62 vs. 38%, respectively; $p = 0.01$) [284]. The OR for the association between atrial fibrillation and OSA (AHI >15) was 3.04 (95% CI 1.24–7.46; $p = 0.02$) after adjustment for confounders. In contrast, a similar prevalence of sleep apnea was observed in patients with lone atrial fibrillation (n = 59) and in gender-, age- and cardiovascular morbidity-matched control patients (n = 56; 32 vs. 29%, respectively; $p = 0.67$) [285]. However, there may have been a recruitment bias for the control group patients, who were included after responding to an invitation letter, of which 43% were not answered.

8.1.1.2 *Prevalence of Atrial Fibrillation in Patients with Sleep Apnea.* Analysis of data from the Sleep Heart Health Study indicated that atrial fibrillation was more common in subjects with SDB (AHI >30, n = 228) than in those without SDB (AHI <5, n = 338; 4.8 vs. 0.9%, respectively; $p = 0.003$) [286]. After adjusting for confounding factors, the OR for SDB and atrial fibrillation was 4.02 (95% CI 1.03–15.74). A retrospective cohort study of 3,542 Olmsted County adults without past or current atrial fibrillation who were referred for an initial diagnostic polysomnogram from 1987 to 2003 [287] revealed the presence of incidental atrial fibrillation in 133 subjects (cumulative probability 14%, 95% CI 9–19%). In subjects <65 years old, independent predictors of incidental atrial fibrillation were a decrease in nocturnal Sao_2 (per 0.5 units log change, HR 3.29, 95% CI 1.35–8.04), BMI, age, male gender and coronary artery disease (fig. 20). Heart failure predicted incidental atrial fibrillation in subjects ≥65 years of age; however, neither OSA nor obesity had a predictive value for atrial fibrillation in this age group. Discrepant findings were observed in older men from the Outcomes of Sleep Disorders in Older Men Study (n = 2,911), where an increasing severity of SDB was associated with a progressive increase in the odds of atrial fibrillation and complex ventricular ectopy (i.e. nonsustained ventricular tachycardia, bigeminy, trigeminy or quadrigeminy) [288]. The highest respiratory disturbance index quartile was associated with increased odds for atrial fibrillation (OR 2.15, 95% CI 1.19–3.89) and complex ventricular ectopy (OR 1.43, 95% CI 1.12–1.82) compared with the lowest quartile. Atrial fibrillation was most strongly associated with CSA, whereas complex ventricular ectopy was most strongly associated with OSA and hypoxia. Therefore, different sleep-related stresses may contribute to atrial and ventricular arrhythmogenesis in older men.

Several studies have shown that atrial fibrillation is more prevalent in heart failure patients with sleep apnea than in those without sleep apnea [119–122]; however, this may be due to CSA rather than OSA [120–122, 289]. For example, atrial fibrillation

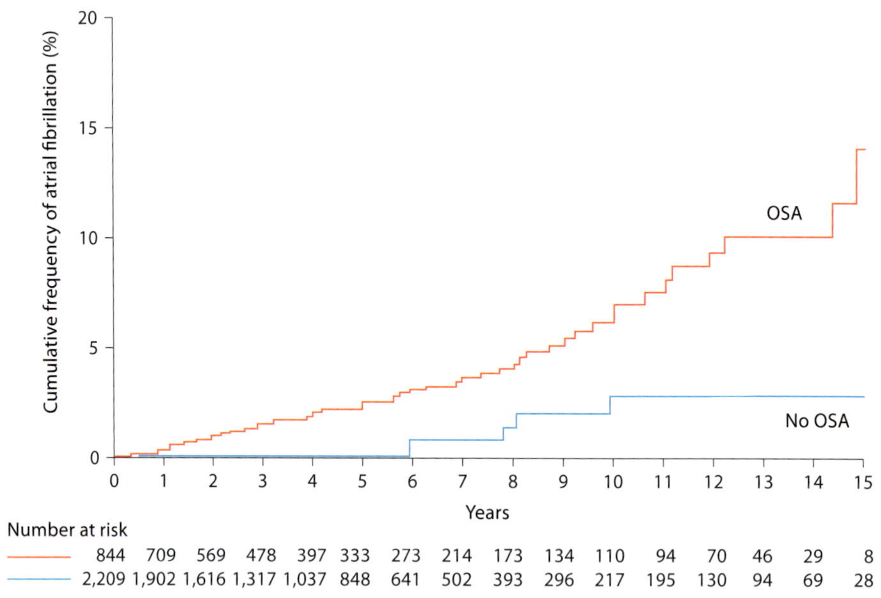

Fig. 20. Incidence of atrial fibrillation based on the presence or absence of OSA. Cumulative frequency curves for incidental atrial fibrillation for subjects <65 years of age with or without OSA during an average 4.7 years of follow-up. p = 0.002. After Gami et al. [287], with permission.

was significantly associated with CSA, but not with OSA, in 450 congestive heart failure patients with and without sleep apnea [120].

8.1.1.3 *Temporal Relationship between SDB and the Occurrence of Atrial Fibrillation.* The causal relationship between OSA and the occurrence of arrhythmias, including atrial fibrillation, was supported by analysis of the Sleep Heart Health Study (n = 2,816) that assessed whether apneas and/or hypopneas were temporally associated with episodes of paroxysmal atrial fibrillation or nonsustained ventricular tachycardia [290]. Fifty-seven participants with a wide range of SDB had 62 arrhythmias (24% paroxysmal atrial fibrillation and 76% nonsustained ventricular tachycardia). The odds of an arrhythmia occurring after a respiratory disturbance were 17.5-fold higher than the odds of an arrhythmia occurring after normal breathing (95% CI 5.3–58.4). However, the absolute rate of arrhythmia associated with respiratory disturbances was low (1 excess arrhythmia per 40,000 respiratory disturbances). Neither hypoxia nor electroencephalogram-defined arousals alone increased the arrhythmia risk. These findings may suggest a direct temporal link between SDB events and the development of these arrhythmias; although the absolute arrhythmia rate was low, the relative risk of paroxysmal atrial fibrillation and nonsustained ventricular tachycardia during sleep was markedly increased shortly after a respiratory disturbance.

8.1.1.4 *Effect of Restoring Sinus Rhythm on OSA Severity in OSA Patients with Atrial Fibrillation.* The severity of sleep apnea did not improve immediately or 4 weeks after restoring sinus rhythm in OSA patients with atrial fibrillation (n = 6) or atrial flutter (n = 10) [291]. This may suggest that atrial fibrillation is not a causative or aggravating condition in sleep apnea.

8.1.1.5 *Effects of CPAP Administration.* The impact of effective CPAP administration on the recurrence of atrial fibrillation within 1 year of electrical cardioversion to sinus rhythm was studied in an observational prospective study [292]. Untreated OSA patients (n = 27), OSA patients with effective CPAP administration (n = 12) and randomly selected postcardioversion control patients (n = 79) were assessed. The recurrence of atrial fibrillation at 1 year in untreated OSA patients was 82%, as opposed to the 42% recurrence in the CPAP-treated OSA group (p = 0.013) and the 53% recurrence in the control patients (p = 0.009). In the untreated OSA patients, the nocturnal fall in Sao_2 was greater (p = 0.034) in those who had a recurrence of atrial fibrillation (n = 20) than in those without recurrence (n = 5). These findings underscore the potential importance of hypoxemia and insufficient CPAP use in the risk of recurrence of atrial fibrillation and suggest that appropriate treatment with CPAP in OSA patients may be associated with a lower recurrence rate of atrial fibrillation. However, it is of note that the number of participants was small, and treatment was not randomly allocated. Patients who had been offered CPAP but did not comply with therapy were included among the untreated OSA patients (this may have introduced a bias between the 2 groups).

8.1.2 Mechanisms Potentially Linking Obstructive Sleep Apnea with Atrial Fibrillation

Cardiac remodeling, hemodynamic and autonomic changes, chronic intermittent hypoxemia and inflammation associated with OSA may potentially contribute to the increased risk for atrial fibrillation in OSA patients. However, this risk is also associated with age, obesity, diabetes mellitus, systemic hypertension, heart failure and coronary artery disease [293–299]. The presence of these confounding variables makes the interpretation of the relationship between OSA and atrial fibrillation difficult. OSA itself may also indirectly increase the risk for atrial fibrillation as it is an independent risk factor for the development of arterial hypertension, which in turn is a risk factor for the occurrence of atrial fibrillation [300, 301].

8.1.2.1 *Oxygen Desaturation.* Oxygen desaturation associated with OSA is an independent predictor for atrial fibrillation in various studies [287, 292, 302]. Nocturnal oxygen desaturation is likely to be an intermediate mechanism linking OSA to the development of atrial fibrillation.

8.1.2.2 *Atrial Remodeling.* OSA patients have an increased left atrial volume compared with BMI-matched control subjects without OSA [130, 275, 303]. In comparison with control subjects matched for age and BMI (n = 50), patients with

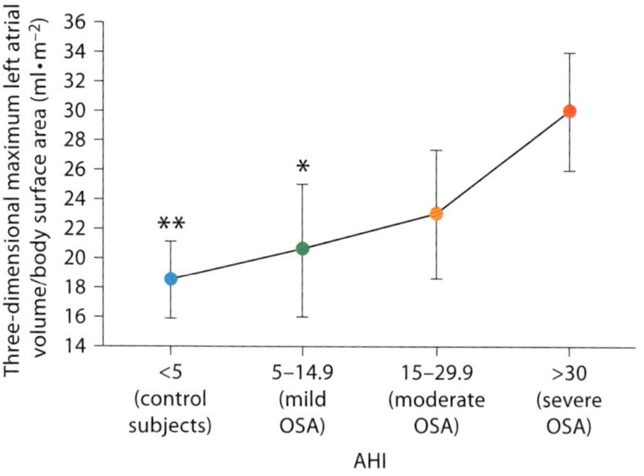

Fig. 21. Left atrial maximum volume indexed for body surface area derived from real-time 3-dimensional echocardiography in OSA patients and control subjects. Left atrial volume indexed for body surface area was significantly greater in patients with severe OSA than in patients with mild OSA (* p = 0.01) and control subjects (** p = 0.001). After Oliveira et al. [130], with permission.

OSA (n = 50) had a larger 3-dimensional maximum left atrial volume indexed to the body surface area (fig. 21), larger atrial volume before contraction and higher active atrial ejection fraction ($p < 0.01$ for all factors cited) [130]. It is suggested that OSA induces a functional burden on the left atrium, resulting in its remodeling. These functional and structural changes were related to diastolic functional impairment, which powerfully predicts incidental nonvalvular atrial fibrillation [304]. The mechanisms by which OSA increases the risk of atrial fibrillation may therefore include diastolic dysfunction and increased left atrial size. The same group compared the effects of 24 weeks of administration of effective CPAP with that of sham CPAP on left atrial function and structure in patients with moderate-to-severe OSA (AHI >20) [305]. In the effective CPAP group, there was an increase in the left atrial passive emptying fraction (the difference between maximal atrial volume and the volume before atrial contraction; 28.8 vs. 46.8%, respectively; $p = 0.01$) and a reduction in the left atrial active emptying fraction (the difference between the volume before atrial contraction and the minimum atrial volume; 42.7 vs. 25.7%, respectively; $p < 0.01$; fig. 22). In the sham group, there were no changes from the baseline to the 24-week echo. This was associated with an improvement in left ventricular diastolic function. Left atrial structural variables were not improved. This suggests that OSA may significantly contribute to atrial dysfunction.

Left atrial dilatation may also be related to obesity, an independent risk factor for atrial fibrillation [294, 295, 297, 298]. A prospective, community-based, observational 13.7-year follow-up study in Framingham, Mass., USA, on 5,282 participants (mean age 57 years) without baseline atrial fibrillation, indicated that obesity was a 1.5-fold increased risk factor for atrial fibrillation ($p = 0.02$ and 0.03 in men

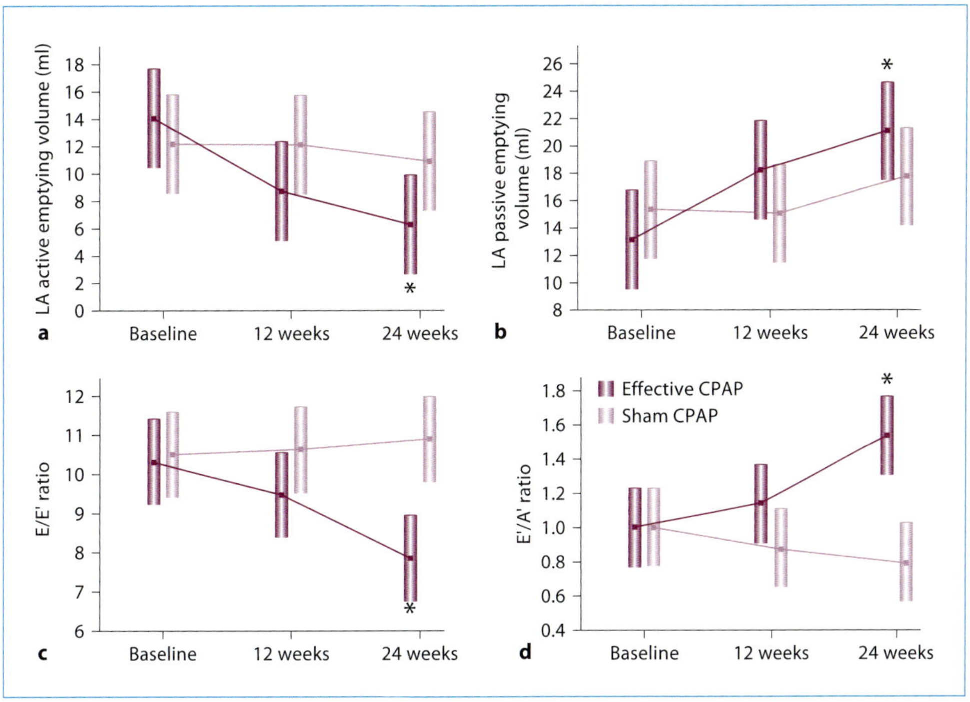

Fig. 22. Left atrial (LA) function (**a**, **b**) and left ventricular diastolic performance (**c**, **d**) throughout 24 weeks of sham or effective CPAP treatment. E/E′ = Ratio of mitral valve early diastolic velocity to mitral annular early diastolic velocity; E′/A′ = ratio of mitral annular early diastolic velocity to late diastolic velocity. * $p < 0.05$, difference from baseline visit. After Oliveira et al. [305], with permission.

and women, respectively), compared with individuals with a normal BMI and after adjustment for clinical and electrocardiographic variables [294]. However, after adjustment for echocardiographic left atrial diameter in addition to clinical risk factors, BMI was no longer associated with atrial fibrillation risk. This suggests that obesity is an important risk factor for atrial fibrillation, which appears to be mediated by left atrial dilatation.

8.1.2.3 Mechanical Consequences of Recurrent Apnea-Ventilation Resumption Cycles during Sleep. The mechanical consequences of recurrent apnea-ventilation resumption cycles during sleep on cardiovascular structures have been hypothesized to contribute to cardiac remodeling, including atrial enlargement [306, 307].

8.1.2.4 Inflammation. An increased systemic inflammation level is associated with OSA [see chapter 2, this vol., pp. 43–66], atrial fibrillation [308] and cardiac remodeling [309]. Whether inflammation is an intermediate mechanism linking OSA to the development of atrial fibrillation through its effect on cardiac remodeling is unknown.

8.1.3 Key Points (table 11)

Table 11.

- The American College of Chest Physicians guidelines for the prevention and management of postoperative atrial fibrillation after cardiac surgery consider that 'undiagnosed sleep apnea is a risk factor for postoperative atrial fibrillation...' and has recommended that '...screening for and treating sleep-disordered breathing as part of the routine preoperative evaluation of cardiac surgical patients may be a useful strategy for preventing postcardiac surgery atrial fibrillation' [347]
- However, the cause-and-effect relationship between OSA and atrial fibrillation and the effect of CPAP therapy on the incidence and recurrence of atrial fibrillation remain to be demonstrated [292]
- The diagnosis and treatment of OSA may be an additional preventive strategy for patients with atrial fibrillation [348]

8.2 *Ventricular Arrhythmias*

8.2.1 Clinical, Epidemiological and Therapeutic Studies

Numerous clinical studies have reported that OSA patients have a greater prevalence of ventricular arrhythmias than non-OSA individuals [286, 310–313]. For example, ventricular ectopy was observed during sleep in 74% of OSA patients, while complex ventricular ectopy (multiform, repetitive or both) was observed in 55% of OSA patients [311]. There was a significant relationship between the premature ventricular complex and Sao_2 when Sao_2 was less than 60%, but not when it was greater than 60% [311]. In addition, 20% of 400 OSA patients had premature ventricular contractions ($>2 \bullet min^{-1}$) [310]; however, other studies have not confirmed these findings [314, 315].

Analysis of data from the Sleep Heart Health Study indicated that nonsustained ventricular tachycardia and complex ventricular ectopy were more common in subjects with SDB (AHI >30, n = 228) than in those without SDB (AHI <5, n = 338): 5.3 versus 1.2% (p = 0.004) for nonsustained ventricular tachycardia; 25.0 versus 14.5% (p = 0.002) for complex ventricular ectopy [286]. Compared to those without SDB and adjusting for age, sex, BMI and prevalent coronary heart disease, SDB patients had 3.4-fold increased odds of nonsustained ventricular tachycardia (95% CI 1.03–11.20) and 1.7-fold increased odds of complex ventricular ectopy (95% CI 1.11–2.74) [286]. In contrast to subjects without known OSA, ventricular arrhythmias appear to predominantly occur during sleep in OSA patients [310, 311, 316–318].

As mentioned above, analysis of the Sleep Heart Health Study indicated that nonsustained ventricular tachycardia is more likely to occur after respiratory disturbance than after normal breathing [290]. When the timing of the occurrence of ventricular ectopy is examined in heart failure patients with either CSA or OSA matched for LVEF, sex and AHI, patients in sinus rhythm who have OSA and with >30 ventricular premature beats • h^{-1} have an increased frequency of ventricular premature beats during stage 2 sleep in the apneic phase than in the hyperpneic phase [318]. In contrast, in CSA patients, these ventricular premature beats occurred more frequently during the hyperpneic phase than the apneic phase. There was no difference in the degree of apnea-related oxygen desaturation between central and obstructive apneas. The difference in ventricular premature beat timing between OSA and CSA patients may be attributable to the differences in timing of arrhythmic stresses in these patients. In heart failure patients with OSA, the treatment of coexisting OSA by CPAP reduced the frequency of ventricular premature beats during sleep [319]. The link between OSA and the risk of ventricular arrhythmias was assessed in chronic heart failure patients with a cardiac resynchronization device with a cardioverter-defibrillator (170 patients with mild or no SDB remained untreated, 113 patients declined ventilation therapy, and 189 patients with moderate-to-severe SDB received either adaptive servoventilation or CPAP) [320]. OSA was independently associated with an increased risk for ventricular arrhythmias (AHI ≥5 • h^{-1}, HR 1.69, 95% CI 1.64–1.75; p = 0.001; AHI ≥15 • h^{-1}, HR 1.69, 95% CI 1.14–2.51; p = 0.02) and appropriate cardioverter-defibrillator therapies (AHI ≥5 • h^{-1}, HR 2.07, 95% CI 1.14–3.77; p = 0.02; AHI ≥15, HR 2.10, 95% CI 1.17–3.78; p = 0.01). Similar findings were also observed for CSA.

8.2.2 Key Points (table 12)

Table 12.

- OSA patients may be at risk of ventricular arrhythmias. This is especially true for patients with severe OSA [226, 310–312] or with coexisting cardiovascular comorbidities
- A causative relationship between OSA and ventricular arrhythmias remains to be demonstrated

8.3 *Bradyarrhythmias*

8.3.1 Clinical, Epidemiological and Therapeutic Studies

8.3.1.1 Clinical and Epidemiological Studies. The prevalences of sinus arrest and 2nd- and 3rd-degree heart block are greater in OSA patients than in individuals without OSA [310, 321–323]. OSA and nocturnal oxygen desaturation severity were associated with a higher risk of bradyarrhythmias [310, 322–325]. A higher prevalence of sinus pauses, but not 2nd-degree heart block, was observed in OSA patients (n = 66) than in control subjects without OSA (n = 81; 9.1 vs. 0%, respectively; p < 0.01) [315]. In contrast, in individuals with and without OSA, a similar prevalence (all p > 0.05) of 2nd-degree atrioventricular block (1.3 vs. 4.1%, respectively) and sinus arrest (5.2 vs. 1.0%, respectively) was observed [314]. In patients with ventricular asystole occurring exclusively during OSA (n = 15), the electrophysiological parameters of sinus node function were normal in 12 patients (80%), and atrioventricular nodal function was normal in 7 patients (47%) [326]. Almost all abnormal findings of sinus node function and atrioventricular nodal function were reversible by the administration of atropine. These findings suggest that prolonged ventricular asystole during OSA may not be due to fixed or anatomical disease of the sinus node or the atrioventricular conduction system, and may instead be related to an increased vagal tone. Analysis of data from the Sleep Heart Health Study revealed no significant differences (all $p > 0.05$) between patients with severe SDB (AHI ≥30, n = 228) and those without SDB (AHI <5, n = 338) in the prevalence of sinus pause (>3 s; 11 vs. 8.6%, respectively), 1st-degree atrioventricular block (25 vs. 22.5%, respectively), type 1 2nd-degree atrioventricular block (1.8 vs. 0.3%, respectively) and type 2 2nd-degree atrioventricular block (2.2 vs. 0.9%, respectively) [286]. The European Multicenter Polysomnographic Study found an excessively high frequency of SDB in patients with pacemakers, where 59% had an AHI ≥10 and 21.2% had an AHI >30 (n = 99) [327]. The SDB was mainly obstructive and associated with few symptoms. The mean Epworth score was in the normal range, suggesting that these patients were less sleepy than is usually noted in OSA. SDB was present in 68% of patients with atrioventricular block. These findings support the systematic assessment for OSA in patients with heart block before considering treatment with pacemakers [327].

8.3.1.2 *Effect of CPAP Administration.* Bradyarrhythmias are significantly reversed with CPAP administration [322, 325, 326, 328]. For example, the effect of CPAP administration on heart block was assessed in 17 patients with OSA and heart block, and revealed that the total number of episodes of heart block during sleep decreased significantly ($p < 0.001$) from 1,575 before therapy to 165 during CPAP. In 12 patients (70.6%), heart block was totally prevented by CPAP. It was suggested that, in patients with heart block, pacemaker treatment should be considered in those without OSA, those with persistent heart block despite CPAP administration or those with poor CPAP compliance [322]. Similar findings were also observed in 16 OSA patients with nocturnal heart block [328]. CPAP treatment was associated with a reduction in the total number of arrhythmias from 651 to 72 ($p < 0.01$); however, in a randomized controlled study of the effect of 4 weeks of effective CPAP versus sham CPAP, there was no significant decrease in arrhythmias, including sinus bradycardia and pauses [329]. Whether CPAP administration should be a first-line treatment of bradyarrhythmias that occur exclusively during OSA in patients with normal electrophysiological characteristics of the sinus node and atrial conduction system needs to be confirmed by further studies [60, 330].

8.3.2 Atrial Pacing and Treatment of Obstructive Sleep Apnea

Atrial pacing at a rate of 15 beats higher than the mean sinus rate significantly reduced the number of episodes of CSA and OSA in one study [331]; however, this was not subsequently confirmed [332–338], and it is now considered that there is no evidence to support atrial overdrive pacing as a treatment option for OSA.

8.3.3 Key Points (table 13)

Table 13.

- Bradyarrhythmias may occur in some OSA patients, especially in those with severe OSA
- Whether patients with bradyarrhythmias need to be routinely assessed for OSA remains to be determined [327]

9 Conclusions and Future Directions

A causal relationship between OSA and hypertension is currently well accepted as there have now been a number of randomized controlled trials showing a lowering of blood pressure with the treatment of OSA (albeit a modest lowering). However, confounders and methodological biases are the main reasons for the lack of definitive conclusions in causality studies between OSA and an increased risk for death and between OSA and other cardiovascular disorders. Longitudinal, randomized, controlled, adequately powered trials, involving well-defined participants and taking into account confounders, are needed to assess clinical cardiovascular endpoints, interactions between OSA and comorbidities, and intermediate pathogenic mechanisms linking OSA and cardiometabolic disorders.

Severe OSA and oxygen desaturation may be required for the development of cardiovascular disorders; therefore, it may be critical to identify cardiac patients with severe OSA and nocturnal oxygen desaturation [339]. Unfortunately, the diagnosis of OSA in cardiac patients may be challenging as excessive BMI or daytime sleepiness may not be evident. OSA symptoms may be difficult to differentiate from fatigue and dyspnea from cardiac causes. Further studies and collaborative guidelines are needed to: (1) define a diagnostic strategy for OSA evaluation in cardiac patients; (2) identify clinical profiles of cardiac patients at risk for OSA in whom OSA evaluation may be routinely recommended; (3) identify early markers of cardiovascular risk associated with OSA, and (4) identify subpopulations at risk of cardiovascular diseases (genetic studies may help to identify these subpopulations).

10 References

1 Friedman O, Logan AG: The price of obstructive sleep apnea-hypopnea: hypertension and other ill effects. Am J Hypertens 2009;22:474–483.

2 He J, Kryger MH, Zorick FJ, Conway W, Roth T: Mortality and apnea index in obstructive sleep apnea: experience in 385 male patients. Chest 1988;94:9–14.

3 Peker Y, Hedner J, Kraiczi H, Loth S: Respiratory disturbance index: an independent predictor of mortality in coronary artery disease. Am J Respir Crit Care Med 2000;162:81–86.

4 Campos-Rodriguez F, Pena-Grinan N, Reyes-Nunez N, De la Cruz-Moron I, Perez-Ronchel J, De la Vega-Gallardo F, Fernandez-Palacin A: Mortality in obstructive sleep apnea-hypopnea patients treated with positive airway pressure. Chest 2005;128:624–633.

5 Gami AS, Howard DE, Olson EJ, Somers VK: Day-night pattern of sudden death in obstructive sleep apnea. N Engl J Med 2005;352:1206–1214.
6 Lavie P, Lavie L, Herer P: All-cause mortality in males with sleep apnoea syndrome: declining mortality rates with age. Eur Respir J 2005;25:514–520.
7 Marin JM, Carrizo SJ, Vicente E, Agusti AG: Long-term cardiovascular outcomes in men with obstructive sleep apnoea-hypopnoea with or without treatment with continuous positive airway pressure: an observational study. Lancet 2005;365:1046–1053.
8 Yaggi HK, Concato J, Kernan WN, Lichtman JH, Brass LM, Mohsenin V: Obstructive sleep apnea as a risk factor for stroke and death. N Engl J Med 2005;353:2034–2041.
9 Buchner NJ, Sanner BM, Borgel J, Rump LC: Continuous positive airway pressure treatment of mild to moderate obstructive sleep apnea reduces cardiovascular risk. Am J Respir Crit Care Med 2007;176:1274–1280.
10 Yumino D, Wang H, Floras JS, Newton GE, Mak S, Ruttanaumpawan P, Parker JD, Bradley TD: Relationship between sleep apnoea and mortality in patients with ischaemic heart failure. Heart 2009;95:819–824.
11 Shah NA, Yaggi HK, Concato J, Mohsenin V: Obstructive sleep apnea as a risk factor for coronary events or cardiovascular death. Sleep Breath 2010;14:131–136.
12 Marshall NS, Wong KK, Liu PY, Cullen SR, Knuiman MW, Grunstein RR: Sleep apnea as an independent risk factor for all-cause mortality: the Busselton Health Study. Sleep 2008;31:1079–1085.
13 Young T, Finn L, Peppard PE, Szklo-Coxe M, Austin D, Nieto FJ, Stubbs R, Hla KM: Sleep disordered breathing and mortality: eighteen-year follow-up of the Wisconsin sleep cohort. Sleep 2008;31:1071–1078.
14 Punjabi NM, Caffo BS, Goodwin JL, Gottlieb DJ, Newman AB, O'Connor GT, Rapoport DM, Redline S, Resnick HE, Robbins JA, Shahar E, Unruh ML, Samet JM: Sleep-disordered breathing and mortality: a prospective cohort study. PLoS Med 2009;6:e1000132.
15 Wang H, Parker JD, Newton GE, Floras JS, Mak S, Chiu KL, Ruttanaumpawan P, Tomlinson G, Bradley TD: Influence of obstructive sleep apnea on mortality in patients with heart failure. J Am Coll Cardiol 2007;49:1625–1631.
16 Kasai T, Narui K, Dohi T, Yanagisawa N, Ishiwata S, Ohno M, Yamaguchi T, Momomura S: Prognosis of patients with heart failure and obstructive sleep apnea treated with continuous positive airway pressure. Chest 2008;133:690–696.
17 Javaheri S, Caref EB, Chen E, Tong KB, Abraham WT: Sleep Apnea Testing and Outcomes in a Large Cohort of Medicare Beneficiaries with Newly Diagnosed Heart Failure. Am J Respir Crit Care Med 2011;183:539–546.
18 Roebuck T, Solin P, Kaye DM, Bergin P, Bailey M, Naughton MT: Increased long-term mortality in heart failure due to sleep apnoea is not yet proven. Eur Respir J 2004;23:735–740.
19 Luo Q, Zhang HL, Tao XC, Zhao ZH, Yang YJ, Liu ZH: Impact of untreated sleep apnea on prognosis of patients with congestive heart failure. Int J Cardiol 2010;144:420–422.
20 Cohen MC, Rohtla KM, Lavery CE, Muller JE, Mittleman MA: Meta-analysis of the morning excess of acute myocardial infarction and sudden cardiac death. Am J Cardiol 1997;79:1512–1516.
21 Doherty LS, Kiely JL, Swan V, McNicholas WT: Long-term effects of nasal continuous positive airway pressure therapy on cardiovascular outcomes in sleep apnea syndrome. Chest 2005;127:2076–2084.
22 Machado MC, Vollmer WM, Togeiro SM, Bilderback AL, Oliveira MV, Leitao FS, Queiroga F Jr, Lorenzi-Filho G, Krishnan JA: CPAP and survival in moderate-to-severe obstructive sleep apnoea syndrome and hypoxaemic COPD. Eur Respir J 2010;35:132–137.
23 Marin JM, Soriano JB, Carrizo SJ, Boldova A, Celli BR: Outcomes in patients with chronic obstructive pulmonary disease and obstructive sleep apnea: the overlap syndrome. Am J Respir Crit Care Med 2010;182:325–331.
24 Kales A, Bixler EO, Cadieux RJ, Schneck DW, Shaw LC 3rd, Locke TW, Vela-Bueno A, Soldatos CR: Sleep apnoea in a hypertensive population. Lancet 1984;ii:1005–1008.
25 Lavie P, Ben-Yosef R, Rubin AE: Prevalence of sleep apnea syndrome among patients with essential hypertension. Am Heart J 1984;108:373–376.
26 Fletcher EC, De Behnke RD, Lovoi MS, Gorin AB: Undiagnosed sleep apnea in patients with essential hypertension. Ann Intern Med 1985;103:190–195.
27 Williams AJ, Houston D, Finberg S, Lam C, Kinney JL, Santiago S: Sleep apnea syndrome and essential hypertension. Am J Cardiol 1985;55:1019–1022.
28 Vardan S, Dunsky MH, Hill NE, Mookherjee S, Smulyan H, Warner RA: Systemic systolic hypertension in the elderly: correlation of hemodynamics, plasma volume, renin, aldosterone, urinary metanephrines and response to thiazide therapy. Am J Cardiol 1986;58:1030–1034.
29 Millman RP, Redline S, Carlisle CC, Assaf AR, Levinson PD: Daytime hypertension in obstructive sleep apnea: prevalence and contributing risk factors. Chest 1991;99:861–866.

30 Worsnop CJ, Naughton MT, Barter CE, Morgan TO, Anderson AI, Pierce RJ: The prevalence of obstructive sleep apnea in hypertensives. Am J Respir Crit Care Med 1998;157:111–115.
31 Logan AG, Perlikowski SM, Mente A, Tisler A, Tkacova R, Niroumand M, Leung RS, Bradley TD: High prevalence of unrecognized sleep apnoea in drug-resistant hypertension. J Hypertens 2001;19: 2271–2277.
32 Carlson JT, Hedner JA, Ejnell H, Peterson LE: High prevalence of hypertension in sleep apnea patients independent of obesity. Am J Respir Crit Care Med 1994;150:72–77.
33 Bartel PR, Loock M, van der Meyden C, Robinson E, Becker P: Hypertension and sleep apnea in black South Africans: a case control study. Am J Hypertens 1995;8:1200–1205.
34 Hla KM, Young TB, Bidwell T, Palta M, Skatrud JB, Dempsey J: Sleep apnea and hypertension: a population-based study. Ann Intern Med 1994;120: 382–388.
35 Young T, Peppard P, Palta M, Hla KM, Finn L, Morgan B, Skatrud J: Population-based study of sleep-disordered breathing as a risk factor for hypertension. Arch Intern Med 1997;157:1746–1752.
36 Grote L, Ploch T, Heitmann J, Knaack L, Penzel T, Peter JH: Sleep-related breathing disorder is an independent risk factor for systemic hypertension. Am J Respir Crit Care Med 1999;160:1875–1882.
37 Lavie P, Herer P, Hoffstein V: Obstructive sleep apnoea syndrome as a risk factor for hypertension: population study. BMJ 2000;320:479–482.
38 Nieto FJ, Young TB, Lind BK, Shahar E, Samet JM, Redline S, D'Agostino RB, Newman AB, Lebowitz MD, Pickering TG: Association of sleep-disordered breathing, sleep apnea, and hypertension in a large community-based study. Sleep Heart Health Study. JAMA 2000;283:1829–1836.
39 Haas DC, Foster GL, Nieto FJ, Redline S, Resnick HE, Robbins JA, Young T, Pickering TG: Age-dependent associations between sleep-disordered breathing and hypertension: importance of discriminating between systolic/diastolic hypertension and isolated systolic hypertension in the Sleep Heart Health Study. Circulation 2005;111:614–621.
40 Peppard PE, Young T, Palta M, Skatrud J: Prospective study of the association between sleep-disordered breathing and hypertension. N Engl J Med 2000;342:1378–1384.
41 O'Connor GT, Caffo B, Newman AB, Quan SF, Rapoport DM, Redline S, Resnick HE, Samet J, Shahar E: Prospective study of sleep-disordered breathing and hypertension: the Sleep Heart Health Study. Am J Respir Crit Care Med 2009;179:1159–1164.
42 Logan A: Sleep-disordered breathing and hypertension. Am J Respir Crit Care Med 2009;179:1082–1083.
43 Peppard PE: Is obstructive sleep apnea a risk factor for hypertension? Differences between the Wisconsin Sleep Cohort and the Sleep Heart Health Study. J Clin Sleep Med 2009;5:404–405.
44 Drager LF, Pereira AC, Barreto-Filho JA, Figueiredo AC, Krieger JE, Krieger EM, Lorenzi-Filho G: Phenotypic characteristics associated with hypertension in patients with obstructive sleep apnea. J Hum Hypertens 2006;20:523–528.
45 Mohsenin V, Yaggi HK, Shah N, Dziura J: The effect of gender on the prevalence of hypertension in obstructive sleep apnea. Sleep Med 2009;10:759–762.
46 Hedner J, Bengtsson-Bostrom K, Peker Y, Grote L, Rastam L, Lindblad U: Hypertension prevalence in obstructive sleep apnoea and sex: a population-based case-control study. Eur Respir J 2006;27:564–570.
47 Baguet JP, Levy P, Barone-Rochette G, Tamisier R, Pierre H, Peeters M, Mallion JM, Pepin JL: Masked hypertension in obstructive sleep apnea syndrome. J Hypertens 2008;26:885–892.
48 Drager LF, Diegues-Silva L, Diniz PM, Bortolotto LA, Pedrosa RP, Couto RB, Marcondes B, Giorgi DM, Lorenzi-Filho G, Krieger EM: Obstructive sleep apnea, masked hypertension, and arterial stiffness in men. Am J Hypertens 2010;23:249–254.
49 Baguet JP, Hammer L, Levy P, Pierre H, Rossini E, Mouret S, Ormezzano O, Mallion JM, Pepin JL: Night-time and diastolic hypertension are common and underestimated conditions in newly diagnosed apnoeic patients. J Hypertens 2005;23:521–527.
50 Hoffstein V, Mateika J. Evening-to-morning blood pressure variations in snoring patients with and without obstructive sleep apnea. Chest 1992;101: 379–384.
51 Suzuki M, Guilleminault C, Otsuka K, Shiomi T: Blood pressure 'dipping' and 'non-dipping' in obstructive sleep apnea syndrome patients. Sleep 1996;19:382–387.
52 Portaluppi F, Provini F, Cortelli P, Plazzi G, Bertozzi N, Manfredini R, Fersini C, Lugaresi E: Undiagnosed sleep-disordered breathing among male nondippers with essential hypertension. J Hypertens 1997;15: 1227–1233.
53 Davies CW, Crosby JH, Mullins RL, Barbour C, Davies RJ, Stradling JR: Case-control study of 24 hour ambulatory blood pressure in patients with obstructive sleep apnoea and normal matched control subjects. Thorax 2000;55:736–740.

54 Ancoli-Israel S, Stepnowsky C, Dimsdale J, Marler M, Cohen-Zion M, Johnson S: The effect of race and sleep-disordered breathing on nocturnal BP 'dipping': analysis in an older population. Chest 2002;122:1148–1155.

55 Møller DS, Lind P, Strunge B, Pedersen EB: Abnormal vasoactive hormones and 24-hour blood pressure in obstructive sleep apnea. Am J Hypertens 2003;16:274–280.

56 Routledge FS, McFetridge-Durdle JA, Dean CR: Night-time blood pressure patterns and target organ damage: a review. Can J Cardiol 2007;23:132–138.

57 Fagard RH, Celis H, Thijs L, Staessen JA, Clement DL, De Buyzere ML, De Bacquer DA: Daytime and nighttime blood pressure as predictors of death and cause-specific cardiovascular events in hypertension. Hypertension 2008;51:55–61.

58 Pierdomenico SD, Lapenna D, Cuccurullo F: Risk of atrial fibrillation in dipper and nondipper sustained hypertensive patients. Blood Press Monit 2008;13: 193–197.

59 Somers VK, Dyken ME, Clary MP, Abboud FM: Sympathetic neural mechanisms in obstructive sleep apnea. J Clin Invest 1995;96:1897–1904.

60 Somers VK, White DP, Amin R, Abraham WT, Costa F, Culebras A, Daniels S, Floras JS, Hunt CE, Olson LJ, Pickering TG, Russell R, Woo M, Young T: Sleep apnea and cardiovascular disease: an American Heart Association/American College of Cardiology Foundation scientific statement from the American Heart Association Council for High Blood Pressure Research Professional Education Committee, Council on Clinical Cardiology, Stroke Council, and Council on Cardiovascular Nursing. In collaboration with the National Heart, Lung, and Blood Institute National Center on Sleep Disorders Research (National Institutes of Health). Circulation 2008;118:1080–1111.

61 Narkiewicz K, Montano N, Cogliati C, van de Borne PJ, Dyken ME, Somers VK: Altered cardiovascular variability in obstructive sleep apnea. Circulation 1998;98:1071–1077.

62 Frattola A, Parati G, Cuspidi C, Albini F, Mancia G: Prognostic value of 24-hour blood pressure variability. J Hypertens 1993;11:1133–1137.

63 Verdecchia P, Angeli F, Borgioni C, Gattobigio R, Reboldi G: Ambulatory blood pressure and cardiovascular outcome in relation to perceived sleep deprivation. Hypertension 2007;49:777–783.

64 Lenz MC, Martinez D: Awakenings change results of nighttime ambulatory blood pressure monitoring. Blood Press Monit 2007;12:9–15.

65 Calhoun DA, Jones D, Textor S, Goff DC, Murphy TP, Toto RD, White A, Cushman WC, White W, Sica D, Ferdinand K, Giles TD, Falkner B, Carey RM: Resistant hypertension: diagnosis, evaluation, and treatment: a scientific statement from the American Heart Association Professional Education Committee of the Council for High Blood Pressure Research. Hypertension 2008;51:1403–1419.

66 Pimenta E, Calhoun DA, Oparil S: Sleep apnea, aldosterone, and resistant hypertension. Prog Cardiovasc Dis 2009;51:371–380.

67 Lavie P, Hoffstein V: Sleep apnea syndrome: a possible contributing factor to resistant hypertension. Sleep 2001;24:721–725.

68 Chobanian AV, Bakris GL, Black HR, Cushman WC, Green LA, Izzo JL Jr, Jones DW, Materson BJ, Oparil S, Wright JT Jr, Roccella EJ: Seventh report of the Joint National Committee on Prevention, Detection, Evaluation, and Treatment of High Blood Pressure. Hypertension 2003;42:1206–1252.

69 Goncalves SC, Martinez D, Gus M, de Abreu-Silva EO, Bertoluci C, Dutra I, Branchi T, Moreira LB, Fuchs SC, de Oliveira AC, Fuchs FD: Obstructive sleep apnea and resistant hypertension: a case-control study. Chest 2007;132:1858–1862.

70 Pratt-Ubunama MN, Nishizaka MK, Boedefeld RL, Cofield SS, Harding SM, Calhoun DA: Plasma aldosterone is related to severity of obstructive sleep apnea in subjects with resistant hypertension. Chest 2007;131:453–459.

71 Ruttanaumpawan P, Nopmaneejumruslers C, Logan AG, Lazarescu A, Qian I, Bradley TD: Association between refractory hypertension and obstructive sleep apnea. J Hypertens 2009;27:1439–1445.

72 Lloberes P, Lozano L, Sampol G, Romero O, Jurado MJ, Rios J, Untoria MD, Tovar JL: Obstructive sleep apnoea and 24-h blood pressure in patients with resistant hypertension. J Sleep Res 2010;19:597–602.

73 Chobanian AV, Bakris GL, Black HR, Cushman WC, Green LA, Izzo JL Jr, Jones DW, Materson BJ, Oparil S, Wright JT Jr, Roccella EJ: The seventh report of the Joint National Committee on Prevention, Detection, Evaluation, and Treatment of High Blood Pressure: the JNC 7 report. JAMA 2003;289:2560–2572.

74 Mancia G, De Backer G, Dominiczak A, Cifkova R, Fagard R, Germano G, Grassi G, Heagerty AM, Kjeldsen SE, Laurent S, Narkiewicz K, Ruilope L, Rynkiewicz A, Schmieder RE, Boudier HA, Zanchetti A, Vahanian A, Camm J, De Caterina R, Dean V, Dickstein K, Filippatos G, Funck-Brentano C, Hellemans I, Kristensen SD, McGregor K, Sechtem U, Silber S, Tendera M, Widimsky P, Zamorano JL, Erdine S, Kiowski W, Agabiti-Rosei E, Ambrosioni E, Lindholm LH, Viigimaa M, Adamopoulos S, Bertomeu V, Clement D, Farsang C, Gaita D, Lip G, Mallion JM, Manolis AJ, Nilsson PM, O'Brien E, Ponikowski P, Redon J, Ruschitzka F, Tamargo J, van Zwieten P, Waeber B, Williams B: 2007 guidelines for the management of arterial hypertension: the task force for the management of arterial hypertension of the European Society of Hypertension (ESH) and of the European Society of Cardiology (ESC). J Hypertens 2007;25:1105–1187.

75 Dimsdale JE, Loredo JS, Profant J: Effect of continuous positive airway pressure on blood pressure : a placebo trial. Hypertension 2000;35:144–147.

76 Faccenda JF, Mackay TW, Boon NA, Douglas NJ: Randomized placebo-controlled trial of continuous positive airway pressure on blood pressure in the sleep apnea-hypopnea syndrome. Am J Respir Crit Care Med 2001;163:344–348.

77 Pepperell JC, Ramdassingh-Dow S, Crosthwaite N, Mullins R, Jenkinson C, Stradling JR, Davies RJ: Ambulatory blood pressure after therapeutic and subtherapeutic nasal continuous positive airway pressure for obstructive sleep apnoea: a randomised parallel trial. Lancet 2002;359:204–210.

78 Campos-Rodriguez F, Grilo-Reina A, Perez-Ronchel J, Merino-Sanchez M, Gonzalez-Benitez MA, Beltran-Robles M, Almeida-Gonzalez C: Effect of continuous positive airway pressure on ambulatory BP in patients with sleep apnea and hypertension: a placebo-controlled trial. Chest 2006;129:1459–1467.

79 Floras JS, Bradley TD. Treating obstructive sleep apnea: is there more to the story than 2 millimeters of mercury? Hypertension 2007;50:289–291.

80 Bradley TD, Floras JS: Obstructive sleep apnoea and its cardiovascular consequences. Lancet 2009;373: 82–93.

81 Barnes M, Houston D, Worsnop CJ, Neill AM, Mykytyn IJ, Kay A, Trinder J, Saunders NA, Douglas McEvoy R, Pierce RJ: A randomized controlled trial of continuous positive airway pressure in mild obstructive sleep apnea. Am J Respir Crit Care Med 2002;165:773–780.

82 Engleman HM, Gough K, Martin SE, Kingshott RN, Padfield PL, Douglas NJ: Ambulatory blood pressure on and off continuous positive airway pressure therapy for the sleep apnea/hypopnea syndrome: effects in 'non-dippers'. Sleep 1996;19:378–381.

83 Norman D, Loredo JS, Nelesen RA, Ancoli-Israel S, Mills PJ, Ziegler MG, Dimsdale JE: Effects of continuous positive airway pressure versus supplemental oxygen on 24-hour ambulatory blood pressure. Hypertension 2006;47:840–845.

84 Marrone O, Romano S, Insalaco G, Bonsignore MR, Salvaggio A, Bonsignore G: Influence of sampling interval on the evaluation of nocturnal blood pressure in subjects with and without obstructive sleep apnoea. Eur Respir J 2000;16:653–658.

85 Hla KM, Skatrud JB, Finn L, Palta M, Young T: The effect of correction of sleep-disordered breathing on BP in untreated hypertension. Chest 2002;122:1125–1132.

86 Becker HF, Jerrentrup A, Ploch T, Grote L, Penzel T, Sullivan CE, Peter JH: Effect of nasal continuous positive airway pressure treatment on blood pressure in patients with obstructive sleep apnea. Circulation 2003;107:68–73.

87 Kohler M, Pepperell JC, Casadei B, Craig S, Crosthwaite N, Stradling JR, Davies RJ: CPAP and measures of cardiovascular risk in males with OSAS. Eur Respir J 2008;32:1488–1496.

88 Coughlin SR, Mawdsley L, Mugarza JA, Wilding JP, Calverley PM: Cardiovascular and metabolic effects of CPAP in obese males with OSA. Eur Respir J 2007;29:720–727.

89 Hui DS, To KW, Ko FW, Fok JP, Chan MC, Ngai JC, Tung AH, Ho CW, Tong MW, Szeto CC, Yu CM: Nasal CPAP reduces systemic blood pressure in patients with obstructive sleep apnoea and mild sleepiness. Thorax 2006;61:1083–1090.

90 Barbé F, Duran-Cantolla J, Capote F, de la Pena M, Chiner E, Masa JF, Gonzalez M, Marin JM, Garcia-Rio F, de Atauri JD, Teran J, Mayos M, Monasterio C, del Campo F, Gomez S, de la Torre MS, Martinez M, Montserrat JM: Long-term effect of continuous positive airway pressure in hypertensive patients with sleep apnea. Am J Respir Crit Care Med 2010; 181:718–726.

91 Robinson GV, Smith DM, Langford BA, Davies RJ, Stradling JR: Continuous positive airway pressure does not reduce blood pressure in nonsleepy hypertensive OSA patients. Eur Respir J 2006;27:1229–1235.

92 Dernaika TA, Kinasewitz GT, Tawk MM: Effects of nocturnal continuous positive airway pressure therapy in patients with resistant hypertension and obstructive sleep apnea. J Clin Sleep Med 2009;5: 103–107.

93 Logan AG, Tkacova R, Perlikowski SM, Leung RS, Tisler A, Floras JS, Bradley TD: Refractory hypertension and sleep apnoea: effect of CPAP on blood pressure and baroreflex. Eur Respir J 2003;21:241–247.

94 Bazzano LA, Khan Z, Reynolds K, He J: Effect of nocturnal nasal continuous positive airway pressure on blood pressure in obstructive sleep apnea. Hypertension 2007;50:417–423.
95 Haentjens P, Van Meerhaeghe A, Moscariello A, De Weerdt S, Poppe K, Dupont A, Velkeniers B: The impact of continuous positive airway pressure on blood pressure in patients with obstructive sleep apnea syndrome: evidence from a meta-analysis of placebo-controlled randomized trials. Arch Intern Med 2007;167:757–764.
96 Giles TL, Lasserson TJ, Smith BH, White J, Wright J, Cates CJ: Continuous positive airways pressure for obstructive sleep apnoea in adults. Cochrane Database Syst Rev 2006;3:CD001106.
97 Alajmi M, Mulgrew AT, Fox J, Davidson W, Schulzer M, Mak E, Ryan CF, Fleetham J, Choi P, Ayas NT: Impact of continuous positive airway pressure therapy on blood pressure in patients with obstructive sleep apnea hypopnea: a meta-analysis of randomized controlled trials. Lung 2007;185:67–72.
98 Barbé F, Mayoralas LR, Duran J, Masa JF, Maimo A, Montserrat JM, Monasterio C, Bosch M, Ladaria A, Rubio M, Rubio R, Medinas M, Hernandez L, Vidal S, Douglas NJ, Agusti AG: Treatment with continuous positive airway pressure is not effective in patients with sleep apnea but no daytime sleepiness: a randomized, controlled trial. Ann Intern Med 2001;134:1015–1023.
99 Chin K, Nakamura T, Takahashi K, Sumi K, Matsumoto H, Niimi A, Fukuhara S, Mishima M: Falls in blood pressure in patients with obstructive sleep apnoea after long-term nasal continuous positive airway pressure treatment. J Hypertens 2006; 24:2091–2099.
100 Malik J, Drake CL, Hudgel DW: Variables affecting the change in systemic blood pressure in response to nasal CPAP in obstructive sleep apnea patients. Sleep Breath 2008;12:47–52.
101 Yoshida K: Effect on blood pressure of oral appliance therapy for sleep apnea syndrome. Int J Prosthodont 2006;19:61–66.
102 Otsuka R, Ribeiro de Almeida F, Lowe AA, Linden W, Ryan F: The effect of oral appliance therapy on blood pressure in patients with obstructive sleep apnea. Sleep Breath 2006;10:29–36.
103 Andren A, Sjoquist M, Tegelberg A: Effects on blood pressure after treatment of obstructive sleep apnoea with a mandibular advancement appliance – a three-year follow-up. J Oral Rehabil 2009;36:719–725.
104 Gotsopoulos H, Kelly JJ, Cistulli PA: Oral appliance therapy reduces blood pressure in obstructive sleep apnea: a randomized, controlled trial. Sleep 2004;27: 934–941.
105 Barnes M, McEvoy RD, Banks S, Tarquinio N, Murray CG, Vowles N, Pierce RJ: Efficacy of positive airway pressure and oral appliance in mild to moderate obstructive sleep apnea. Am J Respir Crit Care Med 2004;170:656–664.
106 Pelttari LH, Hietanen EK, Salo TT, Kataja MJ, Kantola IM: Little effect of ordinary antihypertensive therapy on nocturnal high blood pressure in patients with sleep disordered breathing. Am J Hypertens 1998;11:272–279.
107 Kraiczi H, Hedner J, Peker Y, Grote L: Comparison of atenolol, amlodipine, enalapril, hydrochlorothiazide, and losartan for antihypertensive treatment in patients with obstructive sleep apnea. Am J Respir Crit Care Med 2000;161:1423–1428.
108 Planes C, Foucher A, Leroy M, Dartois N, Juste K, Baillart O, Raffestin B: Effect of celiprolol treatment in hypertensive patients with sleep apnea. Sleep 1999;22:507–513.
109 Grote L, Wutkewicz K, Knaack L, Ploch T, Hedner J, Peter JH: Association between blood pressure reduction with antihypertensive treatment and sleep apnea activity. Am J Hypertens 2000;13:1280–1287.
110 Pepin JL, Tamisier R, Barone-Rochette G, Launois SH, Levy P, Baguet JP: Comparison of continuous positive airway pressure and valsartan in hypertensive patients with sleep apnea. Am J Respir Crit Care Med 2010;182:954–960.
111 Friedman O, Logan AG: Sympathoadrenal mechanisms in the pathogenesis of sleep apnea-related hypertension. Curr Hypertens Rep 2009;11:212–216.
112 Tkacova R, Wang H, Bradley TD: Night-to-night alterations in sleep apnea type in patients with heart failure. J Sleep Res 2006;15:321–328.
113 MacDonald M, Fang J, Pittman SD, White DP, Malhotra A: The current prevalence of sleep disordered breathing in congestive heart failure patients treated with beta-blockers. J Clin Sleep Med 2008;4: 38–42.
114 Oldenburg O, Lamp B, Freivogel K, Bitter T, Langer C, Horstkotte D: Low night-to-night variability of sleep disordered breathing in patients with stable congestive heart failure. Clin Res Cardiol 2008;97: 836–842.
115 Vazir A, Hastings PC, Papaioannou I, Poole-Wilson PA, Cowie MR, Morrell MJ, Simonds AK: Variation in severity and type of sleep-disordered breathing throughout 4 nights in patients with heart failure. Respir Med 2008;102:831–839.
116 Ryan CM, Floras JS, Logan AG, Kimoff RJ, Series F, Morrison D, Ferguson KA, Belenkie I, Pfeifer M, Fleetham J, Hanly PJ, Smilovitch M, Arzt M, Bradley TD: Shift in sleep apnoea type in heart failure patients in the CANPAP trial. Eur Respir J 2010;35: 592–597.

117 Malhotra A, Owens RL: What is central sleep apnea? Respir Care 2010;55:1168–1178.
118 Chan J, Sanderson J, Chan W, Lai C, Choy D, Ho A, Leung R: Prevalence of sleep-disordered breathing in diastolic heart failure. Chest 1997;111:1488–1493.
119 Javaheri S, Parker TJ, Liming JD, Corbett WS, Nishiyama H, Wexler L, Roselle GA: Sleep apnea in 81 ambulatory male patients with stable heart failure: types and their prevalences, consequences, and presentations. Circulation 1998;97:2154–2159.
120 Sin DD, Fitzgerald F, Parker JD, Newton G, Floras JS, Bradley TD: Risk factors for central and obstructive sleep apnea in 450 men and women with congestive heart failure. Am J Respir Crit Care Med 1999;160:1101–1106.
121 Ferrier K, Campbell A, Yee B, Richards M, O'Meeghan T, Weatherall M, Neill A: Sleep-disordered breathing occurs frequently in stable outpatients with congestive heart failure. Chest 2005;128:2116–2122.
122 Javaheri S: Sleep disorders in systolic heart failure: a prospective study of 100 male patients. The final report. Int J Cardiol 2006;106:21–28.
123 Schulz R, Blau A, Borgel J, Duchna HW, Fietze I, Koper I, Prenzel R, Schadlich S, Schmitt J, Tasci S, Andreas S: Sleep apnoea in heart failure. Eur Respir J 2007;29:1201–1205.
124 Paulino A, Damy T, Margarit L, Stoica M, Deswarte G, Khouri L, Vermes E, Meizels A, Hittinger L, d'Ortho MP: Prevalence of sleep-disordered breathing in a 316-patient French cohort of stable congestive heart failure. Arch Cardiovasc Dis 2009;102: 169–175.
125 Yumino D, Wang H, Floras JS, Newton GE, Mak S, Ruttanaumpawan P, Parker JD, Bradley TD: Prevalence and physiological predictors of sleep apnea in patients with heart failure and systolic dysfunction. J Card Fail 2009;15:279–285.
126 Shahar E, Whitney CW, Redline S, Lee ET, Newman AB, Javier Nieto F, O'Connor GT, Boland LL, Schwartz JE, Samet JM: Sleep-disordered breathing and cardiovascular disease: cross-sectional results of the Sleep Heart Health Study. Am J Respir Crit Care Med 2001;163:19–25.
127 Alchanatis M, Paradellis G, Pini H, Tourkohoriti G, Jordanoglou J: Left ventricular function in patients with obstructive sleep apnoea syndrome before and after treatment with nasal continuous positive airway pressure. Respiration 2000;67:367–371.
128 Kraiczi H, Caidahl K, Samuelsson A, Peker Y, Hedner J: Impairment of vascular endothelial function and left ventricular filling: association with the severity of apnea-induced hypoxemia during sleep. Chest 2001;119:1085–1091.
129 Fung JW, Li TS, Choy DK, Yip GW, Ko FW, Sanderson JE, Hui DS: Severe obstructive sleep apnea is associated with left ventricular diastolic dysfunction. Chest 2002;121:422–429.
130 Oliveira W, Campos O, Bezerra Lira-Filho E, Cintra FD, Vieira M, Ponchirolli A, de Paola A, Tufik S, Poyares D: Left atrial volume and function in patients with obstructive sleep apnea assessed by real-time three-dimensional echocardiography. J Am Soc Echocardiogr 2008;21:1355–1361.
131 Arzt M, Young T, Finn L, Skatrud JB, Ryan CM, Newton GE, Mak S, Parker JD, Floras JS, Bradley TD: Sleepiness and sleep in patients with both systolic heart failure and obstructive sleep apnea. Arch Intern Med 2006;166:1716–1722.
132 Ng AC, Freedman SB: Sleep disordered breathing in chronic heart failure. Heart Fail Rev 2009;14:89–99.
133 Wang HQ, Chen G, Li J, Hao SM, Gu XS, Pang JN, Fu XH: Subjective sleepiness in heart failure patients with sleep-related breathing disorder. Chin Med J (Engl) 2009;122:1375–1379.
134 Hastings PC, Vazir A, O'Driscoll DM, Morrell MJ, Simonds AK: Symptom burden of sleep-disordered breathing in mild-to-moderate congestive heart failure patients. Eur Respir J 2006;27:748–755.
135 Nelesen R, Dar Y, Thomas K, Dimsdale JE: The relationship between fatigue and cardiac functioning. Arch Intern Med 2008;168:943–949.
136 Redeker NS, Muench U, Zucker MJ, Walsleben J, Gilbert M, Freudenberger R, Chen M, Campbell D, Blank L, Berkowitz R, Adams L, Rapoport DM: Sleep disordered breathing, daytime symptoms, and functional performance in stable heart failure. Sleep 2010;33:551–560.
137 Kaneko Y, Floras JS, Usui K, Plante J, Tkacova R, Kubo T, Ando S, Bradley TD: Cardiovascular effects of continuous positive airway pressure in patients with heart failure and obstructive sleep apnea. N Engl J Med 2003;348:1233–1241.
138 Johnson CB, Beanlands RS, Yoshinaga K, Haddad H, Leech J, de Kemp R, Burwash IG: Acute and chronic effects of continuous positive airway pressure therapy on left ventricular systolic and diastolic function in patients with obstructive sleep apnea and congestive heart failure. Can J Cardiol 2008; 24:697–704.
139 Mansfield DR, Gollogly NC, Kaye DM, Richardson M, Bergin P, Naughton MT: Controlled trial of continuous positive airway pressure in obstructive sleep apnea and heart failure. Am J Respir Crit Care Med 2004;169:361–366.

140 Egea CJ, Aizpuru F, Pinto JA, Ayuela JM, Ballester E, Zamarron C, Sojo A, Montserrat JM, Barbe F, Alonso-Gomez AM, Rubio R, Lobo JL, Duran-Cantolla J, Zorrilla V, Nunez R, Cortes J, Jimenez A, Cifrian J, Ortega M, Carpizo R, Sanchez A, Teran J, Iglesias L, Fernandez C, Alonso ML, Cordero J, Roig E, Perez F, Muxi A, Gude F, Amaro A, Calvo U, Masa JF, Utrabo I, Porras Y, Lanchas I, Sanchez E: Cardiac function after CPAP therapy in patients with chronic heart failure and sleep apnea: a multicenter study. Sleep Med 2008;9:660–666.
141 Khayat RN, Abraham WT, Patt B, Roy M, Hua K, Jarjoura D: Cardiac effects of continuous and bilevel positive airway pressure for patients with heart failure and obstructive sleep apnea: a pilot study. Chest 2008;134:1162–1168.
142 Smith LA, Vennelle M, Gardner RS, McDonagh TA, Denvir MA, Douglas NJ, Newby DE: Auto-titrating continuous positive airway pressure therapy in patients with chronic heart failure and obstructive sleep apnoea: a randomized placebo-controlled trial. Eur Heart J 2007;28:1221–1227.
143 Bradley TD, Logan AG, Kimoff RJ, Series F, Morrison D, Ferguson K, Belenkie I, Pfeifer M, Fleetham J, Hanly P, Smilovitch M, Tomlinson G, Floras JS: Continuous positive airway pressure for central sleep apnea and heart failure. N Engl J Med 2005;353:2025–2033.
144 Teschler H, Dohring J, Wang YM, Berthon-Jones M: Adaptive pressure support servo-ventilation: a novel treatment for Cheyne-Stokes respiration in heart failure. Am J Respir Crit Care Med 2001;164:614–619.
145 Randerath WJ, Galetke W, Stieglitz S, Laumanns C, Schafer T: Adaptive servo-ventilation in patients with coexisting obstructive sleep apnoea/hypopnoea and Cheyne-Stokes respiration. Sleep Med 2008;9:823–830.
146 Karavidas A, Kapsimalis F, Lazaros G, Markozanes E, Arapi S, Cholidou K, Matzaraki V, Kyrkou K, Tsiachris D, Matsakas E, Pyrgakis V, Alchanatis M: The impact of positive airway pressure on cardiac status and clinical outcomes in patients with advanced heart failure and sleep-disordered breathing: a preliminary report. Sleep Breath 2010, E-pub ahead of print.
147 Koyama T, Watanabe H, Kobukai Y, Makabe S, Munehisa Y, Iino K, Kosaka T, Ito H: Beneficial effects of adaptive servo ventilation in patients with chronic heart failure. Circ J 2010;74:2118–2124.
148 Arias MA, Garcia-Rio F, Alonso-Fernandez A, Mediano O, Martinez I, Villamor J: Obstructive sleep apnea syndrome affects left ventricular diastolic function: effects of nasal continuous positive airway pressure in men. Circulation 2005;112:375–383.
149 Bitter T, Westerheide N, Faber L, Hering D, Prinz C, Langer C, Horstkotte D, Oldenburg O: Adaptive servoventilation in diastolic heart failure and Cheyne-Stokes respiration. Eur Respir J 2010;36:385–392.
150 Gaddam KK, Verma A, Thompson M, Amin R, Ventura H: Hypertension and cardiac failure in its various forms. Med Clin North Am 2009;93:665–680.
151 Kusuoka H, Weisfeldt ML, Zweier JL, Jacobus WE, Marban E: Mechanism of early contractile failure during hypoxia in intact ferret heart: evidence for modulation of maximal Ca^{2+}-activated force by inorganic phosphate. Circ Res 1986;59:270–282.
152 Okuda N, Ito T, Emura N, Suwa M, Hayashi T, Yoneda H, Kitaura Y: Depressed myocardial contractile reserve in patients with obstructive sleep apnea assessed by tissue Doppler imaging with dobutamine stress echocardiography. Chest 2007;131:1082–1089.
153 Franklin KA, Nilsson JB, Sahlin C, Naslund U: Sleep apnoea and nocturnal angina. Lancet 1995;345:1085–1087.
154 Barretto AC, Santos AC, Munhoz R, Rondon MU, Franco FG, Trombetta IC, Roveda F, de Matos LN, Braga AM, Middlekauff HR, Negrao CE: Increased muscle sympathetic nerve activity predicts mortality in heart failure patients. Int J Cardiol 2009;135:302–307.
155 Triposkiadis F, Karayannis G, Giamouzis G, Skoularigis J, Louridas G, Butler J: The sympathetic nervous system in heart failure physiology, pathophysiology, and clinical implications. J Am Coll Cardiol 2009;54:1747–1762.
156 Spaak J, Egri ZJ, Kubo T, Yu E, Ando S, Kaneko Y, Usui K, Bradley TD, Floras JS: Muscle sympathetic nerve activity during wakefulness in heart failure patients with and without sleep apnea. Hypertension 2005;46:1327–1332.
157 Ueno LM, Drager LF, Rodrigues AC, Rondon MU, Braga AM, Mathias W Jr, Krieger EM, Barretto AC, Middlekauff HR, Lorenzi-Filho G, Negrao CE: Effects of exercise training in patients with chronic heart failure and sleep apnea. Sleep 2009;32:637–647.
158 Morgan BJ: Exercise: alternative therapy for heart failure-associated sleep apnea? Sleep 2009;32:585–586.
159 Chiu KL, Ryan CM, Shiota S, Ruttanaumpawan P, Arzt M, Haight JS, Chan CT, Floras JS, Bradley TD: Fluid shift by lower body positive pressure increases pharyngeal resistance in healthy subjects. Am J Respir Crit Care Med 2006;174:1378–1383.

160 Shiota S, Ryan CM, Chiu KL, Ruttanaumpawan P, Haight J, Arzt M, Floras JS, Chan C, Bradley TD: Alterations in upper airway cross-sectional area in response to lower body positive pressure in healthy subjects. Thorax 2007;62:868–872.

161 Su MC, Chiu KL, Ruttanaumpawan P, Shiota S, Yumino D, Redolfi S, Haight JS, Yau B, Lam J, Bradley TD: Difference in upper airway collapsibility during wakefulness between men and women in response to lower-body positive pressure. Clin Sci (Lond) 2009;116:713–720.

162 Su MC, Chiu KL, Ruttanaumpawan P, Shiota S, Yumino D, Redolfi S, Haight JS, Bradley TD: Lower body positive pressure increases upper airway collapsibility in healthy subjects. Respir Physiol Neurobiol 2008;161:306–312.

163 Redolfi S, Yumino D, Ruttanaumpawan P, Yau B, Su MC, Lam J, Bradley TD: Relationship between overnight rostral fluid shift and obstructive sleep apnea in nonobese men. Am J Respir Crit Care Med 2009; 179:241–246.

164 Yumino D, Redolfi S, Ruttanaumpawan P, Su MC, Smith S, Newton GE, Mak S, Bradley TD: Nocturnal rostral fluid shift: a unifying concept for the pathogenesis of obstructive and central sleep apnea in men with heart failure. Circulation 2010;121:1598–1605.

165 Bucca CB, Brussino L, Battisti A, Mutani R, Rolla G, Mangiardi L, Cicolin A: Diuretics in obstructive sleep apnea with diastolic heart failure. Chest 2007;132:440–446.

166 Usui K, Parker JD, Newton GE, Floras JS, Ryan CM, Bradley TD: Left ventricular structural adaptations to obstructive sleep apnea in dilated cardiomyopathy. Am J Respir Crit Care Med 2006;173:1170–1175.

167 Noda A, Okada T, Yasuma F, Nakashima N, Yokota M: Cardiac hypertrophy in obstructive sleep apnea syndrome. Chest 1995;107:1538–1544.

168 White SG, Fletcher EC, Miller CC 3rd: Acute systemic blood pressure elevation in obstructive and nonobstructive breath hold in primates. J Appl Physiol 1995;79:324–330.

169 O'Donnell CP, Ayuse T, King ED, Schwartz AR, Smith PL, Robotham JL: Airway obstruction during sleep increases blood pressure without arousal. J Appl Physiol 1996;80:773–781.

170 Chen L, Scharf SM: Comparative hemodynamic effects of periodic obstructive and simulated central apneas in sedated pigs. J Appl Physiol 1997;83:485–494.

171 Shiomi T, Guilleminault C, Stoohs R, Schnittger I: Leftward shift of the interventricular septum and pulsus paradoxus in obstructive sleep apnea syndrome. Chest 1991;100:894–902.

172 Smith LA, Chong DW, Vennelle M, Denvir MA, Newby DE, Douglas NJ: Diagnosis of sleep-disordered breathing in patients with chronic heart failure: evaluation of a portable limited sleep study system. J Sleep Res 2007;16:428–435.

173 Hayes D Jr, Anstead MI, Ho J, Phillips BA: Insomnia and chronic heart failure. Heart Fail Rev 2009;14: 171–182.

174 Schaffernocker T, Ho J, Hayes D Jr: Sleep-associated movement disorders and heart failure. Heart Fail Rev 2009;14:165–170.

175 Naughton MT: Routine polysomnography is indicated in congestive heart failure. J Clin Sleep Med 2005;1:16–18.

176 Pack AI, Goldberg LR: Routine polysomnography is not indicated in congestive heart failure. J Clin Sleep Med 2005;1:19–22.

177 Dyken ME, Somers VK, Yamada T, Ren ZY, Zimmerman MB: Investigating the relationship between stroke and obstructive sleep apnea. Stroke 1996;27:401–407.

178 Good DC, Henkle JQ, Gelber D, Welsh J, Verhulst S: Sleep-disordered breathing and poor functional outcome after stroke. Stroke 1996;27:252–259.

179 Bassetti C, Aldrich MS, Chervin RD, Quint D: Sleep apnea in patients with transient ischemic attack and stroke: a prospective study of 59 patients. Neurology 1996;47:1167–1173.

180 Bassetti C, Aldrich MS: Sleep apnea in acute cerebrovascular diseases: final report on 128 patients. Sleep 1999;22:217–223.

181 Wessendorf TE, Teschler H, Wang YM, Konietzko N, Thilmann AF: Sleep-disordered breathing among patients with first-ever stroke. J Neurol 2000;247:41–47.

182 Parra O, Arboix A, Bechich S, Garcia-Eroles L, Montserrat JM, Lopez JA, Ballester E, Guerra JM, Sopena JJ: Time course of sleep-related breathing disorders in first-ever stroke or transient ischemic attack. Am J Respir Crit Care Med 2000;161:375–380.

183 Turkington PM, Bamford J, Wanklyn P, Elliott MW: Prevalence and predictors of upper airway obstruction in the first 24 hours after acute stroke. Stroke 2002;33:2037–2042.

184 Sahlin C, Sandberg O, Gustafson Y, Bucht G, Carlberg B, Stenlund H, Franklin KA: Obstructive sleep apnea is a risk factor for death in patients with stroke: a 10-year follow-up. Arch Intern Med 2008; 168:297–301.

185 Johnson KG, Johnson DC: Frequency of sleep apnea in stroke and TIA patients: a meta-analysis. J Clin Sleep Med 2010;6:131–137.

186 Arzt M, Young T, Finn L, Skatrud JB, Bradley TD: Association of sleep-disordered breathing and the occurrence of stroke. Am J Respir Crit Care Med 2005;172:1447–1451.
187 Mooe T, Franklin KA, Holmstrom K, Rabben T, Wiklund U: Sleep-disordered breathing and coronary artery disease: long-term prognosis. Am J Respir Crit Care Med 2001;164:1910–1913.
188 Valham F, Mooe T, Rabben T, Stenlund H, Wiklund U, Franklin KA: Increased risk of stroke in patients with coronary artery disease and sleep apnea: a 10-year follow-up. Circulation 2008;118:955–960.
189 Redline S, Yenokyan G, Gottlieb DJ, Shahar E, O'Connor GT, Resnick HE, Diener-West M, Sanders MH, Wolf PA, Geraghty EM, Ali T, Lebowitz M, Punjabi NM: Obstructive sleep apnea-hypopnea and incident stroke: the Sleep Heart Health Study. Am J Respir Crit Care Med 2010;182:269–277.
190 Sandberg O, Franklin KA, Bucht G, Gustafson Y: Sleep apnea, delirium, depressed mood, cognition, and ADL ability after stroke. J Am Geriatr Soc 2001;49:391–397.
191 Kaneko Y, Hajek VE, Zivanovic V, Raboud J, Bradley TD: Relationship of sleep apnea to functional capacity and length of hospitalization following stroke. Sleep 2003;26:293–297.
192 Parra O, Arboix A, Montserrat JM, Quinto L, Bechich S, Garcia-Eroles L: Sleep-related breathing disorders: impact on mortality of cerebrovascular disease. Eur Respir J 2004;24:267–272.
193 Turkington PM, Allgar V, Bamford J, Wanklyn P, Elliott MW: Effect of upper airway obstruction in acute stroke on functional outcome at 6 months. Thorax 2004;59:367–371.
194 Martinez-Garcia MA, Galiano-Blancart R, Roman-Sanchez P, Soler-Cataluna JJ, Cabero-Salt L, Salcedo-Maiques E: Continuous positive airway pressure treatment in sleep apnea prevents new vascular events after ischemic stroke. Chest 2005;128:2123–2129.
195 Shi YF, Wang YP: Sleep-disordered breathing: impact on functional outcome of ischemic stroke patients. Sleep Med 2009;10:717–719.
196 Dziewas R, Hopmann B, Humpert M, Ritter M, Dittrich R, Schabitz WR, Ringelstein EB, Nabavi DG, Young P: Positional sleep apnea in patients with ischemic stroke. Neurol Res 2008;30:645–648.
197 Wessendorf TE, Wang YM, Thilmann AF, Sorgenfrei U, Konietzko N, Teschler H: Treatment of obstructive sleep apnoea with nasal continuous positive airway pressure in stroke. Eur Respir J 2001;18:623–629.
198 Sandberg O, Franklin KA, Bucht G, Eriksson S, Gustafson Y: Nasal continuous positive airway pressure in stroke patients with sleep apnoea: a randomized treatment study. Eur Respir J 2001;18:630–634.
199 Hsu CY, Vennelle M, Li HY, Engleman HM, Dennis MS, Douglas NJ: Sleep-disordered breathing after stroke: a randomised controlled trial of continuous positive airway pressure. J Neurol Neurosurg Psychiatry 2006;77:1143–1149.
200 Hui DS, Choy DK, Wong LK, Ko FW, Li TS, Woo J, Kay R: Prevalence of sleep-disordered breathing and continuous positive airway pressure compliance: results in Chinese patients with first-ever ischemic stroke. Chest 2002;122:852–860.
201 Bassetti CL, Milanova M, Gugger M: Sleep-disordered breathing and acute ischemic stroke: diagnosis, risk factors, treatment, evolution, and long-term clinical outcome. Stroke 2006;37:967–972.
202 Palombini L, Guilleminault C: Stroke and treatment with nasal CPAP. Eur J Neurol 2006;13:198–200.
203 Bravata DM, Concato J, Fried T, Ranjbar N, Sadarangani T, McClain V, Struve F, Zygmunt L, Knight HJ, Lo A, Richerson GB, Gorman M, Williams LS, Brass LM, Agostini J, Mohsenin V, Roux F, Yaggi HK: Auto-titrating continuous positive airway pressure for patients with acute transient ischemic attack: a randomized feasibility trial. Stroke 2010;41:1464–1470.
204 Martinez-Garcia MA, Soler-Cataluna JJ, Ejarque-Martinez L, Soriano Y, Roman-Sanchez P, Illa FB, Canal JM, Duran-Cantolla J: Continuous positive airway pressure treatment reduces mortality in patients with ischemic stroke and obstructive sleep apnea: a 5-year follow-up study. Am J Respir Crit Care Med 2009;180:36–41.
205 Sacco RL, Adams R, Albers G, Alberts MJ, Benavente O, Furie K, Goldstein LB, Gorelick P, Halperin J, Harbaugh R, Johnston SC, Katzan I, Kelly-Hayes M, Kenton EJ, Marks M, Schwamm LH, Tomsick T: Guidelines for prevention of stroke in patients with ischemic stroke or transient ischemic attack: a statement for healthcare professionals from the American Heart Association/American Stroke Association Council on Stroke: co-sponsored by the Council on Cardiovascular Radiology and Intervention: the American Academy of Neurology affirms the value of this guideline. Circulation 2006;113:e409–e449.

206 Adams HP Jr, del Zoppo G, Alberts MJ, Bhatt DL, Brass L, Furlan A, Grubb RL, Higashida RT, Jauch EC, Kidwell C, Lyden PD, Morgenstern LB, Qureshi AI, Rosenwasser RH, Scott PA, Wijdicks EF: Guidelines for the early management of adults with ischemic stroke: a guideline from the American Heart Association/American Stroke Association Stroke Council, Clinical Cardiology Council, Cardiovascular Radiology and Intervention Council, and the Atherosclerotic Peripheral Vascular Disease and Quality of Care Outcomes in Research Interdisciplinary Working Groups: the American Academy of Neurology affirms the value of this guideline as an educational tool for neurologists. Stroke 2007;38:1655–1711.

207 Hermann DM, Bassetti CL: Sleep-related breathing and sleep-wake disturbances in ischemic stroke. Neurology 2009;73:1313–1322.

208 Davies DP, Rodgers H, Walshaw D, James OF, Gibson GJ: Snoring, daytime sleepiness and stroke: a case-control study of first-ever stroke. J Sleep Res 2003;12:313–318.

209 Arzt M, Young T, Peppard PE, Finn L, Ryan CM, Bayley M, Bradley TD: Dissociation of obstructive sleep apnea from hypersomnolence and obesity in patients with stroke. Stroke 2010;41:e129–e134.

210 Goldstein LB, Adams R, Alberts MJ, Appel LJ, Brass LM, Bushnell CD, Culebras A, Degraba TJ, Gorelick PB, Guyton JR, Hart RG, Howard G, Kelly-Hayes M, Nixon JV, Sacco RL: Primary prevention of ischemic stroke: a guideline from the American Heart Association/American Stroke Association Stroke Council: cosponsored by the Atherosclerotic Peripheral Vascular Disease Interdisciplinary Working Group; Cardiovascular Nursing Council; Clinical Cardiology Council; Nutrition, Physical Activity, and Metabolism Council; and the Quality of Care and Outcomes Research Interdisciplinary Working Group: the American Academy of Neurology affirms the value of this guideline. Stroke 2006;37:1583–1633.

211 Goldstein LB, Bushnell CD, Adams RJ, Appel LJ, Braun LT, Chaturvedi S, Creager MA, Culebras A, Eckel RH, Hart RG, Hinchey JA, Howard VJ, Jauch EC, Levine SR, Meschia JF, Moore WS, Nixon JV, Pearson TA: Guidelines for the primary prevention of stroke. a guideline for healthcare professionals from the American Heart Association/American Stroke Association. Stroke 2011;42:517–584.

212 De Olazabal JR, Miller MJ, Cook WR, Mithoefer JC: Disordered breathing and hypoxia during sleep in coronary artery disease. Chest 1982;82:548–552.

213 Hung J, Whitford EG, Parsons RW, Hillman DR: Association of sleep apnoea with myocardial infarction in men. Lancet 1990;336:261–264.

214 Andreas S, Schulz R, Werner GS, Kreuzer H: Prevalence of obstructive sleep apnoea in patients with coronary artery disease. Coron Artery Dis 1996;7:541–545.

215 Mooe T, Rabben T, Wiklund U, Franklin KA, Eriksson P: Sleep-disordered breathing in women: occurrence and association with coronary artery disease. Am J Med 1996;101:251–256.

216 Mooe T, Rabben T, Wiklund U, Franklin KA, Eriksson P: Sleep-disordered breathing in men with coronary artery disease. Chest 1996;109:659–663.

217 Schafer H, Koehler U, Ewig S, Hasper E, Tasci S, Luderitz B. Obstructive sleep apnea as a risk marker in coronary artery disease. Cardiology 1999;92:79–84.

218 Sanner BM, Konermann M, Doberauer C, Weiss T, Zidek W: Sleep-disordered breathing in patients referred for angina evaluation – association with left ventricular dysfunction. Clin Cardiol 2001;24:146–150.

219 Young T, Peppard PE, Gottlieb DJ: Epidemiology of obstructive sleep apnea: a population health perspective. Am J Respir Crit Care Med 2002;165:1217–1239.

220 Hagenah GC, Gueven E, Andreas S: Influence of obstructive sleep apnoea in coronary artery disease: a 10-year follow-up. Respir Med 2006;100:180–182.

221 Yumino D, Tsurumi Y, Takagi A, Suzuki K, Kasanuki H: Impact of obstructive sleep apnea on clinical and angiographic outcomes following percutaneous coronary intervention in patients with acute coronary syndrome. Am J Cardiol 2007;99:26–30.

222 Steiner S, Schueller PO, Hennersdorf MG, Behrendt D, Strauer BE: Impact of obstructive sleep apnea on the occurrence of restenosis after elective percutaneous coronary intervention in ischemic heart disease. Respir Res 2008;9:50.

223 Philip P, Guilleminault C: ST segment abnormality, angina during sleep and obstructive sleep apnea. Sleep 1993;16:558–559.

224 Schafer H, Koehler U, Ploch T, Peter JH: Sleep-related myocardial ischemia and sleep structure in patients with obstructive sleep apnea and coronary heart disease. Chest 1997;111:387–393.

225 Mooe T, Franklin KA, Wiklund U, Rabben T, Holmstrom K: Sleep-disordered breathing and myocardial ischemia in patients with coronary artery disease. Chest 2000;117:1597–1602.

226 Alonso-Fernandez A, Garcia-Rio F, Racionero MA, Pino JM, Ortuno F, Martinez I, Villamor J: Cardiac rhythm disturbances and ST-segment depression episodes in patients with obstructive sleep apnea-hypopnea syndrome and its mechanisms. Chest 2005;127:15–22.

227 Peled N, Abinader EG, Pillar G, Sharif D, Lavie P: Nocturnal ischemic events in patients with obstructive sleep apnea syndrome and ischemic heart disease: effects of continuous positive air pressure treatment. J Am Coll Cardiol 1999;34:1744–1749.
228 Hamilton GS, Meredith IT, Walker AM, Solin P: Obstructive sleep apnea leads to transient uncoupling of coronary blood flow and myocardial work in humans. Sleep 2009;32:263–270.
229 Mak GS, Kern MJ, Patel PM: Influence of obstructive sleep apnea and treatment with continuous positive airway pressure on fractional flow reserve measurements for coronary lesion assessment. Catheter Cardiovasc Interv 2010;75:207–213.
230 Kuniyoshi FH, Garcia-Touchard A, Gami AS, Romero-Corral A, van der Walt C, Pusalavidyasagar S, Kara T, Caples SM, Pressman GS, Vasquez EC, Lopez-Jimenez F, Somers VK: Day-night variation of acute myocardial infarction in obstructive sleep apnea. J Am Coll Cardiol 2008;52:343–346.
231 Ishibashi Y, Osada N, Sekiduka H, Izumo M, Shimozato T, Hayashi A, Kida K, Yoneyama K, Takahashi E, Suzuki K, Tamura M, Akashi YJ, Inoue K, Omiya K, Miyake F, Izawa K, Watanabe S: Peak time of acute coronary syndrome in patients with sleep disordered breathing. J Cardiol 2009;53:164–170.
232 Sorajja D, Gami AS, Somers VK, Behrenbeck TR, Garcia-Touchard A, Lopez-Jimenez F: Independent association between obstructive sleep apnea and subclinical coronary artery disease. Chest 2008;133:927–933.
233 Turmel J, Series F, Boulet LP, Poirier P, Tardif JC, Rodes-Cabeau J, Larose E, Bertrand OF: Relationship between atherosclerosis and the sleep apnea syndrome: an intravascular ultrasound study. Int J Cardiol 2009;132:203–209.
234 Kim SH, Cho GY, Baik I, Kim J, Kim SJ, Lee JB, Lim HE, Lim SY, Park J, Shin C: Association of coronary artery calcification with obstructive sleep apnea and obesity in middle-aged men. Nutr Metab Cardiovasc Dis 2010;20:575–582.
235 Hanly P, Sasson Z, Zuberi N, Lunn K: ST-segment depression during sleep in obstructive sleep apnea. Am J Cardiol 1993;71:1341–1345.
236 Milleron O, Pilliere R, Foucher A, de Roquefeuil F, Aegerter P, Jondeau G, Raffestin BG, Dubourg O: Benefits of obstructive sleep apnoea treatment in coronary artery disease: a long-term follow-up study. Eur Heart J 2004;25:728–734.
237 Cassar A, Morgenthaler TI, Lennon RJ, Rihal CS, Lerman A: Treatment of obstructive sleep apnea is associated with decreased cardiac death after percutaneous coronary intervention. J Am Coll Cardiol 2007;50:1310–1314.
238 King CR, Knutson KL, Rathouz PJ, Sidney S, Liu K, Lauderdale DS: Short sleep duration and incident coronary artery calcification. JAMA 2008;300:2859–2866.
239 Ayas NT, White DP, Manson JE, Stampfer MJ, Speizer FE, Malhotra A, Hu FB: A prospective study of sleep duration and coronary heart disease in women. Arch Intern Med 2003;163:205–209.
240 Gangwisch JE, Heymsfield SB, Boden-Albala B, Buijs RM, Kreier F, Pickering TG, Rundle AG, Zammit GK, Malaspina D: Short sleep duration as a risk factor for hypertension: analyses of the first National Health and Nutrition Examination Survey. Hypertension 2006;47:833–839.
241 Al Lawati NM, Patel SR, Ayas NT: Epidemiology, risk factors, and consequences of obstructive sleep apnea and short sleep duration. Prog Cardiovasc Dis 2009;51:285–293.
242 Ikehara S, Iso H, Date C, Kikuchi S, Watanabe Y, Wada Y, Inaba Y, Tamakoshi A: Association of sleep duration with mortality from cardiovascular disease and other causes for Japanese men and women: the JACC study. Sleep 2009;32:295–301.
243 Mullington JM, Haack M, Toth M, Serrador JM, Meier-Ewert HK: Cardiovascular, inflammatory, and metabolic consequences of sleep deprivation. Prog Cardiovasc Dis 2009;51:294–302.
244 Ayas NT, White DP, Al-Delaimy WK, Manson JE, Stampfer MJ, Speizer FE, Patel S, Hu FB: A prospective study of self-reported sleep duration and incident diabetes in women. Diabetes Care 2003;26:380–384.
245 Spiegel K, Knutson K, Leproult R, Tasali E, Van Cauter E: Sleep loss: a novel risk factor for insulin resistance and type 2 diabetes. J Appl Physiol 2005;99:2008–2019.
246 Knutson KL: Impact of sleep and sleep loss on glucose homeostasis and appetite regulation. Sleep Med Clin 2007;2:187–197.
247 Van Cauter E, Holmback U, Knutson K, Leproult R, Miller A, Nedeltcheva A, Pannain S, Penev P, Tasali E, Spiegel K: Impact of sleep and sleep loss on neuroendocrine and metabolic function. Horm Res 2007;67(suppl 1):2–9.
248 Tasali E, Leproult R, Spiegel K: Reduced sleep duration or quality: relationships with insulin resistance and type 2 diabetes. Prog Cardiovasc Dis 2009;51:381–391.
249 Meier-Ewert HK, Ridker PM, Rifai N, Regan MM, Price NJ, Dinges DF, Mullington JM: Effect of sleep loss on C-reactive protein, an inflammatory marker of cardiovascular risk. J Am Coll Cardiol 2004;43:678–683.

250 Von Kanel R, Loredo JS, Ancoli-Israel S, Mills PJ, Natarajan L, Dimsdale JE: Association between polysomnographic measures of disrupted sleep and prothrombotic factors. Chest 2007;131:733–739.

251 Arnardottir ES, Mackiewicz M, Gislason T, Teff KL, Pack AI: Molecular signatures of obstructive sleep apnea in adults: a review and perspective. Sleep 2009;32:447–470.

252 Malhotra A, Loscalzo J: Sleep and cardiovascular disease: an overview. Prog Cardiovasc Dis 2009;51: 279–284.

253 Peker Y, Glantz H, Thunstrom E, Kallryd A, Herlitz J, Ejdeback J: Rationale and design of the Randomized Intervention with CPAP in Coronary Artery Disease and Sleep Apnoea–RICCADSA trial. Scand Cardiovasc J 2009;43:24–31.

254 Sampol G, Rodes G, Romero O, Jurado MJ, Lloberes P: Adherence to nCPAP in patients with coronary disease and sleep apnea without sleepiness. Respir Med 2007;101:461–466.

255 Galie N, Hoeper MM, Humbert M, Torbicki A, Vachiery JL, Barbera JA, Beghetti M, Corris P, Gaine S, Gibbs JS, Gomez-Sanchez MA, Jondeau G, Klepetko W, Opitz C, Peacock A, Rubin L, Zellweger M, Simonneau G, Vahanian A, Auricchio A, Bax J, Ceconi C, Dean V, Filippatos G, Funck-Brentano C, Hobbs R, Kearney P, McDonagh T, McGregor K, Popescu BA, Reiner Z, Sechtem U, Sirnes PA, Tendera M, Vardas P, Widimsky P, Al Attar N, Andreotti F, Aschermann M, Asteggiano R, Benza R, Berger R, Bonnet D, Delcroix M, Howard L, Kitsiou AN, Lang I, Maggioni A, Nielsen-Kudsk JE, Park M, Perrone-Filardi P, Price S, Domenech MT, Vonk-Noordegraaf A, Zamorano JL: Guidelines for the diagnosis and treatment of pulmonary hypertension: the task force for the diagnosis and treatment of pulmonary hypertension of the European Society of Cardiology (ESC) and the European Respiratory Society (ERS), endorsed by the International Society of Heart and Lung Transplantation (ISHLT). Eur Heart J 2009;30:2493–2537.

256 Kovacs G, Berghold A, Scheidl S, Olschewski H: Pulmonary arterial pressure during rest and exercise in healthy subjects: a systematic review. Eur Respir J 2009;34:888–894.

257 Chaouat A, Weitzenblum E, Krieger J, Ifoundza T, Oswald M, Kessler R: Association of chronic obstructive pulmonary disease and sleep apnea syndrome. Am J Respir Crit Care Med 1995;151:82–86.

258 Bradley TD, Rutherford R, Grossman RF, Lue F, Zamel N, Moldofsky H, Phillipson EA. Role of daytime hypoxemia in the pathogenesis of right heart failure in the obstructive sleep apnea syndrome. Am Rev Respir Dis 1985;131:835–839.

259 Krieger J, Sforza E, Apprill M, Lampert E, Weitzenblum E, Ratomaharo J: Pulmonary hypertension, hypoxemia, and hypercapnia in obstructive sleep apnea patients. Chest 1989;96:729–737.

260 Weitzenblum E, Krieger J, Apprill M, Vallee E, Ehrhart M, Ratomaharo J, Oswald M, Kurtz D: Daytime pulmonary hypertension in patients with obstructive sleep apnea syndrome. Am Rev Respir Dis 1988;138:345–349.

261 Chaouat A, Weitzenblum E, Krieger J, Oswald M, Kessler R: Pulmonary hemodynamics in the obstructive sleep apnea syndrome: results in 220 consecutive patients. Chest 1996;109:380–386.

262 Weitzenblum E, Chaouat A: Obstructive sleep apnea syndrome and the pulmonary circulation. Ital Heart J 2005;6:795–798.

263 Golbin JM, Somers VK, Caples SM: Obstructive sleep apnea, cardiovascular disease, and pulmonary hypertension. Proc Am Thorac Soc 2008;5:200–206.

264 Sajkov D, McEvoy RD: Obstructive sleep apnea and pulmonary hypertension. Prog Cardiovasc Dis 2009;51:363–370.

265 Sajkov D, Cowie RJ, Thornton AT, Espinoza HA, McEvoy RD: Pulmonary hypertension and hypoxemia in obstructive sleep apnea syndrome. Am J Respir Crit Care Med 1994;149:416–422.

266 Sanner BM, Doberauer C, Konermann M, Sturm A, Zidek W: Pulmonary hypertension in patients with obstructive sleep apnea syndrome. Arch Intern Med 1997;157:2483–2487.

267 Sajkov D, Wang T, Saunders NA, Bune AJ, Neill AM, Douglas Mcevoy R: Daytime pulmonary hemodynamics in patients with obstructive sleep apnea without lung disease. Am J Respir Crit Care Med 1999;159:1518–1526.

268 Bady E, Achkar A, Pascal S, Orvoen-Frija E, Laaban JP: Pulmonary arterial hypertension in patients with sleep apnoea syndrome. Thorax 2000;55:934–939.

269 Alchanatis M, Tourkohoriti G, Kakouros S, Kosmas E, Podaras S, Jordanoglou JB: Daytime pulmonary hypertension in patients with obstructive sleep apnea: the effect of continuous positive airway pressure on pulmonary hemodynamics. Respiration 2001;68:566–572.

270 Hetzel M, Kochs M, Marx N, Woehrle H, Mobarak I, Hombach V, Hetzel J: Pulmonary hemodynamics in obstructive sleep apnea: frequency and causes of pulmonary hypertension. Lung 2003;181:157–166.

271 Arias MA, Garcia-Rio F, Alonso-Fernandez A, Martinez I, Villamor J: Pulmonary hypertension in obstructive sleep apnoea: effects of continuous positive airway pressure: a randomized, controlled cross-over study. Eur Heart J 2006;27:1106–1113.

272 Sajkov D, Wang T, Saunders NA, Bune AJ, McEvoy RD: Continuous positive airway pressure treatment improves pulmonary hemodynamics in patients with obstructive sleep apnea. Am J Respir Crit Care Med 2002;165:152–158.
273 Sanner BM, Konermann M, Sturm A, Muller HJ, Zidek W: Right ventricular dysfunction in patients with obstructive sleep apnoea syndrome. Eur Respir J 1997;10:2079–2083.
274 Dursunoglu N, Dursunoglu D, Kilic M: Impact of obstructive sleep apnea on right ventricular global function: sleep apnea and myocardial performance index. Respiration 2005;72:278–284.
275 Otto ME, Belohlavek M, Romero-Corral A, Gami AS, Gilman G, Svatikova A, Amin RS, Lopez-Jimenez F, Khandheria BK, Somers VK: Comparison of cardiac structural and functional changes in obese otherwise healthy adults with versus without obstructive sleep apnea. Am J Cardiol 2007;99:1298–1302.
276 Tugcu A, Yildirimturk O, Tayyareci Y, Demiroglu C, Aytekin S: Evaluation of subclinical right ventricular dysfunction in obstructive sleep apnea patients using velocity vector imaging. Circ J 2010;74:312–319.
277 Guidry UC, Mendes LA, Evans JC, Levy D, O'Connor GT, Larson MG, Gottlieb DJ, Benjamin EJ: Echocardiographic features of the right heart in sleep-disordered breathing: the Framingham Heart Study. Am J Respir Crit Care Med 2001;164:933–938.
278 Nahmias J, Lao R, Karetzky M: Right ventricular dysfunction in obstructive sleep apnoea: reversal with nasal continuous positive airway pressure. Eur Respir J 1996;9:945–951.
279 Dursunoglu N, Dursunoglu D, Ozkurt S, Gur S, Ozalp G, Evyapan F: Effects of CPAP on right ventricular myocardial performance index in obstructive sleep apnea patients without hypertension. Respir Res 2006;7:22.
280 Magalang UJ, Richards K, McCarthy B, Fathala A, Khan M, Parinandi N, Raman SV: Continuous positive airway pressure therapy reduces right ventricular volume in patients with obstructive sleep apnea: a cardiovascular magnetic resonance study. J Clin Sleep Med 2009;5:110–114.
281 Presberg KW, Dincer HE: Pathophysiology of pulmonary hypertension due to lung disease. Curr Opin Pulm Med 2003;9:131–138.
282 Fanfulla F, Grassi M, Taurino AE, D'Artavilla Lupo N, Trentin R: The relationship of daytime hypoxemia and nocturnal hypoxia in obstructive sleep apnea syndrome. Sleep 2008;31:249–255.
283 Lattimore JD, Wilcox I, Adams MR, Kilian JG, Celermajer DS: Treatment of obstructive sleep apnoea leads to enhanced pulmonary vascular nitric oxide release. Int J Cardiol 2008;126:229–233.
284 Stevenson IH, Teichtahl H, Cunnington D, Ciavarella S, Gordon I, Kalman JM: Prevalence of sleep disordered breathing in paroxysmal and persistent atrial fibrillation patients with normal left ventricular function. Eur Heart J 2008;29:1662–1669.
285 Porthan KM, Melin JH, Kupila JT, Venho KK, Partinen MM: Prevalence of sleep apnea syndrome in lone atrial fibrillation: a case-control study. Chest 2004;125:879–885.
286 Mehra R, Benjamin EJ, Shahar E, Gottlieb DJ, Nawabit R, Kirchner HL, Sahadevan J, Redline S: Association of nocturnal arrhythmias with sleep-disordered breathing: the Sleep Heart Health Study. Am J Respir Crit Care Med 2006;173:910–916.
287 Gami AS, Hodge DO, Herges RM, Olson EJ, Nykodym J, Kara T, Somers VK: Obstructive sleep apnea, obesity, and the risk of incident atrial fibrillation. J Am Coll Cardiol 2007;49:565–571.
288 Mehra R, Stone KL, Varosy PD, Hoffman AR, Marcus GM, Blackwell T, Ibrahim OA, Salem R, Redline S: Nocturnal arrhythmias across a spectrum of obstructive and central sleep-disordered breathing in older men: outcomes of sleep disorders in older men (MrOS sleep) study. Arch Intern Med 2009;169:1147–1155.
289 Leung RS, Huber MA, Rogge T, Maimon N, Chiu KL, Bradley TD: Association between atrial fibrillation and central sleep apnea. Sleep 2005;28:1543–1546.
290 Monahan K, Storfer-Isser A, Mehra R, Shahar E, Mittleman M, Rottman J, Punjabi N, Sanders M, Quan SF, Resnick H, Redline S: Triggering of nocturnal arrhythmias by sleep-disordered breathing events. J Am Coll Cardiol 2009;54:1797–1804.
291 Lissel C, Hennigs S, Hoffmann-Castendiek B, Gardiwal A, Oswald H, Welte T, Klein G: Effect of restoring sinus rhythm on sleep apnea in patients with atrial fibrillation or flutter. Am J Cardiol 2008;102:709–711.
292 Kanagala R, Murali NS, Friedman PA, Ammash NM, Gersh BJ, Ballman KV, Shamsuzzaman AS, Somers VK: Obstructive sleep apnea and the recurrence of atrial fibrillation. Circulation 2003;107:2589–2594.
293 Benjamin EJ, Levy D, Vaziri SM, D'Agostino RB, Belanger AJ, Wolf PA: Independent risk factors for atrial fibrillation in a population-based cohort: the Framingham Heart Study. JAMA 1994;271:840–844.

294 Wang TJ, Parise H, Levy D, D'Agostino RB Sr, Wolf PA, Vasan RS, Benjamin EJ: Obesity and the risk of new-onset atrial fibrillation. JAMA 2004;292:2471–2477.
295 Frost L, Hune LJ, Vestergaard P: Overweight and obesity as risk factors for atrial fibrillation or flutter: the Danish Diet, Cancer, and Health Study. Am J Med 2005;118:489–495.
296 Movahed MR, Hashemzadeh M, Jamal MM: Diabetes mellitus is a strong, independent risk for atrial fibrillation and flutter in addition to other cardiovascular disease. Int J Cardiol 2005;105:315–318.
297 Dublin S, French B, Glazer NL, Wiggins KL, Lumley T, Psaty BM, Smith NL, Heckbert SR: Risk of new-onset atrial fibrillation in relation to body mass index. Arch Intern Med 2006;166:2322–2328.
298 Miyasaka Y, Barnes ME, Gersh BJ, Cha SS, Bailey KR, Abhayaratna WP, Seward JB, Tsang TS: Secular trends in incidence of atrial fibrillation in Olmsted County, Minnesota, 1980 to 2000, and implications on the projections for future prevalence. Circulation 2006;114:119–125.
299 Arias MA, Sanchez AM, Alonso-Fernandez A, Garcia-Rio F: Atrial fibrillation, obesity, and obstructive sleep apnea. Arch Intern Med 2007;167:1552–1553, author reply 1553.
300 Kannel WB, Wolf PA, Benjamin EJ, Levy D: Prevalence, incidence, prognosis, and predisposing conditions for atrial fibrillation: population-based estimates. Am J Cardiol 1998;82:2N–9N.
301 Chugh SS, Blackshear JL, Shen WK, Hammill SC, Gersh BJ: Epidemiology and natural history of atrial fibrillation: clinical implications. J Am Coll Cardiol 2001;37:371–378.
302 Mooe T, Gullsby S, Rabben T, Eriksson P: Sleep-disordered breathing: a novel predictor of atrial fibrillation after coronary artery bypass surgery. Coron Artery Dis 1996;7:475–478.
303 Romero-Corral A, Somers VK, Pellikka PA, Olson EJ, Bailey KR, Korinek J, Orban M, Sierra-Johnson J, Kato M, Amin RS, Lopez Jimenez F: Decreased right and left ventricular myocardial performance in obstructive sleep apnea. Chest 2007;132:1863–1870.
304 Tsang TS, Gersh BJ, Appleton CP, Tajik AJ, Barnes ME, Bailey KR, Oh JK, Leibson C, Montgomery SC, Seward JB. Left ventricular diastolic dysfunction as a predictor of the first diagnosed nonvalvular atrial fibrillation in 840 elderly men and women. J Am Coll Cardiol 2002;40:1636–1644.
305 Oliveira W, Campos O, Cintra F, Matos L, Vieira ML, Rollim B, Fujita L, Tufik S, Poyares D: Impact of continuous positive airway pressure treatment on left atrial volume and function in patients with obstructive sleep apnoea assessed by real-time three-dimensional echocardiography. Heart 2009; 95:1872–1878.
306 Arias MA, Sanchez AM: Obstructive sleep apnea and its relationship to cardiac arrhythmias. J Cardiovasc Electrophysiol 2007;18:1006–1014.
307 Caples SM, Somers VK: Sleep-disordered breathing and atrial fibrillation. Prog Cardiovasc Dis 2009;51: 411–415.
308 Chung MK, Martin DO, Sprecher D, Wazni O, Kanderian A, Carnes CA, Bauer JA, Tchou PJ, Niebauer MJ, Natale A, Van Wagoner DR: C-reactive protein elevation in patients with atrial arrhythmias: inflammatory mechanisms and persistence of atrial fibrillation. Circulation 2001;104:2886–2891.
309 Corradi D, Callegari S, Maestri R, Benussi S, Alfieri O: Structural remodeling in atrial fibrillation. Nat Clin Pract Cardiovasc Med 2008;5:782–796.
310 Guilleminault C, Connolly SJ, Winkle RA: Cardiac arrhythmia and conduction disturbances during sleep in 400 patients with sleep apnea syndrome. Am J Cardiol 1983;52:490–494.
311 Shepard JW Jr, Garrison MW, Grither DA, Dolan GF: Relationship of ventricular ectopy to oxyhemoglobin desaturation in patients with obstructive sleep apnea. Chest 1985;88:335–340.
312 Hoffstein V, Mateika S: Cardiac arrhythmias, snoring, and sleep apnea. Chest 1994;106:466–471.
313 Koshino Y, Satoh M, Katayose Y, Yasuda K, Tanigawa T, Takeyasu N, Watanabe S, Yamaguchi I, Aonuma K. Association of sleep-disordered breathing and ventricular arrhythmias in patients without heart failure. Am J Cardiol 2008;101:882–886.
314 Flemons WW, Remmers JE, Gillis AM: Sleep apnea and cardiac arrhythmias: is there a relationship? Am Rev Respir Dis 1993;148:618–621.
315 Roche F, Xuong AN, Court-Fortune I, Costes F, Pichot V, Duverney D, Vergnon JM, Gaspoz JM, Barthelemy JC: Relationship among the severity of sleep apnea syndrome, cardiac arrhythmias, and autonomic imbalance. Pacing Clin Electrophysiol 2003;26:669–677.
316 Canada WB, Woodward W, Lee G, De Maria A, Low R, Mason DT, Laddu A, Shapiro W: Circadian rhythm of hourly ventricular arrhythmia frequency in man. Angiology 1983;34:274–282.
317 Harbison J, O'Reilly P, McNicholas WT: Cardiac rhythm disturbances in the obstructive sleep apnea syndrome: effects of nasal continuous positive airway pressure therapy. Chest 2000;118:591–595.

318 Ryan CM, Juvet S, Leung R, Bradley TD: Timing of nocturnal ventricular ectopy in heart failure patients with sleep apnea. Chest 2008;133:934–940.
319 Ryan CM, Usui K, Floras JS, Bradley TD: Effect of continuous positive airway pressure on ventricular ectopy in heart failure patients with obstructive sleep apnoea. Thorax 2005;60:781–785.
320 Bitter T, Westerheide N, Prinz C, Hossain MS, Vogt J, Langer C, Horstkotte D, Oldenburg O: Cheyne-Stokes respiration and obstructive sleep apnoea are independent risk factors for malignant ventricular arrhythmias requiring appropriate cardioverter-defibrillator therapies in patients with congestive heart failure. Eur Heart J 2011;32:61–74.
321 Tilkian AG, Guilleminault C, Schroeder JS, Lehrman KL, Simmons FB, Dement WC: Sleep-induced apnea syndrome: prevalence of cardiac arrhythmias and their reversal after tracheostomy. Am J Med 1977;63:348–358.
322 Becker H, Brandenburg U, Peter JH, von Wichert P: Reversal of sinus arrest and atrioventricular conduction block in patients with sleep apnea during nasal continuous positive airway pressure. Am J Respir Crit Care Med 1995;151:215–218.
323 Koehler U, Becker HF, Grimm W, Heitmann J, Peter JH, Schafer H: Relations among hypoxemia, sleep stage, and bradyarrhythmia during obstructive sleep apnea. Am Heart J 2000;139:142–148.
324 Zwillich C, Devlin T, White D, Douglas N, Weil J, Martin R: Bradycardia during sleep apnea: characteristics and mechanism. J Clin Invest 1982;69:1286–1292.
325 Becker HF, Koehler U, Stammnitz A, Peter JH: Heart block in patients with sleep apnoea. Thorax 1998;53(suppl 3):S29–S32.
326 Grimm W, Hoffmann J, Menz V, Kohler U, Heitmann J, Peter JH, Maisch B: Electrophysiologic evaluation of sinus node function and atrioventricular conduction in patients with prolonged ventricular asystole during obstructive sleep apnea. Am J Cardiol 1996;77:1310–1314.
327 Garrigue S, Pepin JL, Defaye P, Murgatroyd F, Poezevara Y, Clementy J, Levy P: High prevalence of sleep apnea syndrome in patients with long-term pacing: the European Multicenter Polysomnographic Study. Circulation 2007;115:1703–1709.
328 Koehler U, Fus E, Grimm W, Pankow W, Schafer H, Stammnitz A, Peter JH: Heart block in patients with obstructive sleep apnoea: pathogenetic factors and effects of treatment. Eur Respir J 1998;11:434–439.
329 Craig S, Pepperell JC, Kohler M, Crosthwaite N, Davies RJ, Stradling JR: Continuous positive airway pressure treatment for obstructive sleep apnoea reduces resting heart rate but does not affect dysrhythmias: a randomised controlled trial. J Sleep Res 2009;18:329–336.
330 Grimm W, Koehler U, Fus E, Hoffmann J, Menz V, Funck R, Peter JH, Maisch B: Outcome of patients with sleep apnea-associated severe bradyarrhythmias after continuous positive airway pressure therapy. Am J Cardiol 2000;86:688–92, A9.
331 Garrigue S, Bordier P, Jais P, Shah DC, Hocini M, Raherison C, Tunon De Lara M, Haissaguerre M, Clementy J: Benefit of atrial pacing in sleep apnea syndrome. N Engl J Med 2002;346:404–412.
332 Luthje L, Unterberg-Buchwald C, Dajani D, Vollmann D, Hasenfuss G, Andreas S: Atrial overdrive pacing in patients with sleep apnea with implanted pacemaker. Am J Respir Crit Care Med 2005;172:118–122.
333 Pepin JL, Defaye P, Garrigue S, Poezevara Y, Levy P: Overdrive atrial pacing does not improve obstructive sleep apnoea syndrome. Eur Respir J 2005;25:343–347.
334 Unterberg C, Luthje L, Szych J, Vollmann D, Hasenfuss G, Andreas S: Atrial overdrive pacing compared to CPAP in patients with obstructive sleep apnoea syndrome. Eur Heart J 2005;26:2568–2575.
335 Simantirakis EN, Schiza SE, Chrysostomakis SI, Chlouverakis GI, Klapsinos NC, Siafakas NM, Vardas PE: Atrial overdrive pacing for the obstructive sleep apnea-hypopnea syndrome. N Engl J Med 2005;353:2568–2577.
336 Krahn AD, Yee R, Erickson MK, Markowitz T, Gula LJ, Klein GJ, Skanes AC, George CF, Ferguson KA: Physiologic pacing in patients with obstructive sleep apnea: a prospective, randomized crossover trial. J Am Coll Cardiol 2006;47:379–383.
337 Sharafkhaneh A, Sharafkhaneh H, Bredikus A, Guilleminault C, Bozkurt B, Hirshkowitz M: Effect of atrial overdrive pacing on obstructive sleep apnea in patients with systolic heart failure. Sleep Med 2007;8:31–36.
338 Baranchuk A, Healey JS, Simpson CS, Redfearn DP, Morillo CA, Connolly SJ, Fitzpatrick M: Atrial overdrive pacing in sleep apnoea: a meta-analysis. Europace 2009;11:1037–1040.
339 Pack AI, Gislason T. Obstructive sleep apnea and cardiovascular disease: a perspective and future directions. Prog Cardiovasc Dis 2009;51:434–451.
340 Vaupel JW, Yashin AI: Heterogeneity's ruses: some surprising effects of selection on population dynamics. Am Stat 1985;39:176–185.
341 Burt VL, Whelton P, Roccella EJ, Brown C, Cutler JA, Higgins M, Horan MJ, Labarthe D: Prevalence of hypertension in the US adult population: results from the Third National Health and Nutrition Examination Survey, 1988–1991. Hypertension 1995;25:305–313.

342 Chobanian AV: Clinical practice: isolated systolic hypertension in the elderly. N Engl J Med 2007;357:789–796.

343 Tkacova R, Rankin F, Fitzgerald FS, Floras JS, Bradley TD: Effects of continuous positive airway pressure on obstructive sleep apnea and left ventricular afterload in patients with heart failure. Circulation 1998;98:2269–2275.

344 Tkacova R, Dajani HR, Rankin F, Fitzgerald FS, Floras JS, Bradley TD: Continuous positive airway pressure improves nocturnal baroreflex sensitivity of patients with heart failure and obstructive sleep apnea. J Hypertens 2000;18:1257–1262.

345 Gibson GJ: Sleep disordered breathing and the outcome of stroke. Thorax 2004;59:361–363.

346 Simonneau G, Robbins IM, Beghetti M, Channick RN, Delcroix M, Denton CP, Elliott CG, Gaine SP, Gladwin MT, Jing ZC, Krowka MJ, Langleben D, Nakanishi N, Souza R. Updated clinical classification of pulmonary hypertension. J Am Coll Cardiol 2009;54:S43–S54.

347 McKeown P, Epstein AE: Future directions: American College of Chest Physicians guidelines for the prevention and management of postoperative atrial fibrillation after cardiac surgery. Chest 2005;128:61S–64S.

348 Arias MA, Alonso-Fernandez A, Garcia-Rio F, Sanchez A, Lopez JM, Pagola C: Obstructive sleep apnea in atrial fibrillation patients. Int J Cardiol 2006;110:426.

Subject Index